4TH EDITION

MCAT*

SAMPLE EXAMS

Stefan Bosworth, Ph.D.
Marion A. Brisk, Ph.D.
Ronald P. Drucker, Ph.D.
Denise Garland, Ph.D.
Edgar M. Schnebel, Ph.D.
Rosie M. Soy, M.A.

THOMSON
ARCO

Australia • Canada • Mexico • Singapore • Spain • United Kingdom • United States

An ARCO Book

ARCO is a registered trademark of Thomson Learning, Inc., and is used herein under license by Peterson's.

About The Thomson Corporation and Peterson's

With revenues of US$7.2 billion, The Thomson Corporation (www.thomson.com) is a leading global provider of integrated information solutions for business, education, and professional customers. Its Learning businesses and brands (www.thomsonlearning.com) serve the needs of individuals, learning institutions, and corporations with products and services for both traditional and distributed learning.

Peterson's, part of The Thomson Corporation, is one of the nation's most respected providers of lifelong learning online resources, software, reference guides, and books. The Education Supersite[SM] at www.petersons.com—the Internet's most heavily traveled education resource—has searchable databases and interactive tools for contacting U.S.-accredited institutions and programs. In addition, Peterson's serves more than 105 million education consumers annually.

For more information, contact Peterson's, 2000 Lenox Drive, Lawrenceville, NJ 08648; 800-338-3282; or find us on the World Wide Web at www.petersons.com/about.

ISSN: International Standard Serial Number information available upon request.
ISBN: 0-7689-0781-0

Printed in the United States of America

10 9 8 7 6 5 4 3 2   02

CONTENTS

THE MEDICAL COLLEGE ADMISSION TEST 1

Who Takes the MCAT and When It Is Given 1

Format and Scoring of the MCAT 1

Description of the MCAT 2

How to Prepare for the MCAT 3

PRACTICE EXAM I 5

Answer Sheet Practice Exam I 7

Verbal Reasoning 15

Physical Sciences 29

Writing Sample 41

Biological Sciences 44

Practice Exam I Answer Key 59

Practice Exam I Explanatory Answers 60

PRACTICE EXAM II 77

Answer Sheet Practice Exam II 79

Verbal Reasoning 87

Physical Sciences 103

Writing Sample 116

Biological Sciences 119

Practice Exam II Answer Key 134

Practice Exam II Explanatory Answers 135

PRACTICE EXAM III 151

Answer Sheet Practice Exam III 153

Verbal Reasoning 161

Physical Sciences 176

Writing Sample 188

Biological Sciences 191

Practice Exam III Answer Key 206

Practice Exam III Explanatory Answers 207

PRACTICE EXAM IV 223

Answer Sheet Practice Exam III 225

Verbal Reasoning 233

Physical Sciences 251

Writing Sample 269

Biological Sciences 272

Practice Exam IV Answer Key 290

Practice Exam IV Explanatory Answers 291

Periodic Table of the Elements

1	2	3	4	5	6	7	8	9	10	11	12	13	14	15	16	17	18
1 H 1.008																	2 He 4.003
3 Li 6.941	4 Be 9.012											5 B 10.81	6 C 12.01	7 N 14.01	8 O 16.00	9 F 19.00	10 Ne 20.18
11 Na 22.99	12 Mg 24.31											13 Al 26.98	14 Si 28.09	15 P 30.97	16 S 32.06	17 Cl 35.45	18 Ar 39.95
19 K 39.10	20 Ca 40.08	21 Sc 44.96	22 Ti 47.90	23 V 50.94	24 Cr 52.00	25 Mn 54.94	26 Fe 55.85	27 Co 58.93	28 Ni 58.70	29 Cu 63.55	30 Zn 65.38	31 Ga 69.72	32 Ge 72.59	33 As 74.92	34 Se 78.96	35 Br 79.90	36 Kr 83.80
37 Rb 85.47	38 Sr 87.62	39 Y 88.91	40 Zr 91.22	41 Nb 92.91	42 Mo 95.94	43 Tc (98)	44 Ru 101.1	45 Rh 102.9	46 Pd 106.4	47 Ag 107.9	48 Cd 112.4	49 In 114.8	50 Sn 118.7	51 Sb 121.8	52 Te 127.6	53 I 126.9	54 Xe 131.3
55 Cs 132.9	56 Ba 137.3	57 La* 138.9	71 Hf 178.5	73 Ta 180.9	74 W 183.9	75 Re 186.2	76 Os 190.2	77 Ir 192.2	78 Pt 195.1	79 Au 197.0	80 Hg 200.6	81 Tl 204.4	82 Pb 207.2	83 Bi 209.0	84 Po (209)	85 At (210)	86 Rn (222)
87 Fr (223)	88 Ra 226.0	89 Ac** (227)	104 Unq (261)	105 Unp (262)	106 Unh (263)	107 Uns (262)	108 Uno (265)	109 Une (267)									

*Lanthanides (Rare Earths)

58 Ce 140.1	59 Pr 140.9	60 Nd 144.2	61 Pm (145)	62 Sm 150.4	63 Eu 152.0	64 Gd 157.3	65 Tb 158.9	66 Dy 162.5	67 Ho 164.9	68 Er 167.3	69 Tm 168.9	70 Yb 173.0	71 Lu 175.0

**Actinides (Transuranium)

90 Th 232.0	91 Pa (231)	92 U 238.0	93 Np (237)	94 Pu (244)	95 Am (243)	96 Cm (247)	97 Bk (247)	98 Cf (251)	99 Es (252)	100 Fm (257)	101 Md (258)	102 No (259)	103 Lr (260)

Labels: Alkaline earth metals · Halogens · Transition Metals · Nonmetals · Metals

THE MEDICAL COLLEGE ADMISSION TEST

WHO TAKES THE MCAT AND WHEN IT IS GIVEN

The Medical College Admission Test (MCAT) is required for admission to virtually every medical school in the United States and Canada. In addition, it is either required or recommended by many schools of veterinary medicine.

The MCAT is used as one means of evaluating an applicant's chances of success in medical school. Admission committees also review grades, letters of reference, and the medical school application essay before deciding which candidates will be called for an interview for medical school admission. Success on the MCAT will greatly enhance your chances of being accepted to medical school.

The MCAT exam is given twice a year: once in April and once in August. Registration materials are available at the premed office of most colleges, or you can write to MCAT Program Office at P.O. Box 4056, Iowa City, Iowa 52243.

You may take the MCAT as many times as you like. However, scores from previous MCATs will be furnished to the medical schools you apply to and may affect your chances of being accepted. If you want to take the exam more than three times, you must request permission in writing from the American Association of Medical Colleges.

The MCAT score you receive is good for five years. After that, you will be required to take the exam again. Candidates are encouraged to take the MCAT in the spring of their junior year in order to meet medical school application deadlines. However, you may take the MCAT at any time during your academic career.

FORMAT AND SCORING OF THE MCAT

The MCAT exam is divided into four sections, which are administered as follows:

Section 1   Verbal Reasoning—65 questions, 85 minutes
              (10-minute break)
Section 2   Physical Sciences—77 questions, 100 minutes
              (60-minute lunch break)
Section 3   Writing Sample—2 essays, 60 minutes
              (10-minute break)
Section 4   Biological Sciences—77 questions, 100 minutes

The exam begins at 8 am and ends at approximately 5:30 pm.

You will receive four separate scores for your MCAT exam, one score for each section. The Verbal Reasoning, Physical Sciences, and Biological Sciences scores are reported on a scale ranging from 1 to 15, with 1 being the lowest and 15 the highest. The Writing Sample score is converted to an alphabetic scale ranging from a low of J to a high of T. Each letter represents the sum of two separate scores for each Writing Sample item.

The range of acceptable scores varies greatly from school to school. Some schools consider a score of 4 acceptable and others consider only scores of 10 or more acceptable. In a recent survey of medical school admission officers, the average response for the lowest acceptable score was 7.

DESCRIPTION OF THE MCAT

The four sections of the MCAT are quite different from past MCAT exams and are quite different from each other. Let's examine them one by one.

Verbal Reasoning. The Verbal Reasoning section of the MCAT is similar to the reading section of the old exam, but both the articles and the questions cover a broader range of topics and skills. The Verbal Reasoning test consists of several 500- to 600-word passages taken from the humanities, the social sciences, and the natural sciences. Each passage is followed by 6 to 10 multiple-choice questions based on the information presented. All the information necessary to answer the questions is found in the passages. No prior subject matter knowledge is needed to answer any questions in this test.

Verbal reasoning questions are designed to measure your ability to understand, evaluate, and apply information presented in prose passages. You may be asked to recognize information that supports a writer's thesis and to evaluate additional information that does not support the writer's argument. You may be asked to evaluate the strengths and weaknesses of a particular author's arguments or to use information given in a passage to solve other, similar problems. You may be asked what effect new information might have on the conclusions of specific passages and how broad conclusions, explanation, and hypotheses can be applied.

Physical Sciences. The Physical Sciences section of the MCAT covers inorganic chemistry and physics. The knowledge required for this section of the exam includes the basic concepts covered in first-year courses in general chemistry and physics. The problem-solving questions require math knowledge up to and including pre-calculus as well as some basic statistics.

The Physical Science test consists of 10 to 11 problem sets with 4 to 8 questions based on each set. In addition, the test includes 15 questions that are independent of any passage and independent of each other.

The specific concepts covered include the following: acids and bases, atomic and nuclear structure, bonding, electrochemistry, electronic circuits, electrostatics and electromagnetism, electronic structure and the periodic table, equilibrium and momentum, fluids and solids, force and motion, gravitation, light and geometrical optics, phases and phase equilibria, rate processes in chemical reactions, kinetics and equilibrium, solution chemistry, sound, stoichiometry, thermodynamics and thermochemistry, translational motion, wave characteristics and periodic motion, and work and energy.

While there is no longer a quantitative section on the MCAT exam, many of the concepts that were covered in the quantitative section are now included in the physical and biological sciences sections.

Writing Sample. The Writing Sample in the new MCAT is based on the experimental writing section that has been used on previous MCATs. This section consists of two 30-minute essays on specific topics presented on the test. Each writing sample item consists of a statement followed by three writing tasks. The first task is to explain the statement. The second task is to provide an example illustrating a viewpoint opposite to the statement given. And the third task is to discuss how the conflict between these two opposing statements might be resolved.

Your essays will be reviewed by two readers who look for your ability to organize an answer, explain the statement, develop a central concept, synthesize conflicting concepts and ideas, and express yourself clearly and correctly.

The essay topics will not cover controversial subjects such as religion or politics, nor will they be medical topics or topics that require prior knowledge.

Any school to which you send your MCAT scores will receive your writing score. Copies of your essays will be sent to any medical school that requests them.

Biological Sciences. The Biological Sciences section tests the basic concepts covered in first-year biology and genetics as well as concepts covered in the first semester of organic chemistry. In addition, the problem solving questions may require knowledge of statistics, particularly as it applies to genetics and environmental concepts.

Like the Physical Sciences test, the Biological Sciences test consists of 10 to 11 problem sets with 4 to 8 questions based on each set. Each test also includes 15 independent multiple-choice questions.

The specific concepts covered include the following: amines; biological molecules; circulatory, lymphatic, and immune systems; digestive and excretory systems; evolution; generalized eukaryotic cell; genetics; hydrocarbons; microbiology; molecular biology; enzymes and cellular metabolism; DNA and protein synthesis; muscle and skeletal systems; nervous and endocrine systems; organic covalent bonding; oxygen-containing compounds; reproductive systems; respiration systems; separations and purifications; skin systems; specialized eukaryotic cells; and the use of spectroscopy in structural identification.

HOW TO PREPARE FOR THE MCAT

The best preparation for the MCAT starts months before the exam and follows a rigorous course of review and study. For those who wish to begin by seeing what the exam is like and perhaps trying a practice test, this book provides the four full-length practice exams complete with explanatory answers. Visit www.petersons.com bookstore to find more Arco and Peterson's MCAT review books.

Use the scoring guide on the next page to give yourself some indication as to how well you have done on the practice exams. The guide should help you to identify your areas of weakness so that you can direct your study where it will do you the most good. You might also want to highlight your score on each successive practice exam to keep track of your increasing expertise on the MCAT. Do be aware, however, that this guide is only an approximation. This is NOT the actual scoring mechanism used on the MCAT. The range of raw scores contributing to each scaled score is adjusted with each administration of the MCAT to take into account variations in difficulty of questions.

Verbal Reasoning		Physical Sciences		Biological Sciences	
Raw Score	**Scaled Score**	**Raw Score**	**Scaled Score**	**Raw Score**	**Scaled Score**
0–6	1	0–9	1	0–8	1
7–14	2	10–17	2	9–17	2
15–21	3	18–28	3	18–29	3
22–28	4	29–34	4	30–34	4
29–34	5	35–39	5	35–40	5
35–38	6	40–45	6	41–46	6
39–43	7	46–49	7	47–51	7
44–48	8	50–56	8	52–58	8
49–53	9	57–61	9	59–64	9
54–56	10	62–65	10	65–68	10
57–59	11	66–69	11	69–70	11
60–61	12	70–72	12	71–72	12
62–63	13	73–74	13	73–74	13
64	14	75–76	14	75–76	14
65	15	77	15	77	15

PRACTICE EXAM I

	Time
Verbal Reasoning Questions 1–65	85 minutes
Physical Sciences Questions 66–142	100 minutes
Writing Sample 2 Essays	60 minutes
Biological Sciences Questions 143–219	100 minutes

ANSWER SHEET
PRACTICE EXAM I

VERBAL REASONING

1. Ⓐ Ⓑ Ⓒ Ⓓ
2. Ⓐ Ⓑ Ⓒ Ⓓ
3. Ⓐ Ⓑ Ⓒ Ⓓ
4. Ⓐ Ⓑ Ⓒ Ⓓ
5. Ⓐ Ⓑ Ⓒ Ⓓ
6. Ⓐ Ⓑ Ⓒ Ⓓ
7. Ⓐ Ⓑ Ⓒ Ⓓ
8. Ⓐ Ⓑ Ⓒ Ⓓ
9. Ⓐ Ⓑ Ⓒ Ⓓ
10. Ⓐ Ⓑ Ⓒ Ⓓ
11. Ⓐ Ⓑ Ⓒ Ⓓ
12. Ⓐ Ⓑ Ⓒ Ⓓ
13. Ⓐ Ⓑ Ⓒ Ⓓ
14. Ⓐ Ⓑ Ⓒ Ⓓ
15. Ⓐ Ⓑ Ⓒ Ⓓ
16. Ⓐ Ⓑ Ⓒ Ⓓ
17. Ⓐ Ⓑ Ⓒ Ⓓ
18. Ⓐ Ⓑ Ⓒ Ⓓ
19. Ⓐ Ⓑ Ⓒ Ⓓ
20. Ⓐ Ⓑ Ⓒ Ⓓ
21. Ⓐ Ⓑ Ⓒ Ⓓ
22. Ⓐ Ⓑ Ⓒ Ⓓ
23. Ⓐ Ⓑ Ⓒ Ⓓ
24. Ⓐ Ⓑ Ⓒ Ⓓ
25. Ⓐ Ⓑ Ⓒ Ⓓ
26. Ⓐ Ⓑ Ⓒ Ⓓ
27. Ⓐ Ⓑ Ⓒ Ⓓ
28. Ⓐ Ⓑ Ⓒ Ⓓ
29. Ⓐ Ⓑ Ⓒ Ⓓ
30. Ⓐ Ⓑ Ⓒ Ⓓ
31. Ⓐ Ⓑ Ⓒ Ⓓ
32. Ⓐ Ⓑ Ⓒ Ⓓ
33. Ⓐ Ⓑ Ⓒ Ⓓ
34. Ⓐ Ⓑ Ⓒ Ⓓ
35. Ⓐ Ⓑ Ⓒ Ⓓ
36. Ⓐ Ⓑ Ⓒ Ⓓ
37. Ⓐ Ⓑ Ⓒ Ⓓ
38. Ⓐ Ⓑ Ⓒ Ⓓ
39. Ⓐ Ⓑ Ⓒ Ⓓ
40. Ⓐ Ⓑ Ⓒ Ⓓ
41. Ⓐ Ⓑ Ⓒ Ⓓ
42. Ⓐ Ⓑ Ⓒ Ⓓ

43. Ⓐ Ⓑ Ⓒ Ⓓ
44. Ⓐ Ⓑ Ⓒ Ⓓ
45. Ⓐ Ⓑ Ⓒ Ⓓ
46. Ⓐ Ⓑ Ⓒ Ⓓ
47. Ⓐ Ⓑ Ⓒ Ⓓ
48. Ⓐ Ⓑ Ⓒ Ⓓ
49. Ⓐ Ⓑ Ⓒ Ⓓ
50. Ⓐ Ⓑ Ⓒ Ⓓ
51. Ⓐ Ⓑ Ⓒ Ⓓ
52. Ⓐ Ⓑ Ⓒ Ⓓ
53. Ⓐ Ⓑ Ⓒ Ⓓ
54. Ⓐ Ⓑ Ⓒ Ⓓ
55. Ⓐ Ⓑ Ⓒ Ⓓ
56. Ⓐ Ⓑ Ⓒ Ⓓ
57. Ⓐ Ⓑ Ⓒ Ⓓ
58. Ⓐ Ⓑ Ⓒ Ⓓ
59. Ⓐ Ⓑ Ⓒ Ⓓ
60. Ⓐ Ⓑ Ⓒ Ⓓ
61. Ⓐ Ⓑ Ⓒ Ⓓ
62. Ⓐ Ⓑ Ⓒ Ⓓ
63. Ⓐ Ⓑ Ⓒ Ⓓ
64. Ⓐ Ⓑ Ⓒ Ⓓ
65. Ⓐ Ⓑ Ⓒ Ⓓ

PHYSICAL SCIENCES

66. Ⓐ Ⓑ Ⓒ Ⓓ
67. Ⓐ Ⓑ Ⓒ Ⓓ
68. Ⓐ Ⓑ Ⓒ Ⓓ
69. Ⓐ Ⓑ Ⓒ Ⓓ
70. Ⓐ Ⓑ Ⓒ Ⓓ
71. Ⓐ Ⓑ Ⓒ Ⓓ
72. Ⓐ Ⓑ Ⓒ Ⓓ
73. Ⓐ Ⓑ Ⓒ Ⓓ
74. Ⓐ Ⓑ Ⓒ Ⓓ
75. Ⓐ Ⓑ Ⓒ Ⓓ
76. Ⓐ Ⓑ Ⓒ Ⓓ
77. Ⓐ Ⓑ Ⓒ Ⓓ
78. Ⓐ Ⓑ Ⓒ Ⓓ
79. Ⓐ Ⓑ Ⓒ Ⓓ
80. Ⓐ Ⓑ Ⓒ Ⓓ
81. Ⓐ Ⓑ Ⓒ Ⓓ
82. Ⓐ Ⓑ Ⓒ Ⓓ
83. Ⓐ Ⓑ Ⓒ Ⓓ
84. Ⓐ Ⓑ Ⓒ Ⓓ
85. Ⓐ Ⓑ Ⓒ Ⓓ
86. Ⓐ Ⓑ Ⓒ Ⓓ
87. Ⓐ Ⓑ Ⓒ Ⓓ
88. Ⓐ Ⓑ Ⓒ Ⓓ
89. Ⓐ Ⓑ Ⓒ Ⓓ
90. Ⓐ Ⓑ Ⓒ Ⓓ
91. Ⓐ Ⓑ Ⓒ Ⓓ
92. Ⓐ Ⓑ Ⓒ Ⓓ
93. Ⓐ Ⓑ Ⓒ Ⓓ
94. Ⓐ Ⓑ Ⓒ Ⓓ
95. Ⓐ Ⓑ Ⓒ Ⓓ
96. Ⓐ Ⓑ Ⓒ Ⓓ
97. Ⓐ Ⓑ Ⓒ Ⓓ
98. Ⓐ Ⓑ Ⓒ Ⓓ
99. Ⓐ Ⓑ Ⓒ Ⓓ
100. Ⓐ Ⓑ Ⓒ Ⓓ
101. Ⓐ Ⓑ Ⓒ Ⓓ
102. Ⓐ Ⓑ Ⓒ Ⓓ
103. Ⓐ Ⓑ Ⓒ Ⓓ
104. Ⓐ Ⓑ Ⓒ Ⓓ
105. Ⓐ Ⓑ Ⓒ Ⓓ
106. Ⓐ Ⓑ Ⓒ Ⓓ
107. Ⓐ Ⓑ Ⓒ Ⓓ

BIOLOGICAL SCIENCES

108. Ⓐ Ⓑ Ⓒ Ⓓ	143. Ⓐ Ⓑ Ⓒ Ⓓ	192. Ⓐ Ⓑ Ⓒ Ⓓ
109. Ⓐ Ⓑ Ⓒ Ⓓ	144. Ⓐ Ⓑ Ⓒ Ⓓ	193. Ⓐ Ⓑ Ⓒ Ⓓ
110. Ⓐ Ⓑ Ⓒ Ⓓ	145. Ⓐ Ⓑ Ⓒ Ⓓ	194. Ⓐ Ⓑ Ⓒ Ⓓ
111. Ⓐ Ⓑ Ⓒ Ⓓ	146. Ⓐ Ⓑ Ⓒ Ⓓ	195. Ⓐ Ⓑ Ⓒ Ⓓ
112. Ⓐ Ⓑ Ⓒ Ⓓ	147. Ⓐ Ⓑ Ⓒ Ⓓ	196. Ⓐ Ⓑ Ⓒ Ⓓ
113. Ⓐ Ⓑ Ⓒ Ⓓ	148. Ⓐ Ⓑ Ⓒ Ⓓ	197. Ⓐ Ⓑ Ⓒ Ⓓ
114. Ⓐ Ⓑ Ⓒ Ⓓ	149. Ⓐ Ⓑ Ⓒ Ⓓ	198. Ⓐ Ⓑ Ⓒ Ⓓ
115. Ⓐ Ⓑ Ⓒ Ⓓ	150. Ⓐ Ⓑ Ⓒ Ⓓ	199. Ⓐ Ⓑ Ⓒ Ⓓ
116. Ⓐ Ⓑ Ⓒ Ⓓ	151. Ⓐ Ⓑ Ⓒ Ⓓ	200. Ⓐ Ⓑ Ⓒ Ⓓ
117. Ⓐ Ⓑ Ⓒ Ⓓ	152. Ⓐ Ⓑ Ⓒ Ⓓ	201. Ⓐ Ⓑ Ⓒ Ⓓ
118. Ⓐ Ⓑ Ⓒ Ⓓ	153. Ⓐ Ⓑ Ⓒ Ⓓ	202. Ⓐ Ⓑ Ⓒ Ⓓ
119. Ⓐ Ⓑ Ⓒ Ⓓ	154. Ⓐ Ⓑ Ⓒ Ⓓ	203. Ⓐ Ⓑ Ⓒ Ⓓ
120. Ⓐ Ⓑ Ⓒ Ⓓ	155. Ⓐ Ⓑ Ⓒ Ⓓ	204. Ⓐ Ⓑ Ⓒ Ⓓ
121. Ⓐ Ⓑ Ⓒ Ⓓ	156. Ⓐ Ⓑ Ⓒ Ⓓ	205. Ⓐ Ⓑ Ⓒ Ⓓ
122. Ⓐ Ⓑ Ⓒ Ⓓ	157. Ⓐ Ⓑ Ⓒ Ⓓ	206. Ⓐ Ⓑ Ⓒ Ⓓ
123. Ⓐ Ⓑ Ⓒ Ⓓ	158. Ⓐ Ⓑ Ⓒ Ⓓ	207. Ⓐ Ⓑ Ⓒ Ⓓ
124. Ⓐ Ⓑ Ⓒ Ⓓ	159. Ⓐ Ⓑ Ⓒ Ⓓ	208. Ⓐ Ⓑ Ⓒ Ⓓ
125. Ⓐ Ⓑ Ⓒ Ⓓ	160. Ⓐ Ⓑ Ⓒ Ⓓ	209. Ⓐ Ⓑ Ⓒ Ⓓ
126. Ⓐ Ⓑ Ⓒ Ⓓ	161. Ⓐ Ⓑ Ⓒ Ⓓ	210. Ⓐ Ⓑ Ⓒ Ⓓ
127. Ⓐ Ⓑ Ⓒ Ⓓ	162. Ⓐ Ⓑ Ⓒ Ⓓ	211. Ⓐ Ⓑ Ⓒ Ⓓ
128. Ⓐ Ⓑ Ⓒ Ⓓ	163. Ⓐ Ⓑ Ⓒ Ⓓ	212. Ⓐ Ⓑ Ⓒ Ⓓ
129. Ⓐ Ⓑ Ⓒ Ⓓ	164. Ⓐ Ⓑ Ⓒ Ⓓ	213. Ⓐ Ⓑ Ⓒ Ⓓ
130. Ⓐ Ⓑ Ⓒ Ⓓ	165. Ⓐ Ⓑ Ⓒ Ⓓ	214. Ⓐ Ⓑ Ⓒ Ⓓ
131. Ⓐ Ⓑ Ⓒ Ⓓ	166. Ⓐ Ⓑ Ⓒ Ⓓ	215. Ⓐ Ⓑ Ⓒ Ⓓ
132. Ⓐ Ⓑ Ⓒ Ⓓ	167. Ⓐ Ⓑ Ⓒ Ⓓ	216. Ⓐ Ⓑ Ⓒ Ⓓ
133. Ⓐ Ⓑ Ⓒ Ⓓ	168. Ⓐ Ⓑ Ⓒ Ⓓ	217. Ⓐ Ⓑ Ⓒ Ⓓ
134. Ⓐ Ⓑ Ⓒ Ⓓ	169. Ⓐ Ⓑ Ⓒ Ⓓ	218. Ⓐ Ⓑ Ⓒ Ⓓ
135. Ⓐ Ⓑ Ⓒ Ⓓ	170. Ⓐ Ⓑ Ⓒ Ⓓ	219. Ⓐ Ⓑ Ⓒ Ⓓ
136. Ⓐ Ⓑ Ⓒ Ⓓ	171. Ⓐ Ⓑ Ⓒ Ⓓ	
137. Ⓐ Ⓑ Ⓒ Ⓓ	172. Ⓐ Ⓑ Ⓒ Ⓓ	
138. Ⓐ Ⓑ Ⓒ Ⓓ	173. Ⓐ Ⓑ Ⓒ Ⓓ	
139. Ⓐ Ⓑ Ⓒ Ⓓ	174. Ⓐ Ⓑ Ⓒ Ⓓ	
140. Ⓐ Ⓑ Ⓒ Ⓓ	175. Ⓐ Ⓑ Ⓒ Ⓓ	
141. Ⓐ Ⓑ Ⓒ Ⓓ	176. Ⓐ Ⓑ Ⓒ Ⓓ	
142. Ⓐ Ⓑ Ⓒ Ⓓ	177. Ⓐ Ⓑ Ⓒ Ⓓ	
	178. Ⓐ Ⓑ Ⓒ Ⓓ	
	179. Ⓐ Ⓑ Ⓒ Ⓓ	
	180. Ⓐ Ⓑ Ⓒ Ⓓ	
	181. Ⓐ Ⓑ Ⓒ Ⓓ	
	182. Ⓐ Ⓑ Ⓒ Ⓓ	
	183. Ⓐ Ⓑ Ⓒ Ⓓ	
	184. Ⓐ Ⓑ Ⓒ Ⓓ	
	185. Ⓐ Ⓑ Ⓒ Ⓓ	
	186. Ⓐ Ⓑ Ⓒ Ⓓ	
	187. Ⓐ Ⓑ Ⓒ Ⓓ	
	188. Ⓐ Ⓑ Ⓒ Ⓓ	
	189. Ⓐ Ⓑ Ⓒ Ⓓ	
	190. Ⓐ Ⓑ Ⓒ Ⓓ	
	191. Ⓐ Ⓑ Ⓒ Ⓓ	

Writing Sample 1

END OF PART 1

Writing Sample 2

_____

_____

_____

_____

_____

_____

_____

_____

_____

_____

_____

_____

_____

_____

_____

_____

_____

_____

_____

_____

_____

_____

_____

_____

_____

_____

END OF PART 2

VERBAL REASONING

Time: 85 Minutes
Questions 1–65

Directions: There are nine passages in this test. Each passage is followed by questions based on its content. After reading a passage, choose the one best answer to each question and indicate your selection by blackening the corresponding space on your answer sheet.

Passage I (Questions 1–8)

The deliberate violation of constituted law (civil disobedience) is never morally justified if the law being violated is not the prime target or focal point of the protest. Although our government maintains the prin-
(5) ciple of the Constitution by providing methods for and protection of those engaged in individual or group dissent, the violation of law simply as a technique of demonstration constitutes rebellion.

Civil disobedience is, by definition, a violation
(10) of the law. The theory of civil disobedience recognizes that its actions, regardless of their justification, must be punished. However, disobedience of laws not the subject of dissent, but merely used to dramatize dissent, is regarded as morally as well as legally unac-
(15) ceptable. It is only with respect to those laws that offend the fundamental values of human life that moral defense of civil disobedience can be rationally supported.

The assumption that a law is a valid target of civil
(20) disobedience is filled with moral and legal responsibility that cannot be taken lightly. To be morally justified in such a stance, one must be prepared to submit to legal prosecution for violation of the law and accept the punishment if the attack is unsuccessful. One should
(25) even demand that the law be enforced and then be willing to acquiesce in the ultimate judgment of the courts. As members of an organized society, we benefit from our government and our Constitution. If we challenge the law and our challenge is not vindicated, our im-
(30) plied duty is to accept the verdict.

For a just society to exist, the principle of tolerance must be accepted, both by the government in regard to properly expressed individual dissent and by the individual toward legally established majority ver-
(35) dicts. No individual has a monopoly on freedom and all must tolerate opposition. Dissenters must accept dis-
sent from their dissent, giving it all the respect they claim for themselves. To disregard this principle is to make civil disobedience not only legally wrong but
(40) morally unjustifiable.

1. It can be inferred from the article that the author's attitude toward civil disobedience when properly conducted is one of:

   A. contempt.
   B. respect.
   C. shock.
   D. enthusiasm.

2. The author regards the violation of law simply as a technique to dramatize dissent as:

   A. unlawful.
   B. morally wrong.
   C. acceptable if changing the Constitution.
   D. an act of rebellion.

3. According to the author of the article, the violation of constituted law (civil disobedience) is never morally justified unless:

   A. a greater good is being fought for.
   B. the law being broken is the law that the people involved want changed.
   C. the act of civil disobedience has taken over an important moral issue.
   D. the saving of human life is involved.

4. The author says that in order to be morally responsible for an act of civil disobedience, an individual must:

    I. completely understand the law he or she is breaking.
    II. realize the law that he or she is trying to change may not be changed by the act of civil disobedience.
    III. be willing to be arrested and be prosecuted for his or her act of civil disobedience.

    A. I only
    B. III only
    C. I and II only
    D. II and III only

5. According to the article, in order for society to exist:

    A. people must be tolerant of government and not break laws.
    B. government must have enormous power to control people.
    C. government must be tolerant of people and people must be tolerant of government.
    D. the relationship between the governed and the government must be balanced.

6. According to the author, civil disobedience is justifiable only when:

    A. other methods to change a law have been tried and have failed.
    B. the law that people are trying to change offends fundamental values of human life.
    C. the law that people are trying to change is a violation of the Constitution.
    D. a group has decided that rebellion is the only course open to them.

7. The use of individual or group dissent in our society is interpreted by the author as a:

    A. privilege.
    B. right.
    C. violation of the law.
    D. means to test governmental control.

8. The article points out that in accordance with the theory of civil disobedience, one who supports civil disobedience should be prepared to:

    A. be punished.
    B. accept praise.
    C. be reviled.
    D. become ostracized.

Passage II (Questions 9–16)

Contemporary astronomy is ordinarily at least as much of an observational as a theoretical science. Sooner or later on the basis of observation and analysis, what astronomers detect finds its way into theory,
(5) or the theory is modified to accept it.

Neutrino astronomy doesn't fit this pattern. Its highly developed body of theory grew for 30 years without any possibility of verification. Despite the construction, finally, of a string of elaborate observatories, some
(10) buried in the earth from southern India to Utah to South Africa, the last five years as well have produced not a single, validated observation of an extraterrestrial neutrino.

It is a testament to the persistence of the neutrino
(15) astronomers and the strength of their theoretical base that their intensive search for these ghost particles goes on.

The neutrino is a particle with a vanishingly small mass and no charge. Having no charge, it does not in-
(20) teract with the fields around which most particle detection experiments are built; it can be detected only inferentially, by identifying the debris left from its rare interaction with matter.

Even such indirect observations need elaborate
(25) and highly sensitive equipment that wasn't in place until about five years ago. The goal is worth the effort, however: once detected, extraterrestrial neutrinos will provide solid, firsthand information on the sources and conditions that spawned them.
(30) Scientists are sure of this in light of results of sophisticated experiments already conducted on neutrino reactions in particle accelerators and other earthbound apparatus. These experiments have been refined rigorously over the years and are the basis of neutrino
(35) theory, which is an integral part of modern physics.

The existence of neutrinos was first postulated in the early 1930s, in order to explain a form of radioactive decay in which a beta particle—an electron—is emitted. Certain quantities that physicists insist should
(40) be the same after an interaction as before—momentum, energy, and angular momentum—could be con-

served only if another particle of zero charge and negligible mass were emitted.

9. The normal pattern of research in astronomy according to the article is to:

   A. develop theories through the process of analytical reasoning and then make observations to see if the theory works.
   B. observe and then, after many observations, try to develop a theory that explains the observations.
   C. develop a theory and then use observations to prove the theory.
   D. conduct experimental research to validate unproven theories.

10. According to the article, equipment for studying extraterrestrial neutrinos has been available:

    A. since the 1930s.
    B. for 25 years.
    C. for the last five years.
    D. for the last 15 years.

11. It can be inferred from the article that neutrino theory was first developed as a result of which one of the following laws?

    A. Magnetism
    B. Conservation
    C. Inertial
    D. Motion

12. One reason neutrinos are hard to find according to the article is that they are:

    I. positively charged.
    II. negatively charged.
    III. neither positively nor negatively charged.

    A. I only
    B. II only
    C. I and II only
    D. III only

13. According to the article, the theory of extraterrestrial neutrinos is based on:

    A. a great number of observations.
    B. the use of earthbound equipment to detect neutrinos.
    C. a theory that was first developed in the 1930s based on astronomical observations made at that time.
    D. a theory that has been sustained even though no extraterrestrial neutrino has ever been observed.

14. Observing neutrinos is worth the effort according to the article because:

    A. this discovery will prove that developing a theory about something before we observe it is a valid idea.
    B. observing neutrinos will give us considerable knowledge of what spawned them.
    C. if we can observe neutrinos, we will be able to build better telescopes.
    D. we will understand neutrons better.

15. Three quantities that physicists say should be the same after an interaction as before are:

    A. electrons, protons, and neutrons.
    B. magnetism, force, and energy.
    C. neutrinos, atoms, and molecules.
    D. momentum, energy, and angular motion.

16. According to the article, neutrino theory is a basic part of:

    A. physics.
    B. physical Chemistry.
    C. astronomy.
    D. molecular Biology.

Passage III (Questions 17–24)

Many poets who appreciate and admire Mr. Swinburne's genius cannot help regretting that he should ever have descended from the serene heights of poetry into the arena of criticism. Creation and analy-
(5) sis are two very different things; and poetic inspiration is often divorced from the sanity of judgment. It is very easy to pardon the excess of a poet's imagination; but we cannot overlook the absence of common sense and impartiality in a writer who claims to be regarded as a
(10) literary critic.

Mr. Swinburne's criticism is characterized by an utter want of proportion and an aggressive dogmatism which finds vent in offensive and vituperative language quite unsuited to the dignity of literature. . .
(15) A careful comparison of *Essays and Studies* with another volume published about eleven years later, under the title of *Miscellanies,* shows that their author has either deliberately or unconsciously contradicted many of the opinions he had previously expressed.
(20) No doubt, Mr. Swinburne has read the best portion of modern literature. He is filled with apparently genuine admiration for lesser-known Elizabethan dramatists, and he has done a service by pointing out some of their praiseworthy characteristics. But even in this
(25) work of utility, there is an element of false criticism, for some of the weakest plays of Ford and Webster are lauded by him as great and immortal dramas. Mr. Swinburne, when he writes about Victor Hugo, cannot be taken seriously; he is a Hugomaniac, and when he
(30) refers to either *L'Homme qui Rit* or *L'Annee Terrible,* he can only express himself in the superlative degree. Indeed, nearly all that he has written about this rather overrated representative of the French romanticist school is little better than hysterical declamation.
(35) True poet though he be, Mr. Swinburne has none of the faculties that are properly termed judicial. In his entire estimates of the merits and demerits of other men of genius (for undoubtedly he is himself a man of genius) he is too one-sided, too extravagant, too unre-
(40) strained. Literature is, perhaps, with him a consuming passion, and for that very reason he may not be able to discuss it with calmness or moderation. This fact, however, remains; his judgments upon books and their authors are the very reverse of impartial, and it is mani-
(45) fest that Nature never intended him for a critic.

17. It can be inferred that the author of this article believes that two characteristics of a good critic are:

   A. imagination and the ability to use vituperative language.
   B. dogmatism and passion.
   C. love of romantic literature and love of poetry.
   D. common sense and impartiality.

18. According to the author, Mr. Swinburne is a good:

   I. poet.
   II. playwright.
   III. critic.

   A. I only
   B. I and II only
   C. II and III only
   D. III only

19. The author states that a comparison between Mr. Swinburne's *Essays and Studies* and *Miscellanies* shows the two volumes to be:

   A. consistent with each other.
   B. well connected with each other.
   C. inconsistent with each other in many respects.
   D. complementary to each other.

20. According to the author, Mr. Swinburne's criticisms can be described as all of the following **EXCEPT:**

   A. unrestrained.
   B. calm and detached.
   C. one-sided.
   D. offensive.

21. The author states that Mr. Swinburne's criticisms are very:

   A. impartial.
   B. knowledgeable.
   C. poetic.
   D. partial.

22. It can be inferred from the article that the author does not think highly of:

A. Elizabethan writers.
B. French romanticism.
C. Mr. Swinburne's knowledge of literature.
D. neoclassical writers.

23. It may be inferred from the passage that the author considers Mr. Swinburne's literary talents as a critic to be:

A. praiseworthy.
B. an ideal difficult to aspire to.
C. biased and censorious.
D. a model for future literary critics.

24. The example of Mr. Swinburne as a biased literary critic implies that:

A. his creative literary talents were squandered on writing only criticism.
B. his literary reviews were taken seriously by the public at the time.
C. most of the literature he reviewed tended to be mediocre and dull.
D. he mistakenly assumed his writing talents could also extend to literary criticism.

Passage IV (Questions 25–31)

A proper, English-born minister, George Wharton James seemed out of his element when he arrived in the still-wild West in 1881. But James became fascinated by the endangered Native American culture he
(5) saw in California and neighboring Arizona.

Before his death in 1923, James wrote more than forty books chronicling the region and its Mojavi, Yavapai, and Havasupai tribes. A prolific photographer, he also took thousands of photographs documenting
(10) the daily lives and customs of the peoples he saw. After his death, James' unique pictorial history of the region was donated to the Southwest Museum in Los Angeles, a nonprofit educational institution founded in 1907 to preserve and interpret the art, artifacts, and
(15) documentary material of the prehistoric and historic cultures of the Americas.

But many of James' best pictures—just like the vanishing society he photographed—now are in danger. They and thousands of other pictures could liter-
(20) ally turn to dust without quick action to preserve them. With help from the National Endowment for the Humanities, the Southwest Museum is trying to protect the visual memory of the region and make the pictures more accessible to historians and researchers.

(25) "There is very little documentation of that period remaining," says Daniela P. Moneta, the museum's head librarian and director of its film preservation project. "Much of it has already been destroyed."

Moneta explains that James and many other pho-
(30) tographers of the early 1900s often used a nitrate-based film to capture the culture of native Americans facing the onslaught of American settlers. Within decades, however, the nitrate-based film begins to deteriorate. Ultimately, it can crumble into powder. The early pho-
(35) tographers, notes Moneta, "just didn't realize it would deteriorate so quickly."

The threatened degeneration poses a major problem for historians of the period. The museum's extensive collection contains thousands of fragile negatives,
(40) taken between 1900 and 1940, of important ethnographic and archaeological documentation of California, the Southwest, and Meso-america. The photo library is a treasure house for researchers—particularly those living in the West—since it contains vintage prints
(45) which show the crafts, costume, dances, ceremonies, dwellings, and daily life of the native Americans. "The library includes unique images not contained in other photo archives," notes Moneta.

In addition to the George Wharton James collec-
(50) tion, the museum's photo treasure chest includes such rare items as negatives of the dress and culture of the Cupeno and Luiseno Indians of Southern California in the early 1900s, scenes of the Seminole and Choctaw tribes in the Southeastern United States, pictures of daily
(55) life among the Pueblo and other tribes in Arizona and New Mexico, documentation of the Mayan ruins in Yucatan, and photos taken by the Southwest Museum staff during archaeological excavations in California, Nevada, and Colorado.

(60) The more than eleven thousand nitrate-based negatives in the museum's collection "are still in good condition," says Moneta, but experts have already detected early warning signals of deterioration. "The negatives could turn to powder before we know it," she notes,
(65) adding the museum's anxiety over the film has increased greatly in the past five years.

For several decades, the negatives were kept in a cool storage area within the museum. But in 1981, a nitrate film expert with the San Diego Historical Soci-
(70) ety recommended that the deteriorating negatives be moved out of the museum because they could soon begin to emit destructive gaseous fumes and could even explode.

In 1983, the negatives were shipped out to a re-
(75) mote storage warehouse approved by the Los Angeles Fire Department. Now, the negatives are not only relatively inaccessible to researchers, but are threatened with even more rapid deterioration because the storage facility lacks temperature and humidity controls.

(80)   With help from the National Endowment for the Humanities, the museum plans to save the film by converting it into "interpositives" on safety-based film, which then can be stored in the museum for easy access by researchers. The interpositives will be similar to a positive *(85)* print of the negative on paper, but it will be of finer quality, and less detail will be lost in the copying process. "Having a positive image of the negatives available will make the collection more usable and therefore more valuable to researchers," says Moneta.

25. According to the article, George Wharton James was important because he was:

   I. one of the first settlers in the Southwest.
   II. an expert in film preservation.
   III. an important photographer of Native American cultures of the Southwest.

   A. I and III only
   B. II only
   C. III only
   D. II and III only

26. The Southwestern Museum has:

   A. the only visual documentation of Native American culture of the early 1900s.
   B. very little experience with film preservation.
   C. converted all its nitrate negatives to interpositives.
   D. eleven thousand nitrate negatives that are threatened with deterioration.

27. The article states that many of James' best photographs are in danger because:

   A. the kind of film he used deteriorates over time.
   B. they are not in the possession of the Southwestern Museum.
   C. visitors to the museum have been careless with the photographs and have damaged them.
   D. the museum lacks space to care for the photos and is forced to store them at facilities far from the museum.

28. George Wharton James came to the United States in:

   A. 1804.
   B. 1826.
   C. 1874.
   D. 1881.

29. The article implies that the Southwestern Museum was unable to save many of the nitrate negatives because:

   A. the negatives were deteriorating so rapidly it was virtually impossible to save them.
   B. loss of funding from various sources had forced the museum to abandon its search for alternative methods.
   C. a San Diego Historical Society expert on nitrate film was critical of the museum's method of handling the negatives.
   D. the costs of preserving nitrate negatives were so exorbitant.

30. Which of the following is the best explanation of the value of James' pictures to be drawn from the article?

   A. They preserve a unique pictorial history of a number of Native American tribes of the Southwest.
   B. The deterioration of the negatives proves the inefficiency of early photographic film despite the value of their cultural contribution.
   C. They are interesting artifacts of a forgotten culture.
   D. James was an important, leading religious authority whose influence is remembered.

31. According to the article, which of the following statements is true about photography in the period from the 1880s to the 1920s?

   A. So many photographs were taken during this time that it is not crucial to save all of the negatives.

   B. So few photographs were taken during this time that it is essential that all of James' photographs be saved.

   C. Although few photographs were taken during this period, James' photos were of such poor quality that they are not worth the expense of saving them.

   D. No effective method for saving nitrate negatives was available then and none has yet been developed.

Passage V (Questions 32–37)

It would grieve me to seem unjust toward a writer to whom I have long felt very specially attracted—and this by no means only because of a pious although perhaps more or less apocryphal bond. Yet, the highest
(5) praise, which it seems right to bestow upon Thomas Heywood, is that which was happily expressed by Tieck when he described him as the "model of a light and rapid talent." Carried, it may be, by fortune or by choice from the tranquil court of Peterhouse to a very differ-
(10) ent scene of intellectual effort, he worked during a long and laborious life with an energy in itself deserving of respect, and manifestly also with a facility attesting no ordinary natural endowment. His creative power was, however, of that secondary order which is content with
(15) accommodating itself to conditions imposed by the prevailing tastes of the day. It may be merely his prenticed hand that he tried on a dramatic reproduction of chronicles and popular storybooks; but though even here the simplicity of his workmanship was due to a
(20) natural directness of touch by no means to be confounded with rudeness of hand, he cannot be said to have done much to revive a species which though still locally popular was already doomed to decay. . . Of humor he had his share—or he would have been no
(25) master of pathos; but he cannot be said to have excelled in humorous characterization; there is as a rule little individuality in his comic figures at large, and his clowns, although good examples of their kind, are made to order. Indeed, the inferior sort of wit—which of all
(30) writers, dramatists most readily acquire as a literary accomplishment—his practiced inventiveness displays with the utmost abundance; of all the Elizabethan playwrights he is one of the most unwearied, and to my mind one of the most intolerable punsters. In outward
(35) form, he is nearly as Protean as in choice of subject and

of treatment; his earlier plays more especially abound with rimes; in general, fluent verse and easy prose are freely intermixed. But—apart from the pathetic force of particular passages and scenes, and a straightforward
(40) naturalness which lends an irresistible charm to a writer as it does to a friend in real life—his strength lies in a dramatic insight which goes far toward the making of a master of the playwright's art, while it has undoubtedly been possessed by some not entitled to rank as
(45) dramatic poets.

32. It can be inferred that the author of the article thinks that Thomas Heywood was:

   A. a great poet.
   B. a very poor playwright.
   C. a very insightful playwright.
   D. an average poet.

33. The period of time in which Thomas Heywood wrote was the:

   A. present.
   B. Elizabethan.
   C. nineteenth century.
   D. eighteenth century.

34. The author's attitude toward Thomas Heywood is one of:

   A. admiration.
   B. ridicule.
   C. criticism.
   D. dislike.

35. According to the author of the article, Thomas Heywood's greatest strength as a writer was his:

   A. humor.
   B. pathos.
   C. dramatic insight.
   D. comic figures.

36. The main theme of the article is Heywood's:

   A. emotional lifestyle.
   B. sense of humor.
   C. creative powers.
   D. reputation as an intolerable punster.

37. It can be inferred from the article that the author believes that a truly great writer must be able to:

    I. develop universal themes that will live through the ages.

    II. develop characters with which the audience can identify.

    III. rise above the taste of the times rather than cater to them.

    A. I only
    B. III only
    C. I and II only
    D. II and III only

Passage VI (Questions 38–45)

During the past four decades the fishery scientists of the West have studied the dynamics of fish populations with the objective of determining the relationship between the amount of fishing and the sustainable
(5) catch. They have developed a substantial body of theory that has been applied successfully to a large number of animal populations and has led to significant improvement in the management of some of the major marine fisheries.
(10) The theory has been developed for single-species populations with man as a predator. Much of it is based on the Darwinian concept of a constant overpopulation of young that is reduced by density-dependent mortality resulting from intraspecific competition. The
(15) unfished population tends toward a maximum equilibrium size and proportions of large, old individuals. As fishing increases, both population size and proportions of large, old individuals are reduced. Fishing mortality eventually takes the place of most natural mortality. If
(20) the amount of fishing is increased too much, the individuals will tend to be taken before realizing their potential growth, and total yield will be reduced. The maximum sustainable yields can be taken at an intermediate population size that in some populations is
(25) about one-third to one-half the unfished population size.
G. V. Nikolskii, of Moscow State University, develops his theory from a different approach. He is a non-Darwinian and is (he says) a nonmathematician; rather he considers himself an ecologist and a morpholo-
(30) gist. He argues that Darwin's concept of constant overpopulation has led to the neglect of the problem of protecting spawners and young fish. He argues also that Darwin's concept of a variety as an incipient species

has led to extensive mathematical analysis of racial char-
(35) acteristics without an understanding of the adaptive significance of the characters. Nikolskii considers the main laws of population dynamics to be concerned with the succession of generations; their birth, growth, and death. The details are governed by the relative states of adap-
(40) tation and environmental change. The mass and age structure of a population are the result of adaptation to the food supply. The rate of growth of individuals, the time of sexual maturity, and the accumulation of reserves vary according to the food supply. These fac-
(45) tors, in turn, influence the success of reproduction in ways that tend to bring the size of the population into balance with its food supply.

38. Fishing experts have been studying the dynamics of fish populations with the goal of discovering:

    A. the conditions under which fish survive best.
    B. how environmental change affects fish populations.
    C. how different species of fish interact.
    D. the maximum sustainable level of fishing that will keep the fish population constant.

39. According to Nikolskii, the rate of growth of individuals and the time of sexual maturity is based on:

    I. food supply.
    II. how many males are in the population.
    III. number of predators.

    A. I only
    B. I and II only
    C. III only
    D. II and III only

40. The research done by western scientists is based on:

    A. mathematical concepts.
    B. concepts of space and density.
    C. Darwinian concepts of constant overpopulation of the young.
    D. non-Darwinian concepts of ecology.

41. G. V. Nikolskii believes that the Darwinians have failed to take into account:

    A. the size of the body of water the fish live in.

    B. whether the fish are fresh-water or salt-water fish.

    C. the impact of other predators besides man.

    D. how to protect spawners and young fish.

42. The article states that this kind of marine research has been done by western scientists over the last:

    A. decade.

    B. four decades.

    C. two decades.

    D. five decades.

43. Nikolskii considers the main laws of population dynamics to be concerned with:

    A. size, age, and genetic traits.

    B. the succession of generations, number of predators, and rate of habitat destruction.

    C. the succession of generations; their birth, growth, and death.

    D. ecology, evolution, and death.

44. It can be inferred from the article that one main difference between the Darwinians and Nikolskii is the:

    A. influence that the food supply will have on the success of a fish population's maintaining its level.

    B. role of the environment on a fish population's ability to sustain itself.

    C. role that predators other than man play.

    D. mass of the body of water that the fish inhabit.

45. According to Nikolskii, mass and age structure of populations are the result of:

    A. the number of predators in the environment.

    B. whether the fish is environmentally well adapted.

    C. adaptation to the food supply.

    D. size of the species of fish.

Passage VII (Questions 46–51)

The cultural life of modern democratic societies is a pluralistic enterprise. Fortunately, no central direction is imposed on the creation of art and ideas. Instead, we see an apparently limitless number of forces *(5)* competing in a dynamic struggle of creation and consumption.

Precisely because modern democratic society is so diverse, a peculiar component of our cultural situation—criticism—has emerged. So powerful, indeed, *(10)* is this force in today's society that we are undoubtedly justified in asking, "who will criticize the critic?" Before we can criticize the critic, however, we must try to understand what he does.

The first task of the critic is to see the work of art *(15)* and describe its qualities and attributes as clearly as possible. This is the task of elucidation, and it is fundamental to all criticism worthy of the name. Yet, the task of elucidation is not easily separable from another important function of criticism, evaluation. Even the most *(20)* objectively conceived critical elucidation is bound to contain signs of a judgment. Therefore, so as not to conceal this admixture of description and judgment, critical evaluation is best performed as honestly as possible with reasoned arguments and detailed examples.

(25) In our own time, when all of the institutions of society—the museums, the media, the universities, the galleries, the collectors, and all government agencies concerned with the arts—are prejudiced in favor of whatever is deemed on any grounds new and innova- *(30)* tive in the arts, the challenge to criticism is monumental.

The question in a democratic society is not whether criticism has a role to play; that is taken for granted. The real question concerns, rather, the respon- *(35)* sibility of criticism to defend the integrity of art against all encroachments—especially, in our day, the ideological encroachments. By concentrating in the most disinterested way on its traditional tasks of elucidation and evaluation, criticism will make its necessary contribu- *(40)* tion to the life of art and the freedom of the spirit.

46. It can be inferred that the author's major point in the article is that:

    A. critics stifle creativity.

    B. criticism of art tends to keep art traditional.

    C. the most important role of critics is to define art.

    D. the critic's role is to defend art's integrity against all encroachments.

47. The author believes that critics:

    I. have a difficult but important task in a democratic society.

    II. need to be controlled by the government so that their evaluation of art will be fair.

    III. should play a part in our societies whether the societies are democratic or dictatorial.

    A. I only
    B. II only
    C. I and II only
    D. II and III only

48. According to the author, because of the great power critics have, their criticism should be performed:

    A. in a totally objective manner.
    B. with reasoned arguments and detailed examples.
    C. with comparisons to other criticism of the same work.
    D. in a manner that is balanced and fair to all concerned.

49. It would be reasonable to infer from the article that the writer believes that critics are likely to look more positively at art that is:

    A. traditional.
    B. in a museum's exhibit.
    C. new and innovative.
    D. able to appeal to a wide audience.

50. According to the article, the first task of the critic is:

    A. objectivism.
    B. evaluation.
    C. elucidation.
    D. criticism.

51. According to the article, in which type of society can criticism flourish?

    A. Oligarchy
    B. Totalitarian
    C. Dictatorial
    D. Democratic

Passage VIII (Questions 52–58)

After a century, the message first enunciated by John Muir is sinking in: "When you dip your hand into nature, you find that everything is connected to everything else." But until recently, few comprehended the
(5) implications of the naturalist's words.

The message first found institutional expression on a global scale in the 1972 United Nations Conference on the Human Environment at Stockholm. Their 130 nations solemnly acknowledged a mutual obliga-
(10) tion in maintaining a livable global environment. They promulgated a host of recommendations for steps that should be taken. But they created no comprehensive mechanism or procedure for realizing the measures recommended. Some important measures have been imple-
(15) mented. But meanwhile new environmental problems with global ramifications have surfaced faster than problems have been resolved.

It has taken an ominously accelerating succession of calamities, accidents, and incipient crises—the
(20) diminishing stratospheric ozone layer and the Greenhouse Effect, Chernobyl and Bhopal, desertification and deforestation, famines and oil spills—to remind us forcefully that the implications of Muir's words and the good intentions of Stockholm have not been effec-
(21) tively heeded.

Although Americans tend to bask in the notion that we are environmentally progressive, in truth the United States is in many ways a mirror of global environmental problems—a story of too little and too late,
(22) of disarray and confusion, of human welfare treated as a shuttlecock or left to the problematical mercies of "the marketplace."

The United States did move quickly, as the Environmental Revolution dawned in the late 1960s, to en-
(23) act constructive measures: the epochal National Environmental Policy Act; laws to abate air and water pollution and even noise; laws to deal with solid waste, to protect wildlife, to save coasts from degradation; and more. But the ensuing years have painfully demon-
(24) strated that environmental quality is much easier sought than achieved. Although we have been spending roughly $85 billion a year—$340 per capita—on pollution controls, we are far short of our goals of clean air and water. Disposal of everyday solid waste has
(25) become a nightmare. Raw sewage and worse despoil our shores.

The United States exemplifies the worldwide conflict of interests standing in the way of environmental reforms: the conflict between professed desires for en-
(26) vironmental quality versus an addiction to lifestyles that are environmentally destructive in every aspect, from industrial activity to forest destruction and the reckless use of chemicals. Lack of a coherent national energy

(30) policy has contributed to problems extending from the Alaska oil spill to Detroit auto manufacturing, and from acid rain in the Adirondacks to a stymied nuclear power industry from coast to coast.

In the last decade, a wave of environmental popu-
(35) lism has swept across Western Europe. Under the loose generic appellation "the Greens," the movement has become an important political force in a score of nations, drawing support from both the left and the right. Greens have been elected to legislative bodies in West
(40) Germany, France, Italy, Austria, Luxembourg, Switzerland, Belgium, Finland, and Portugal. Some 3,000 Greens have been counted in the federal, state, and local legislative bodies in West Germany alone. "Environmentalists have become Europe's most formidable
(45) and best-organized pressure group," a correspondent wrote in June.

Despite the long prevalence in America of old-line organizations like the Sierra Club and the Audubon Society, the Green movement is getting a
(50) portentous foothold in the United States. Its original spawning ground in New England is reported to have expanded to 200 chapters throughout the country.

In recent public opinion surveys, two Americans out of three said they believed that "protecting the en-
(55) vironment is so important that requirements and standards cannot be too high, and the continued environmental improvements must be made regardless of cost."

With such environmental populism gathering such momentum, it seems only a matter of time, and
(60) not too long a time, until it brings significant changes in national lifestyles that are *conspicuously* inimical to environmental quality. Such conspicuous habits include demands for gas-guzzling cars, a voracious pattern of energy consumption, throwaway consumerism, *recre-*
(65) *ational* vehicles designed to ravage deserts, the equation of growth with good, and all the rest.

The Green Wave that is changing the face of politics in Europe has the potential to do the same thing in other parts of the world—knitting the political muscle
(70) and consolidating the all-important consensus.

52. John Muir said, "When you dip your hand into nature, you find that everything is connected to everything else." The reader could assume the author uses this quote to emphasize:

A. the beauty of nature.
B. the interrelationship of different components of the environment.
C. a commitment to clean air.
D. the need for international action to save the environment.

53. Although the United States likes to bask in the notion that we are environmentally progressive, the author suggests that:

A. we have, in fact, been environmentally reactionary.
B. we have failed to appropriate funds for pollution control.
C. while we were progressive in the late 1960s and early 1970s, we reversed our stand in the late 1970s and 1980s.
D. while we have been progressive, we have not done enough.

54. It would be reasonable to infer from the article that the author believes which of the following?

I. The United States has played a very positive role in the environmental movement.
II. The United States must follow the example of Europe in passing more aggressive environmental legislation.
III. While the rest of the world has done a lot about the environment, the United States has lagged behind.

A. I only
B. III only
C. I and II only
D. II and III only

55. On the basis of this article, it would be reasonable to say that:

A. our lifestyles are developing in a way appropriate to helping the environment.
B. based on the money the United States is spending on the environment, we can expect that rapid improvement in the environmental quality of life will occur in the near future.
C. the United States does not have environmental problems similar to those of the rest of the world.
D. though most Americans claim a strong commitment to improving the environment, our lifestyles are often harmful to it.

56. Greens have been elected to the legislatures of all of the following countries **EXCEPT**:

A. Germany.
B. the United States.
C. Belgium.
D. France.

57. The author attributes the relatively slow growth of the Green movement in the United States to which of the following causes?

A. Americans are always reluctant to follow European trends.
B. Americans tend to pursue a lifestyle that abuses rather than preserves the environment.
C. The movement provides insufficient political power.
D. The movement appeals only to nature lovers.

58. According to the article, the United States spends:

A. 65 billion dollars a year protecting the environment.
B. $340 per person a year protecting the environment.
C. $330 per capita protecting the environment.
D. 75 billion dollars a year to protect the environment.

Passage IX (Questions 59–65)

The way we live is profoundly affected by our climate. When and where we farm, how much we heat and cool our homes, how we obtain our water—all depend on the climate we experience. Climate determines
(5) whether we have a bumper crop or a shortage. It affects the severity of our pollution problems. It determines where the sea meets the shore and the makeup of our forests and our wetlands.

Everyone contributes to greenhouse gas concen-
(10) trations. The activities leading to rising concentrations of greenhouse gases occur in every country in the world. In some it may be the burning of wood for heating and cooking. In others, it may be automobile use. But both the source of the problem and its impacts are global in
(15) scope. No one country dominates in the emission of greenhouse gases, and any country that takes action to control emissions will achieve only limited success if other countries do not follow suit. It is thus necessary that, if action needs to be taken, it should be taken on a
(20) global scale with the participation of as many countries as possible for a sustained period of time.

While we know that much is at stake if the climate changes, there is uncertainty concerning the rate and magnitude of climate change. This poses a major
(25) dilemma since the longer we wait before taking action, the larger the amount of warming we will have to live in. Already, we have seen an increase in greenhouse gas concentrations which means that some climate change may be inevitable. Since there is a great deal of
(30) year-to-year variation in climate from purely natural causes, it will also be difficult to detect the early signs of a global warming. If we wait until we can actually measure warming before we take action, then we may have to live with warmings for many generations, since
(35) it takes many years before emission reductions could have an impact on atmospheric concentrations and the climate system.

In short, global climate change is an issue with potentially profound consequences for mankind and na-
(40) ture. Limiting climate change would require sustained concerted action by many nations for a long period of time.

Given these facts, a number of actions must urgently be undertaken. We must continue to build our
(45) scientific research capabilities and to develop an international scientific consensus on the nature of the climate change problem—the kind of consensus that can endure changes in governments and incorporate a wide number of nations. This international understanding of
(50) the problem is necessary before effective policy responses can be developed.

Yet, we do not have the luxury of sitting on our hands while a scientific consensus emerges. Rather, the United States and other countries should begin to think (55) of ways to reduce greenhouse gas emissions, in the event that it ultimately proves necessary to do so. The source of these reductions would be different for every country. For one, it may be changing land-use patterns to reduce tropical deforestation. For another, it may be (60) improving energy efficiency. In many cases, actions that may be found to be effective in reducing greenhouse gas concentrations may make sense on their own, for totally independent reasons. For example, reducing production of chlorofluorocarbons (CFCs) will slow the (65) depletion of the stratospheric ozone layer and have the ancillary benefit of potentially limiting global warming.

Finally, we must improve our understanding of the effects of warming in case we find that we need to (70) adapt to climate changes. Since greenhouse gas emissions have already increased, some amount of adaptation may be necessary even if we limited emissions today. Moreover, if concerted action on an international level is to be undertaken, then a consensus must emerge (75) on the seriousness of the climate change problem. Only through internationally coordinated research on the impacts of climate change can this be accomplished.

59. The author argues that if action is to be taken on the greenhouse effect, it must be taken:

A. by those countries that contribute most to the greenhouse effect.
B. by those countries that use high concentrations of fossil fuels.
C. by those countries that can best afford to take action.
D. on a global scale.

60. The article suggests various approaches to achieving global control of increased greenhouse gas emissions. Which of the following is NOT a suggested approach?

A. Change the source of reduction of greenhouse gas emissions in cooperating countries.
B. Allow individual nations to have the option of initiating any approaches to solving climate change problems.
C. Utilize varied methods of adaptation even if limited emissions are reduced.
D. Reach a consensus on the seriousness of the problem and undertaking concerted action on an international level.

61. According to the author, the major dilemma as to what action to take concerning global warming is that:

A. if we wait till we are sure how much warming will take place, we may have to live with the effects of global warming for generations.
B. we do not really have any clear idea of what action we should take.
C. any action taken will hamper developing countries.
D. too much global warming has already taken place for action to be of significant value.

62. The author discusses the effect of climate on all of the following aspects of our lives **EXCEPT**:

A. how much food we can grow.
B. how much we heat and cool our houses.
C. the kind of clothing we buy.
D. how we obtain water.

63. The author believes that if we wait for the final results of scientific research before acting to control greenhouse gas emissions:

A. we will not have the consensus required to enact the necessary changes.
B. it may be too late to reverse the greenhouse effect.
C. the level of chlorofluorocarbons will be too high.
D. the rain forest will be gone and we will not be able to replace it.

64. The tone of the article stresses the urgent need to address global climate change:

A. through international cooperative efforts at decreasing greenhouse gas emissions.
B. by limiting greenhouse gas emissions through an international scientific consensus.
C. through United States leadership working with international governments.
D. through coordinated research leading to understanding of the problem and some degree of adaptation on an international level.

65. According to the article, which of the following actions should be taken in order to effect a global reduction of greenhouse gas emissions?

  I. A global cooperative organization should be formed to provide appropriate measures.

  II. The United States should assume the responsibility of providing leadership.

  III. The United Nations should sponsor a global cooperative action.

  A. I only
  B. III only
  C. I and II only
  D. II and III only

END OF TEST 1.

IF YOU FINISH BEFORE THE TIME IS UP, YOU MAY CHECK YOUR WORK ON THIS TEST ONLY.

PHYSICAL SCIENCES

Time: 100 Minutes
Questions 66–142

Directions: This test contains 77 questions. Most of the questions consist of a descriptive passage followed by a group of questions related to the passage. For these questions, study the passage carefully and then choose the best answer to each question in the group. Some questions in this test stand alone. These questions are independent of any passage and independent of each other. For these questions, too, you must select the one best answer. Indicate all your answers by blackening the corresponding circles on your answer sheet.

A periodic table is provided at the beginning of this book. You may consult it whenever you wish.

Passage I (Questions 66–73)

The figure below shows a photograph obtained when light from a low-pressure hydrogen lamp is passed through a spectrometer.

← wavelength (nm)

Energy

Two scientists offer their views on the interpretation of these lines.

Scientist 1: These "spectral lines" point to the existence of quantized energy levels in the hydrogen atom. The lines at different wavelengths represent photons emitted after an electron has been promoted to a higher level in the atom, and then relaxed down to either the ground state or a low-lying excited state.

By converting the wavelengths to energies, we can construct the following diagram showing the energy levels that must exist in the atom:

Scientist 2: My colleague has missed an important alternative explanation, which I am certain is the correct one. Hydrogen does not have discrete energy levels; rather, the glass in the spectrometer used to measure the wavelength has *peculiar gaps in its transmission properties*—it only allows certain colors through.

66. What is the approximate ratio of the longest to the shortest wavelength shown?

   A. −0.5
   B. 0.5
   C. 1.2
   D. 1.7

67. The wavelengths shown are given in nanometers (nm), where 1 nm = 10^{-9} m. Which of the following represents the shortest-wavelength spectral line shown in meters?

    A. 3.89×10^{-11} m
    B. 3.89×10^{-9} m
    C. 3.89×10^{-7} m
    D. 3.89×10^{-6} m

68. In Scientist 1's view, the shortest wavelength transition represents the:

    A. transition of lowest energy difference.
    B. transition of highest energy difference.
    C. most intense transition.
    D. transition most likely to occur.

69. Which relation would Scientist 1 use to convert wavelength to energy *most directly?*

    A. $E = h\nu$
    B. $E = hc/\lambda$
    C. $c = \nu\lambda$
    D. $E_n = -k/n^2$

70. For Scientist 1, a transition in hydrogen having $\lambda = 610$ nm would be:

    A. impossible.
    B. obscured by the transitions around it.
    C. found between the transitions at 656 nm and 486 nm.
    D. found to represent higher energy transitions than those for 656 nm.

71. Scientist 2 views the transition at 434 nm as:

    A. the only one possible in the region between 420 and 480 nm.
    B. not accurately determined.
    C. originating in the glass in the spectrometer.
    D. made visible by the glass in the spectrometer.

72. Scientist 2's views would be reinforced by which of the following?

    I. The finding that other atoms gave similar emission spectra in the same spectrometer.
    II. The finding that other atoms gave different emission spectra in the same spectrometer.
    III. Evidence that the spectrometer contained hydrogen atoms.

    A. I only
    B. II only
    C. III only
    D. I and II only

73. Another researcher analyzes the light from a tungsten filament lamp using the same spectrometer, and finds that a broad spectrum of wavelengths are present in the region from 400 to 650 nm, with no sharp lines. These findings support:

    A. Scientist 1's position.
    B. Scientist 2's position.
    C. both positions.
    D. neither position.

Passage II (Questions 74–79)

A chemist wishes to separate a mixture containing 0.1 M Zn^{2+} ions and 0.1 M Pb^{2+} ions. She decides to use the difference in K_{sp}'s of the metal sulfides (see Table 1) to effect the separation.

Table 1

Salt	K_{sp}
ZnS	1×10^{-21}
PbS	8×10^{-28}

The chemist predicts the following results (Table 2).

Table 2

ion	[S^{2-}] needed to precipitate
Zn^{2+}	$1 \times 10^{-20}\ M$
Pb^{2+}	$8 \times 10^{-27}\ M$

In preparing sulfide solutions, the chemist makes use of the following relation for the H_2S system:

$$[H^+]^2[S^{2-}] = 1 \times 10^{-23}$$

74. If a small quantity of sulfide ion is introduced into the mixture of Zn^{2+} and Pb^{2+}, what will precipitate first?

    A. ZnS
    B. PbS
    C. Both ZnS and PbS
    D. Neither will precipitate

75. Which of the following expressions should the chemist use to calculate the concentration of sulfide at which PbS will precipitate?

    A. $[S^{2-}] = (8 \times 10^{-28})^{\frac{1}{2}}$
    B. $[S^{2-}] = (8 \times 10^{-28})/(0.1)$
    C. $[S^{2-}] = (8 \times 10^{-28})^2/(0.1)$
    D. $[S^{2-}] = (8 \times 10^{-28})/(0.1)^2$

76. The chemist wonders how difficult it will be to prepare the dilute solutions of sulfide indicated in Table 2. How many S^{2-} ions per cubic centimeter are represented in the solution indicated in the first row of the table?

    A. 1×10^{-20}
    B. 6×10^{-20}
    C. 6
    D. 6000

77. The chemist must now determine a means of preparing a highly dilute solution of sulfide, and she decides to use the H_2S system. The relation already given for H_2S implies that:

    A. high pH leads to low $[S^{2-}]$.
    B. low pH leads to low $[S^{2-}]$.
    C. pH is not necessarily related to $[S^{2-}]$.
    D. none of the above

78. What is the value of $[S^{2-}]$ when pH is 2.0?

    A. $1 \times 10^{-19} M$
    B. $5 \times 10^{-24} M$
    C. $2.5 \times 10^{-23} M$
    D. $2.0 M$

79. At what value of $[H^+]$ will ZnS precipitate?

    A. $0.0032 M$
    B. $0.032 M$
    C. $0.32 M$
    D. $3.2 M$

Passage III (Questions 80–85)

A student wishes to determine the solubility of $Mg(OH)_2$ under various conditions.

Experiment 1

The student dissolves some of the compound in water and finds $[Mg^{2+}]$ in the saturated solution to be 1.65×10^{-4}.

Experiment 2

The student dissolves enough $Mg(OH)_2$ in $0.1 M$ NaOH to make a saturated solution.

Experiment 3

The student prepares a saturated solution of $Mg(OH)_2$ in a solution that is buffered to pH 5 .

80. From Experiment 1, the student concludes that the solubility of the salt is:

    A. 1.65×10^{-4}
    B. 3.3×10^{-4}
    C. $(1.65 \times 10^{-4})^2$
    D. $(1.65 \times 10^{-4})^3$

81. Based on LeChatelier's Principle, how will the solubility of the compound in $0.1 M$ NaOH compare to the solubility of the compound in water?

    A. It will be less.
    B. It will be the same.
    C. It will be greater.
    D. It cannot be determined.

82. Which of the following expressions would allow the student to solve for the approximate concentration of Mg^{2+} in the alkaline solution? (Note that K_{sp} is the solubility product for $Mg(OH)_2$.)

    A. $[Mg^{2+}](.1) = K_{sp}$
    B. $[Mg^{2+}]^2(.1) = K_{sp}$
    C. $[Mg^{2+}](.1)^2 = K_{sp}$
    D. $[Mg^{2+}](.2)^2 = K_{sp}$

83. The student decides to measure the solubility of the salt in strong acid solution, as in Experiment 3. How would the solubility in acid compare to the solubility in the basic solution, as in Experiment 2?

    A. It would be less.
    B. It would be about the same.
    C. It would be greater.
    D. It cannot be determined.

84. Which of the following expressions could be used to calculate the solubility of $Mg(OH)_2$ prepared in Experiment 3?

    A. $[Mg^{2+}](1.0) = K_{sp}$
    B. $[Mg^{2+}](1.0)^2 = K_{sp}$
    C. $[Mg^{2+}](1.0 \times 10^{-14}) = K_{sp}$
    D. $[Mg^{2+}](1.0 \times 10^{-14})^2 = K_{sp}$

85. Which of the following can the student conclude?

    I. K_{sp} is pH-dependent.
    II. The solubility of $Mg(OH)_2$ is pH-dependent.
    III. The pH-dependence of this solubility serves as a model for all other magnesium salts.

    A. I only
    B. II only
    C. III only
    D. I and II only

Passage IV (Questions 86–91)

A student wants to know the molecular weight of a substance that is liquid at room temperature but a gas at 100° C.

She pours some of the liquid into an open, 400-mL flask, heats the flask to 100° C for several minutes, then cools the flask to room temperature. She finds that the condensed liquid in the flask weighs 0.900 g. The barometric pressure is 750 torr.

The student then calculates that the number of moles of gas in the sample is 0.0129. She further calculates that the molar mass of the sample must be 72.1 g/mol.

However, her instructor tells her that the molar mass of the sample is actually 24.0 g/mol.

86. Once the substance in the flask is vaporized, how do changes in temperature affect the number of moles of gas in the flask (assuming the flask to be open and the pressure and volume to be constant)?

    A. The number of moles increases as T increases.
    B. The number of moles decreases as T increases.
    C. The number has no relation to T.
    D. It depends on the substance.

87. Which of the following expressions did the student use to calculate the number of moles of gas in the flask at 100° C?

    A. (750)(.400)/(.0821)(100)
    B. (750/760)(.400)/(.0821)(100)
    C. (750/760)(.400)/(.0821)(373)
    D. (750/760)(.400)/(.0821)(273)

88. Which of the following expressions did the student use to calculate the molecular weight of the gas in the flask?

    A. (.900)/(.0129)
    B. (.0129)(.900)
    C. (.0129)/(.90)
    D. (.900) + (.0129)

89. Which of the following errors might help to explain the difference between the molecular weight calculated by the student and the figure given by the instructor?

    A. Instead of being completely filled with gas, the flask contained some air.
    B. The temperature of the sample was actually higher than 100° C.
    C. The temperature of the sample was actually lower than 100° C.
    D. The volume of the flask was actually less than 400 mL.

90. The student decides to investigate whether the discrepancy in molecular weight measurements is due to molecules that bind together to form aggregates in the gas phase. If such aggregated molecules occurred in the gas sample, which of the following would be affected?

    I. The number of independent particles
    II. The total weight of the gas
    III. The average speed of the molecules

    A. I only
    B. II only
    C. III only
    D. I and III only

91. If aggregation were the cause of the discrepancy in molecular weight, how many molecules must bind together on average to result in the observed molecular weight of 72.1 g/mol?

    A. 2
    B. 3
    C. 4
    D. 5

Passage V (Questions 92–96)

Two theories for predicting the rate of a chemical reaction are given below. As you read them, look for both their similarities and their differences. Then answer the questions that follow.

Theory 1

The rate of a chemical reaction is defined to be the number of moles per liter of a specified reactant that is consumed per unit of time. Because reactants must collide in order for a reaction to occur, it might seem that reaction rates would depend upon the concentration of reactants—since the more reactants are present, the greater the likelihood of a reaction. This is, in fact, the case, as the following example shows.

For the reaction

$$N_2O_5 \rightarrow 2NO_2 + 1/2\ O_2$$

the rate is proportional to the amount of N_2O_5 present. We may express this fact as a "rate law":

$$\text{rate} = k\ [N_2O_5]$$

where k is the rate constant.

A more complicated reaction will have a more complicated rate law. For the reaction

$$2NO + O_2 \rightarrow 2NO_2$$

the rate law will be

$$\text{rate} = k\ [NO]^2[O_2]^1$$

where the powers in the rate law reflect the coefficients of the reactants in the chemical equation. This relationship between numbers of reactant molecules and exponents in the rate law is a general one.

Theory 2

Theory 1 is very often true, for it expresses the reasonable insight that the greater the concentration of reactants, the greater the likelihood of a reaction. It has a great shortcoming, however, in its assumption that all reactions proceed in one fell swoop rather than in several steps. Let us take an example, using the letters A, B, and C, to represent molecules. In the reaction

$$A + 2B \rightarrow C$$

Theory 1 predicts a rate law of

$$\text{rate} = k[A][B]^2$$

But suppose the reaction actually proceeds in two stages, with the first one being

$$A + B \rightarrow AB$$

followed by

$$AB + B \rightarrow C$$

Let us also suppose that the first stage is much slower than the second, perhaps taking thousands of times as long. Then the rate of the overall process will essentially be the same as the rate of the first stage, which is given by

$$\text{rate} = k\ [A][B]$$

in contrast to Theory 1's prediction. Theory 2 implies, then, that we must understand the details of the reaction, including the relative speed of the various subreactions, in order to predict a rate law. Theory 1 is not totally wrong, just incomplete.

92. Theory 1 relates the:

    A. rate of a reaction to the concentration of products.
    B. rate of a reaction to the concentration of reactants.
    C. relative amounts of reactants to each other.
    D. rate of a reaction to the individual rates of various stages of that reaction.

93. According to Theory 1, which of the following expresses the rate of this reaction?

    $$3M + 2N \rightarrow 4P$$

    A. $k\,[M][N]$
    B. $k\,[M]^3[N]^2$
    C. $k\,[M]^3[N]^2[P]^4$
    D. $k\,([M]^3 + [N]^2)$

94. According to a proponent of Theory 2:

    A. Theory 1 can never give a correct prediction for a rate law.
    B. Theory 1 will give a correct result if the reactant coefficients are all equal to 1.
    C. Theory 1 will give a correct result for a single-stage reaction.
    D. Theory 1 is in error because it claims that collisions are necessary for reactions to take place.

95. A chemist studies the rate of the reaction

    $$2NO_2 + F_2 \rightarrow 2NO_2F$$

    According to Theory 1, which of the following would **not** affect the rate of the reaction?

    A. Increasing the concentration of NO_2.
    B. Decreasing the concentration of F_2.
    C. Doubling the concentration of NO_2 while cutting the concentration of F_2 by a factor of 2.
    D. Increasing the concentration of NO_2F.

96. The chemist suspects that the reaction given in Question 95 proceeds in two stages:

    $$NO_2 + F_2 \rightarrow NO_2F + F \text{ (Stage 1)}$$
    $$F + NO_2 \rightarrow NO_2F \text{ (Stage 2)}$$

    According to Theory 2, if Stage 1 is much slower than Stage 2, then the overall reaction rate:

    A. will be determined by the rate of Stage 1.
    B. will be determined by the rate of Stage 2.
    C. will be determined by the rate of Stage 1 minus that of Stage 2.
    D. cannot be determined unless the rate law is measured experimentally.

Passage VI (Questions 97–104)

We have seen that when a salt dissolves in pure water, the expression for K_{sp} can be used to solve for the concentration of the ions. For example, for AgCl,

$$K_{sp} = [Ag^+][Cl^-]$$

Since in pure water, every silver or chloride ion results from a dissociation, either concentration may be used to calculate the solubility.

The situation is different if there is another source of either ion. **The table on page 35 gives** solubility data for various salts in pure water (column 3) and for a solution containing 0.1 mol/L of the cation in the original salt. For example, for $BaSO_4$, the last column refers to solubility in $0.1\,M\,Ba^{2+}$.

97. The pair of salts with the least and greatest solubility in pure water, respectively, are:

    A. PbS and $CaSO_4$.
    B. PbS and BaF_2.
    C. BaF_2 and PbS.
    D. $CaSO_4$ and PbS.

98. The solubility of $Pb(OH)_2$ in the presence of 0.1 M cation is:

    A. greater than the K_{sp} by a factor of 10.
    B. less than the K_{sp} by a factor of 10.
    C. less than the solubility in pure water by a factor of 10.
    D. greater than the solubility in pure water by a factor of 10.

Salt	K_{sp}	Solubility (pure H_2O)	Solubility (0.1 M cation)
$BaSO_4$	1.1×10^{-10}	1.0×10^{-5}	1.1×10^{-9}
$BaCO_3$	1.6×10^{-9}	4.0×10^{-5}	1.6×10^{-8}
$CaSO_4$	2.4×10^{-5}	4.9×10^{-3}	2.4×10^{-4}
CaF_2	1.7×10^{-6}	3.5×10^{-4}	1.7×10^{-5}
PbS	7×10^{-29}	8.4×10^{-15}	7×10^{-28}
$PbSO_4$	1.3×10^{-8}	1.1×10^{-4}	1.3×10^{-7}
BaF_2	1.7×10^{-6}	7.5×10^{-3}	1.7×10^{-5}
$Pb(OH)_2$	2.8×10^{-16}	4.1×10^{-6}	2.8×10^{-15}
$Fe(OH)_2$	1.6×10^{-15}	7.4×10^{-6}	1.6×10^{-14}
$Cu(IO_3)_3$	1.3×10^{-7}	5.1×10^{-3}	1.3×10^{-6}

99. The solubility of a given salt in pure water is:

 A. less than in the 0.1 M solution of the cation.
 B. greater than in the 0.1 M solution of the cation.
 C. sometimes less, sometimes greater, than in the 0.1 M solution of the cation.
 D. equal to the solubility in the solution of the cation.

100. The solubility of a given salt in the 0.1 M cation solution can be calculated as which of the following?

 A. $(K_{sp})^{1/2}$
 B. $(0.10)K_{sp}$
 C. $K_{sp}/(0.10)$
 D. The square root of the solubility in pure water

101. Which of the following is closest to the ratio of the smallest K_{sp} shown in the chart to the largest?

 A. 10^{24}
 B. 10^{-24}
 C. 10^{12}
 D. 10^{-12}

102. Which of the lead salts listed produces the greatest concentration of Pb^{2+} when added in excess to pure water?

 A. PbS
 B. $PbSO_4$
 C. $Pb(OH)_2$
 D. All the salts produce the same concentration.

103. Excess BaF_2 is added to pure water; then $Ba(NO_3)_2$ is added until the solution is 0.1 M in Ba^{2+}. Which of the following is true?

 A. BaF_2 dissolves after the addition of barium nitrate.
 B. The solubility product of BaF_2 drops as the barium nitrate is added.
 C. BaF_2 precipitates as the barium nitrate is added.
 D. $Ba(NO_3)$ precipitates at the last step.

104. Solution A is 0.1 M in both $Ba(NO_3)_2$ and $Ca(NO_3)_2$. To 1.0 L of solution A, a student adds 1.0 mL of 0.1 M Na_2SO_4. What will be the result?

 A. Precipitation of $BaSO_4$
 B. Precipitation of $CaSO_4$
 C. Precipitation of both $BaSO_4$ and $CaSO_4$
 D. None of the above

Passage VII (Questions 105–109)

A worker on the third floor of a building under construction needs to remove a 100-kg block of steel. The worker, whose body mass is 70 kg, pushes the block along the level floor at a constant velocity covering 8 m in 4 s. The force applied on the block is 200 N. When the block reaches the edge of the building, it falls off. It tumbles 8 meters, accidentally strikes a stake partially embedded in the ground, and drives the stake completely into the ground.

105. What is the weight of the steel block?

 A. 9.8×10^{-2} N
 B. 4.9×10^{-2} N
 C. 4.9×10^{2} N
 D. 9.8×10^{2} N

106. Which statement is most accurate about the force of friction exerted while the block is pushed along the floor?

 A. F_{friction} is greater than 200 N.
 B. F_{friction} is less than 200 N.
 C. F_{friction} is exactly equal to 200 N.
 D. F_{friction} can not be determined from the data given.

107. What is the work done by the man in pushing the block?

 A. 1600 J
 B. 400 J
 C. 50 J
 D. 25 J

108. What is the approximate velocity of the block just before striking the stake?

 A. 9.80 m/s
 B. 2.00 m/s
 C. 12.5 m/s
 D. 16.0 m/s

109. What is the approximate kinetic energy of the block just before striking the stake?

 A. 3263 J
 B. 7840 J
 C. 8500 J
 D. 12,000 J

Passage VIII (Questions 110–114)

An electrical technician constructs a circuit that consists of three resistors, R_1, R_2, and R_3 of 30 Ω, 60 Ω, and 40 Ω, respectively, and a voltage source, V. The circuit diagram for the set up is:

With an ammeter the technician measures the amount of current at point A.

110. If the amount of current measured at point A is 2.0 amperes, what is the rate at which R_2 uses electrical energy?

 A. 30 W
 B. 60 W
 C. 240 W
 D. 180 W

111. What is the amount of heat developed in R_2 in 3 seconds?

 A. 720 J
 B. 120 J
 C. 360 J
 D. 40 J

112. What is the voltage drop across the 30 Ω resistor, R_1?

 A. 60 V
 B. 120 V
 C. 180 V
 D. 240 V

113. What is the voltage of the potential difference source V?

 A. 60 V
 B. 120 V
 C. 240 V
 D. 360 V

114. The voltage source, V, has an internal resistance of 4 Ω. What is its electromotive force (emf)?

   A. 384 V
   B. 336 V
   C. 356 V
   D. 364 V

Passage IX (Questions 115–118)

In order to compare the refractive properties of various liquid substances, a researcher constructs the apparatus illustrated below. It consists of two adjacent chambers, 1 and 2, with walls and partitions made from very thin glass so that the effects of the glass on the refraction of light passing through the chambers is negligible. One chamber is filled with a reference liquid for which the refractive index is known. Water is a typical reference liquid. The refractive index for water, $n_{H2O} = 1.33$. The liquid to be tested is then placed in the second chamber. The apparatus is surrounded by the air in the laboratory.

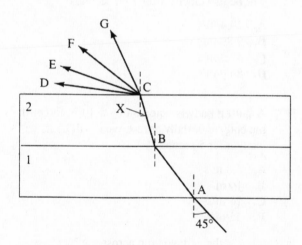

The researcher then shines a beam of light through the two liquids and traces its path. The angle of incidence of the beam on the first wall of the apparatus (chamber 1) is 45°. (sin 45° = 0.707. Sin 30° = 0.500.)

115. In the diagram, several possible rays for the light beam exiting from chamber 2 into the air are indicated. Which ray best represents the actual exit path of the beam?

   A. D
   B. E
   C. F
   D. G

116. What is the speed of light in water?

   A. 1.13×10^3 m/s
   B. 2.26×10^8 m/s
   C. 3.00×10^8 m/s
   D. 3.99×10^8 m/s

117. If the refractive index of the unknown liquid in chamber 2 is 2.00, which of the statements below most accurately describes the angle of incidence, x, of the beam on the wall between the unknown liquid in chamber 2 and the air?

   A. It is less than 30°.
   B. It is exactly 30°.
   C. It is greater than 30° but less than 45°.
   D. It is exactly 45°.

118. What is the sine of the critical angle between the unknown liquid in chamber 2 and the air?

   A. 0.500
   B. 0.707
   C. 1.00
   D. 2.00

Passage X (Questions 119–123)

A Nebraska telephone company lineman needs to determine the size of copper wire that can best withstand the typical buildup of ice on the wires during the winter. He takes a sample that is 240 meters long and 2.0 mm in diameter. He simulates the net effect of the ice by applying a 628-N force to one of the wires so that the line of action of the force coincides with the axis of the wire. The length after stretching the wire is 240.24 m. When the force is removed, the wire returns to its original length.

119. What is the stress on the wire?

    A. 2.00×10^8 N/m^2
    B. 2.00×10^8 J
    C. 314 N/m^2
    D. 314

120. What is the strain on the wire?

    A. 0.24 m
    B. 1.0×10^{-3} N/m^2
    C. 0.24
    D. 1.0×10^{-3}

121. What is the estimated elastic modulus for copper?

    A. 2.0×10^{11} N/m^2
    B. 314 N/m^2
    C. 480 N/m^2
    D. 2.0×10^5 N/m^2

122. The elastic modulus for copper is called the:

    A. Shear modulus.
    B. Bulk modulus.
    C. Young's modulus.
    D. Unit modulus.

123. The reaction of the wire to the removal of the force is called the:

    A. elastic limit.
    B. breaking point.
    C. elasticity.
    D. tensile strength.

Questions 124–142 are independent of any passage and independent of each other.

124. The speed of sound in air at a given temperature is 360 m/s. What is the shortest closed-end pipe that will produce an air column length that can resonate at a frequency of 450 Hz?

    A. 20 cm
    B. 80 cm
    C. 90 cm
    D. 125 cm

125. What is the acceleration of a falling stone whose velocity increases from 80 m/s to 100 m/s in 2 seconds?

    A. 0.10 m/s^2
    B. 10 m/s^2
    C. 10 m/s
    D. 90 m/s^2

126. A ball is thrown vertically upward with an initial velocity of 40.0 meters per second. What will be its velocity after 2.00 seconds?

    A. 20.4 m/s
    B. 9.80 m/s
    C. 49.0 m/s
    D. 80.0 m/s

127. A 2.0-kg body is acted on by a 10-N force. If the body is initially at rest, what will be its velocity after 5 seconds?

    A. 5.0 m/s
    B. 10 m/s
    C. 20 m/s
    D. 25 m/s

128. A sample of 22.5 g of NiCl$_2$ (molar mass = 219 g/mol) reacts completely with a sufficient amount of NH3 and NaBr to form Ni(NH$_3$)$_2$Br$_2$Cl$_2$ (molar mass = 323 g/mol). Which of the following expressions gives the number of moles of product that are formed?

    A. 22.5/58.7
    B. 22.5/219
    C. (22.5) (323)
    D. (22.5/219) (323)

129. Which is the correct electron-dot formula for H_2O_2?

 A. H:Ö::Ö:H

 B. H:Ö::O:H

 C. H:O::Ö:H

 D. H:Ö : Ö:H

130. Which of the following is closest to the pH of a mixture containing 1.0 mole each of formic acid (whose K_a is 1.8×10^{-4}) and potassium formate?

 A. 0.1
 B. 2
 C. 4
 D. 7

131. If 1.0 mole each of graphite at 350K ($C_p = 8.63$ J/mol deg) and water at 273K ($C_p = 4.18$ J/mol deg) are put together in an insulated container, which of the following gives the final temperature (T) of the water in degrees C?

 A. $(8.63)(350 + T) = (4.18)(273 + T)$
 B. $(8.63)(350 - T) = (4.18)(T - 273)$
 C. $(4.18)(350 - T) = (8.63)(T - 273)$
 D. $T = (8.63 - 4.18)/(350 - 273)$

132. A 0th order reaction requires 5 minutes for the original concentration of its reactant to drop from 0.180 M to 0.090 M. How much additional time, in minutes, will be required for the reactant concentration to decline to 0.045 M?

 A. 2.5
 B. 5
 C. 7.5
 D. 10

133. A "3-minute egg" cooked in Boston might require extra cooking time in:

 A. Denver, because of the higher boiling point of the water at Denver's higher altitude.
 B. Death Valley, because of the higher boiling point of the water at Death Valley's lower altitude.
 C. Denver, because of the lower boiling point of the water at high altitude.
 D. Death Valley, because of the lower boiling point of the water at low altitude.

134. An electron in a hydrogen atom is excited to a state where $l = 2$ and $n = 4$. This state is referred to as:

 A. $2p$.
 B. $4s$.
 C. $2d$.
 D. $4d$.

135. Which of the following thermodynamic quantities determines the spontaneity of a chemical reaction?

 A. ΔE
 B. ΔH
 C. ΔS
 D. ΔG

136. What is the force between two 10-μC charges separated by a distance of 10 cm?

 A. 1.0×10^{-8} N
 B. 90 N
 C. 30 N
 D. -30 N

137. A heating device requires 1200 watts of power when supplied by a 120-volt source. What is the resistance of this device?

 A. 12 Ω
 B. 10 Ω
 C. 6 Ω
 D. 0.10 Ω

138. The light emitted from an incandescent source follows the inverse square law of intensity. By what factor does the brightness change if the source is moved from 6 ft away from an observer to 3 ft away from the observer?

 A. The brightness doubles.
 B. The brightness quadruples.
 C. The brightness is halved.
 D. The brightness is quartered.

139. What radiation is emitted during the following decay process?

$$^{226}_{88}\text{Ra} \rightarrow {}^{222}_{86}\text{Rn} + x$$

A. α decay
B. β decay
C. Neutron emission
D. Positron emission

140. A 20 Ω and a 40 Ω resistor are connected in series with a voltage source as shown below

20 Ω

40 Ω

If the current through the 20 Ω-resistor is 2.0 A, what is the voltage drop across the 40 Ω resistor?

A. 40 V
B. 80 V
C. 120 V
D. 400 V

141. How many neutrons are produced in the following nuclear reaction?

$$^{235}_{92}\text{U} + {}^{1}_{0}n \rightarrow {}^{144}_{56}\text{Ba} + {}^{89}_{36}\text{Kr} + X{}^{1}_{0}n$$

A. 1
B. 2
C. 3
D. 4

142. A 6-N and an 8-N force act on the same point of a body, but at right angles to each other. What is the resultant force?

A. 2 N
B. 7 N
C. 10 N
D. 14 N

END OF TEST 2.

**IF YOU FINISH BEFORE THE TIME IS UP, YOU MAY
CHECK YOUR WORK ON THIS TEST ONLY.**

WRITING SAMPLE

Time: 60 Minutes
2 Essays

Directions: This test consists of two parts. You will have 30 minutes to complete each part. During the first 30 minutes, you may work on Part 1 only. During the second 30 minutes, you may work on Part 2 only. You will have three pages for each essay answer, but you do not have to fill all three pages. Be sure to write legibly; illegible essays will not be scored.

Part 1

Consider this statement:

Know the truth and it shall set you free.

Write a unified essay in which you perform the following tasks. Explain what you think the above statement means. Describe a specific situation in which knowing the truth does NOT set you free. Discuss what you think determines whether knowledge of the truth allows one to be free.

DO NOT START THE NEXT TOPIC UNTIL THE TIME IS UP.

Part 2

Consider this statement:

He has not learned the first lesson of life who does not everyday surmount a fear.

Write a unified essay in which you perform the following tasks. Explain what you think the above statement means. Describe a specific situation in which the first lesson of life does NOT involve conquering a fear. Discuss what you think determines whether life is or is not governed by a daily conquest of fear.

END OF SECTION 3.

DO NOT RETURN TO PART 1.

BIOLOGICAL SCIENCES

Time: 100 Minutes
Questions 143–219

Directions: This test contains 77 questions. Most of the questions consist of a descriptive passage followed by a group of questions related to the passage. For these questions, study the passage carefully and then choose the best answer to each question in the group. Some questions in this test stand alone. These questions are independent of any passage and independent of each other. For these questions, too, you must select the one best answer. Indicate all your answers by blackening the corresponding circles on your answer sheet.

A periodic table is provided at the beginning of the book. You may consult it whenever you wish.

Passage I (Questions 143–149)

Enzymes act as biological catalysts that help speed up reactions by lowering the activation energy needed to bring reactants to their "transition state." In this unstable condition, bonds can break and the reaction proceeds. The reaction itself is often described in the following way:

$$E + S \rightarrow ES \rightarrow P + E$$

E = Enzyme   ES = Enzyme-Substrate
                                     Complex
S = Substrate(s)   P = Product(s)

Enzymes can carry out their catalytic functions only with particular substrates, and only under particular environmental (pH, temperature, etc.) conditions. This characteristic of enzymes is referred to as enzyme specific-

ity. The enzyme specificity in four different enzymes is shown in the figure below.

(A)

(B)

143. Enzymes X and Y in the figure are both protein-digesting enzymes found in humans. Where would they most likely be at work?

   A. X in the mouth; Y in the small intestine
   B. X in the small intestine; Y in the mouth
   C. X in the stomach; Y in the small intestine
   D. X in the small intestine; Y in the stomach

144. Which statement is true concerning enzymes X and Y?

   A. They could not possibly be at work in the same part of the body at the same time.
   B. They have different temperature ranges at which they work best.
   C. At a pH of 4.5, enzyme X works slower than enzyme Y.
   D. At their appropriate pH ranges, both enzymes work equally fast.

145. What conclusion may be drawn concerning enzymes A and B?

   A. Neither enzyme is likely to be a human enzyme.
   B. Enzyme A is more likely to be a human enzyme.
   C. Enzyme B is more likely to be a human enzyme.
   D. Both enzymes are likely to be human enzymes.

146. At which temperatures might enzymes A and B both work?

   A. Above 40°C
   B. Below 50°C
   C. Above 50°C and below 40°C
   D. Between 40°C and 50°C

147. An enzyme-substrate complex can form when the substrate(s) binds to the active site of the enzyme. Which environmental condition might alter the conformation of an enzyme in the figure to the extent that its substrate is unable to bind?

   A. Enzyme A at 40°C
   B. Enzyme B at pH 2
   C. Enzyme X at pH 4
   D. Enzyme Y at 37°C

148. At 35°, the rate of the reaction catalyzed by enzyme A begins to level off. Which hypothesis best explains this observation?

   A. The temperature is too far below optimum.
   B. The enzyme has become saturated with substrate.
   C. Both A and B
   D. Neither A nor B

149. In which of the following environmental conditions would digestive enzyme Y be unable to bring its substrate(s) to the transition state?

   A. At any temperature below optimum
   B. At any pH where the rate of reaction is not maximum
   C. At any pH lower than 5.5
   D. At any temperature higher than 37°C

Passage II (Questions 150–156)

A set of experiments was performed to examine the effects of ultraviolet radiation (UV) on the bacterium, *E.coli*. It is known that purines and pyrimidines absorb UV radiation at 260 nanometers (nm). Fewer colonies suggests that cells have died, while smaller colonies suggests that growth has been inhibited.

Experiment 1

The undersides of two glass petri dishes (A and B) were divided in half (each dish divided into sides 1 and 2) using a marking pencil. Melted agar and nutrients were poured into the dishes and allowed to harden. A sample of bacterial culture was streaked across the entire surface of each dish before covering with the glass lid. Treatment was as follows: With the lid removed, dish A was radiated with UV (260 nm) on side 1 only, while dish B was radiated with green light (550 nm) on side 1 only. Both dishes were then covered and incubated in a dark container.

Experiment 2

The procedures used in Experiment 1 were repeated except that the dishes were exposed to regular incandescent light for 20 minutes before being incubated in a dark container.

The results of both experiments are summarized in the table on page 46.

Number and Characteristics of Bacterial Colonies

	Dish *A*		Dish *B*	
	Side 1	Side 2	Side 1	Side 2
Experiment 1	5 large 5 small	30 large	31 large	29 large
Experiment 2	10 large 10 small	29 large	30 large	30 large

150. The results of Experiment 1 demonstrate that UV light (260 nm):

   A. can inhibit growth in *E. coli*.
   B. can kill *E. coli*.
   C. Both A and B
   D. Neither A nor B

151. A total of 40 colonies on Dish *A* can be observed in Experiment 1. Which statement is true concerning these colonies?

   A. Of the colonies exposed to UV light, 25 percent show the effects of radiation.
   B. Exposure to UV light results in one-third the number of colonies that result in bacteria not exposed to UV light.
   C. Two-thirds of the colonies on the plate were not affected by exposure to UV light.
   D. Exposure to UV light results in one-eighth of all cells dying.

152. Based on the results of both experiments, what conclusions can be drawn about the effects of green light on bacterial colony formation?

   A. It has no effects when bacteria are incubated in the dark.
   B. It has no effects when bacteria are incubated in the light.
   C. Both A and B
   D. Neither A nor B

153. Identify the control(s) in this set of experiments.

   A. Side 1 of Dish *A*
   B. Side 2 of Dish *B*
   C. Side 1 of both Dish *A* and Dish *B*
   D. Side 2 of both Dish *A* and Dish *B*

154. Which hypothesis is a reasonable interpretation of results observed when comparing Dish *A* in both experiments?

   A. Exposure to incandescent light helps magnify the effects of UV damage.
   B. Exposure to incandescent light helps repair the effects of UV damage.
   C. Exposure to UV light does twice as much damage as exposure to incandescent light.
   D. Exposure to UV light does one-half the damage of exposure to incandescent light.

155. UV light probably affects what part(s) of the bacterium?

   A. Most covalent molecules in the cell wall
   B. Proteins in the membrane
   C. DNA in the chromosome
   D. All of the above

156. Experiment 1 was repeated without removing the glass lid prior to UV radiation. The results in Dish *A* were as follows: After incubation, Side 1 had 29 large colonies and Side 2 had 30 large colonies. What do these results suggest when compared to data from the earlier experiments?

   A. UV radiation has no effect on bacterial colony formation.
   B. UV radiation can inhibit growth but it does not kill.
   C. Glass has no effect on bacterial colony formation.
   D. Glass blocks the effects of UV radiation.

Passage III (Questions 157–162)

The small intestine is one of many organs that has endocrine functions in addition to its more familiar roles in the body. By producing such hormones as intestinal gastrin, gastric inhibitory peptide (GIP), secretin, and cholecystokinin, the small intestine regulates the activities of neighboring digestive organs and their secretions.

The thymus gland secretes thymosin, a protein hormone that stimulates the maturation and differentiation of T-lymphocytes. These cells of the immune system provide cell-mediated immunity, which not only includes attacks on infectious agents, but on infected cells as well.

Other endocrine-producing structures include the pineal gland, the kidney, and the heart. In response to light stimuli entering the eye, the pineal gland (located in the brain) releases melatonin, which is believed to play a role in regulating daily circadian rhythms. The kidney regulates red blood cell production through the secretion of erythropoietin. The heart, by secreting atrial natriuretic factor (ANF), helps regulate blood pressure, salt, and water balance.

157. The factor(s) that these structures have in common is that they:

A. are all glands.
B. release chemicals into the blood.
C. secretory function is regulated by the hypothalamus.
D. All of the above

158. An indirect effect of erythropoietin is the increase in blood volume that accompanies increased red blood cell production. This, in turn, helps raise blood pressure. In contrast, ANF helps lower blood pressure by increasing the kidney's:

A. reabsorption of sodium and excretion of water.
B. reabsorption of water and excretion of sodium.
C. reabsorption of sodium and water.
D. excretion of sodium and water.

159. Secretin acts as a signal to the pancreas to release bicarbonate ions through the pancreatic duct. The release of secretin is itself stimulated because:

A. acidic chyme arrives in the small intestine.
B. digestive pancreatic enzymes require a slightly alkaline environment.
C. Both A and B
D. Neither A nor B

160. When cells from the pineal gland of various vertebrates are cultured in a dish under conditions of darkness, they release melatonin in a cyclic pattern. This suggests that:

A. the pineal cells themselves have an intrinsic rhythmic property.
B. melatonin production varies proportionately with light and dark cycles.
C. melatonin production is not cyclic during daylight.
D. pineal tissue probably has neural connections with the hypothalamus.

161. Thymosin can directly:

A. respond to specific foreign antigens and bind to receptors on invading organisms.
B. destroy infected host cells.
C. produce chemical (humoral) antibodies.
D. None of the above

162. Cholecystokinin stimulates the gall bladder to release bile when fats arrive in the small intestine. While in the gall bladder, bile can become overly concentrated and gallstones may form. If this necessitates removal of the gallbladder, which of the following statements is true?

A. Fats can no longer be emulsified before digestion in the small intestine.
B. Bile can still reach the small intestine from the liver.
C. Fats can no longer be digested.
D. None of the above

Passage IV (Questions 163–169)

The immune response is part of the body's "specific defense system." Two aspects of this defense mechanism are the primary and secondary immune responses. When the body is first exposed to a foreign antigen (primary immune response), B-lymphocytes or B-cells, as well as macrophages, come in contact with the antigen. When the macrophages digest the antigen-bearing agent and display the antigen on their surface, T-helper cells (one kind of T-cell) become activated. The T-helper cells assist other types of T-cells in responding to the agent and interact with B-cells, causing some of them to differentiate into antibody-secreting plasma cells. Such humoral antibodies (immunoglobulins) can be produced and released by plasma cells for many weeks as other effector components of the immune system help destroy the invading organisms. During this time, the host suffers through various symptoms (depending on the invader), but in addition, sensitized memory cells are produced that can remain dormant for decades. Upon second exposure to the same antigen, the memory cells (various T-cells and B-cells) can give rise to clones of appropriate effector cells much more rapidly than the first time; this is a secondary immune response.

The figure below characterizes both primary and secondary responses.

163. On approximately which day would the peak of the secondary immune response to antigen B occur?

  A. 40
  B. 56
  C. 63
  D. 70

164. According to the figure, which answer most closely approximates the number of days between the initial exposure to a foreign antigen and the peak primary immune response?

  A. Less than 5 days
  B. Less than 12 days
  C. Less than 19 days
  D. Less than 28 days

165. Which answer most closely approximates how many more antibodies the peak secondary immune response produces in comparison to the peak primary response?

  A. More than 10 times as many
  B. More than 100 times as many
  C. More than 1,000 times as many
  D. More than 10,000 times as many

166. Referring to the passage, what types of cells are the macrophages, and by what process do they help fight off invading organisms?

  A. Red blood cells/hemolysis
  B. White blood cells/phagocytosis
  C. Platelets/coagulation (clotting)
  D. White blood cells/agglutination

167. The ability of our immune system to carry out a "secondary immune response" provides a direct theoretical basis for:

  A. how cells differentiate.
  B. regeneration technology.
  C. vaccine technology.
  D. most recessive lethal genes.

168. The AIDS virus (HIV) can infect T-helper cells, preventing them from functioning properly and often killing them. Which aspect(s) of the body's defenses will be affected by the virus?

  A. Primary immune response
  B. Secondary immune response
  C. Both A and B
  D. Neither A nor B

169. Which conclusion can be drawn concerning the danger at hand if a serious allergy to a drug such as penicillin is discovered during initial treatment?

A. When the drug is administered a second time, the patient's allergic response can be even more severe.
B. When the drug is administered a second time, the patient should be able to receive the benefits even faster.
C. Both A and B
D. Neither A nor B

Passage V (Questions 170–175)

Loss of muscular movement may be caused by numerous agents including microorganisms, poisons, and both environmental and genetic factors that manifest themselves by interfering with normal function. Changes in function can occur at various locations that contribute to muscular activity, such as the motor neurons, neuromuscular junctions, and within the muscle cells themselves.

170. *Clostridium botulinum* is the bacterium associated with botulism, a disease that leads to flaccid paralysis. The organism prevents the release of acetylcholine by motor neurons at the neuromuscular junction. The physiological effect of this action is to:

A. prevent repolarization of the sarcolemma.
B. prevent depolarization of the sarcolemma.
C. inhibit the active transport needed to return calcium to the sarcoplasmic reticulum.
D. inhibit neurons of the sympathetic autonomic nervous system.

171. The polio virus can infect and destroy cell bodies located in the anterior horn of the spinal cord. These motor neurons are vital because they stimulate:

A. the part of the brain that controls voluntary movement.
B. receptors found in freely movable joints.
C. skeletal muscles.
D. interneurons along circuits leading to the cerebrum.

172. When athletes overexert themselves on hot days, they often suffer immobility from painful muscle cramping. Which of the following is a reasonable hypothesis to explain such cramps?

A. Muscle cells do not have enough ATP for normal muscle relaxation.
B. Excessive sweating has affected the salt balance within the muscles.
C. Prolonged contractions have temporarily interrupted blood flow to parts of the muscle.
D. All of the above

173. Myasthenia gravis is a heritable disorder in which autoantibodies (antibodies to one's own tissues) bind to receptors at the motor end plate. This disease *directly* affects:

A. motor neurons.
B. brain cells.
C. muscle insertions.
D. neuromuscular junctions.

174. Multiple sclerosis is another disease associated with an autoimmune response. Antibodies cause the destruction of myelin sheaths in the central nervous system. This affects:

A. axons in the brain and spinal cord.
B. axons and dendrites in the brain only.
C. axons and dendrites in the brain and spinal cord.
D. axons in the brain, spinal cord, and spinal nerves.

175. Duchenne muscular dystrophy is a sex-linked recessive disorder associated with severe deterioration of muscle tissue. The gene for the disease:

A. is inherited by males from their mothers.
B. should be more common in females than in males.
C. Both A and B
D. Neither A nor B

Passage VI (Questions 176–181)

The role of chlorophyll, a light-absorbing pigment, in photosynthesis was investigated in a pair of experiments. Pigment was extracted from a leaf preparation and examined using paper chromatography and spectrophotometric techniques.

Experiment 1

In order to analyze the composition of leaf extract, a sample of the pigment was applied near the bottom of a strip of chromatographic filter paper and allowed to dry. This was repeated a number of times to ensure that an adequate amount of pigment was present. The strip was suspended in a test tube containing the solvent acetone. As the experiment proceeded, the acetone soaked into the filter paper and slowly moved up across the pigment sample, eventually reaching the top of the paper. This technique is designed to separate substances in a mixture based on differences in their tendency to adhere to the material over which they are passed (adsorption), as well as on their solubility in the solvent used. Substances with color can easily be detected on the paper. The experiment revealed three separate bands of color on the filter paper: a green band, a yellow-green band, and an orange band.

Experiment 2

Samples of each band were examined using a spectrophotometer. This instrument can send light of various wavelengths (375 nm to 750 nm) through a sample. For each wavelength, the amount of light passing through (percentage of transmittance) can be monitored and then converted to absorbance. Absorbance is a measure of the amount of light absorbed as it passes through a sample. Unless light is absorbed, the energy in the light cannot be utilized. A sample's absorption spectrum indicates the range of its ability to absorb different wavelengths of

light. The absorption spectra of all three samples are shown in the figure below.

Absorption spectrum

176. Which statement is true concerning the paper chromatography technique used in Experiment 1?

- **A.** All other factors being equal, the most soluble substance travels fastest and will likely be highest on the paper.
- **B.** All other factors being equal, the substance with the greatest adsorptive tendency will likely be highest on the paper.
- **C.** Both A and B
- **D.** Neither A nor B

177. The most reasonable hypothesis that addresses the results of Experiment 1 is which of the following?

- **A.** The chlorophyll extract may contain three different pigments.
- **B.** Chlorophyll has three different solubility/ adsorption patterns.
- **C.** The chlorophyll applied to the filter paper was not allowed to dry properly.
- **D.** Chlorophyll can have three different conformations.

178. As seen in the figure, the three samples from Experiment 1 have different absorption spectra. Which of the following statements is correct?

    A. Each substance shows at least two different absorbance peaks of 40 percent or higher.
    B. Substance A shows a low level of transmittance across a broad range of wavelengths.
    C. Each pigment shows an absorbance peak at both ends of the spectrum.
    D. Substance B shows its greatest absorption in the blue range of wavelengths.

179. Which colors of light are most likely utilized in photosynthesis by substance A?

    A. Blue-green
    B. Blue-green and red
    C. Violet-blue and red
    D. Violet-blue and orange

180. What do the results of Experiment 2 suggest about the question "Why are green plants green"?

    A. The light wavelengths utilized by each pigment mix to form green.
    B. The pigments absorb green.
    C. The pigments do not absorb green.
    D. Green light is the most utilized light in photosynthesis.

181. Which hypothesis best interprets the presence of more than one pigment in green leaves?

    A. The ability of different pigments to use the same wavelengths equally well makes photosynthesis more efficient.
    B. Making small amounts of more than one pigment is energetically less expensive than making a large amount of the same pigment.
    C. When light is absorbed by more than one pigment, heat can be dissipated in the plant more easily.
    D. The ability of different pigments to use different wavelengths makes photosynthesis more efficient.

Passage VII (Questions 182–187)

Phenylalanine is an amino acid that is necessary in small amounts for proper human nutrition. The normal metabolism of this substance requires the enzyme phenylalanine hydroxylase. The ability to produce the enzyme is controlled by an autosomal dominant trait. Approximately one in 15,000 whites in the United States is born without the capacity to produce the enzyme due to a homozygous recessive condition called phenylketonuria (PKU). In people with PKU, phenylalanine accumulates in the blood, and phenylpyruvic acid accumulates in the urine—giving it a distinctive odor. High levels of phenylalanine in the brain and spinal fluid during the first weeks after birth causes mental retardation in PKU individuals. Since PKU can be identified by a blood test at birth, dietary treatment can be administered to prevent this damage. If placed on a low-phenylalanine diet for the first few years of life, symptoms can be avoided.

182. If a couple, both heterozygous for PKU, have a child, what is the probability that the child will have *at least one normal allele?*

    A. 100 percent
    B. 75 percent
    C. 50 percent
    D. 0 percent

183. If the same couple were to have two children, what is the probability that *both children* will be carriers (heterozygotes) of the disease?

    A. 100 percent
    B. 75 percent
    C. 50 percent
    D. 25 percent

184. A woman, homozygous for PKU, was successfully treated after birth to avoid symptoms of the disorder. If she becomes pregnant, why must similar precautions be taken to control her diet again?

   A. The fetus must have the genotype for the disorder.
   B. High levels of phenylalanine in her blood can cause brain damage in the fetus, regardless of its genotype.
   C. High levels of phenylalanine in her blood can stimulate her body to overproduce phenylalanine hydroxylase, which causes damage in the fetus.
   D. Phenylpyruvic acid in her urine can cause damage to the fetus.

185. Polydactyly (extra toes or fingers) is an autosomal dominant trait. Identify the correct statement concerning this trait.

   A. All children of homozygotes must have the trait.
   B. Affected children must have at least one affected parent.
   C. Seventy-five percent of the children of two heterozygote parents must have the trait.
   D. All of the above

186. Holandric traits are Y-linked. Which of the following statements is correct concerning such traits?

   A. Holandric traits will only appear in males.
   B. Every holandric gene that is present will be expressed.
   C. Both A and B
   D. Neither A nor B

187. Amyotrophic lateral sclerosis (Lou Gehrig's Disease) is caused by an autosomal recessive gene. Which of the following statements is correct concerning family members of individuals with this disorder?

   A. If not affected themselves, both parents of an affected individual have to be carriers.
   B. If not affected themselves, all siblings of an affected individual must be carriers.
   C. Both A and B
   D. Neither A nor B

Passage VIII (Questions 188–193)

Tautomers are compounds that differ in their arrangement of atoms and undergo rapid equilibrium reactions. An example is enol-keto tautomerism:

$$-\overset{|}{C}=\overset{|}{C}-OH \rightleftharpoons -\overset{|}{C}-\overset{|}{\underset{H}{C}}=O$$

Because the equilibrium lies to the right, usually the reactions that produce the enol tautomer end up mostly with the keto form. The rearrangement takes place because of the polarity of the O-H bond, which enables H^+ to separate readily from oxygen:

$$-\overset{|}{C}=\overset{|}{C}-OH \rightleftharpoons -\overset{|}{C}=\overset{|}{C}-O^{\ominus}$$

$$-\overset{|}{\underset{H}{C}}-\overset{|}{C}=O \rightleftharpoons -\overset{|}{C}-\overset{|}{C}=O + H^+$$

When the H^+ returns, it can join with the negatively charged carbon in the anion or go back to the oxygen. However, when H^+ attaches to carbon it tends to stay on much longer, favoring the keto tautomer.

188. Adding one mole of water to one mole of acetylene produces mostly:

   A. vinyl alcohol.
   B. a diol.
   C. acetaldehyde.
   D. acetone.

189. Which of the following statements best explains why the above equilibrium favors the keto form?

   A. Ketones are, in general, more stable than alcohols.
   B. Ketones are stronger acids.
   C. Equilibrium favors the weaker acid.
   D. Equilibrium favors the stronger acid.

190. Phenol is favored over its keto form:

$$\langle\bigcirc\rangle\!-\!OH \rightleftarrows \langle\bigcirc\rangle\!=\!O$$

Which of the following statements best explains this exception?

A. Weaker acids tend to form from stronger acids.

B. Extra stability associated with the aromatic phenyl ring makes phenol more stable.

C. Oxygen does not have an octet in the keto form.

D. Enols tend to be favored over their keto tautomers.

191. Another example of tautomerism is the enamine-imine equilibrium system:

The acidic proton on the enamine form is attached to:

A. R′.
B. C—2.
C. N.
D. C—1.

192. Carbonyl compounds react with 1° and 2° amines by nucleophilic addition. The addition product then undergoes dehydration. Which pair of reactions best describes these reactions?

A.

B.

C.

D.

193. Which of the following enamines does not form an imine tautomer?

A.

$$CH_2=C-N-CH_3$$

with CH_3H above

B.

$$CH_2=C-N-CH_3$$

with H H above

C.

$$H-C=C-N-CH_3$$

with CH_3CH_3H above

D.

$$H-C=C-N-CH_3$$

with CH_3H CH_3 above

Passage IX (Questions 194–199)

A student titrates one liter of a $1.0\ M$ amino acid solution, which is acidified with HCl with a NaOH solution. He plots pH versus moles of NaOH added to give the following graph:

194. The titration curve indicates that the amino acid is:

A. triprotic.
B. diprotic.
C. a base.
D. monoprotic.

195. The amino acid can be identified by comparing:

A. the first full neutralization point with pK_{a1}.
B. the second full neutralization point with pK_{a2}.
C. the isoelectric point (pI) with pK_{a1}.
D. the pK_{a1} and pK_{a2} of the amino acid with the pH after addition of 0.5 mol and 1.5 mol of NaOH.

196. At which isoelectric point (pH) does the amino acid have a dipolar or zwitterioric form?

A. 6.10
B. 2.40
C. 7.00
D. 9.80

197. Which of the following is the predominant form of the amino acid after 0.60 mol of NaOH is added?

A.

$$H_2N-\overset{\overset{\displaystyle H}{|}}{\underset{\underset{\displaystyle R}{|}}{C}}-\overset{\overset{\displaystyle O}{\|}}{C}-O^{\ominus}$$

B.

$$\overset{\oplus}{H_3N}-\overset{\overset{\displaystyle H}{|}}{\underset{\underset{\displaystyle R}{|}}{C}}-\overset{\overset{\displaystyle O}{\|}}{C}-OH$$

C.

$$\overset{\oplus}{H_3N}-\overset{\overset{\displaystyle H}{|}}{\underset{\underset{\displaystyle R}{|}}{C}}-\overset{\overset{\displaystyle O}{\|}}{C}-\overset{\ominus}{O}$$

D.

$$H_2N-\overset{\overset{\displaystyle H}{|}}{\underset{\underset{\displaystyle R}{|}}{C}}-\overset{\overset{\displaystyle O}{\|}}{C}-OH$$

198. After 2.0 mol of NaOH is added, the pH of the solution is:

A. higher than pI.
B. lower than pI but lower than pK_{a2}.
C. higher than pK_{a2}.
D. lower than pK_{a1}.

199. A buffer solution is produced after the addition of how much NaOH?

A. 1.0 mol
B. 1.5 mol
C. 2.0 mol
D. 2.5 mol

Passage X (Questions 200–204)

An organic chemistry student conducts a free radical reaction by exposing a mixture of 2-methylpropane and Br_2 to light. She separates the products and obtains the NMR spectrum of a dibromo substituted propane. The spectrum contains two singlets with a peak ratio of 3:1.

200. The NMR spectrum is of:

A. 1,1-dibromo-2-methylpropane.
B. 1,3-dibromo-2-methylpropane.
C. 1,2-dibromo-2-methylpropane.
D. 2-bromo-2-methylpropane.

201. A dehydrohalogenation reaction produces 2-methyl-3-bromo-1-propane. How many signals will its NMR spectrum contain?

A. 4
B. 3
C. 2
D. 1

202. The NMR spectrum of 1,1-dideutero-2-methyl-3-bromo-1-propane contains:

A. a quartet and a triplet.
B. two singlet peaks.
C. three singlet peaks.
D. a singlet, a quartet, and a triplet.

203. The effect of bromine on the chemical shift of a proton bonded to the same carbon is to:

A. move the absorption downfield.
B. move the absorption upfield.
C. cause a singlet peak to split into a doublet peak.
D. increase the intensity of the peak.

204. Which of the following statements is FALSE?

A. The area under an NMR signal depends on the number of protons causing the signal.
B. Splitting of NMR signals is caused by nearby protons.
C. Equivalent protons have the same chemical shift.
D. Only protons give rise to NMR spectra.

Questions 205–219 are independent of any passage and independent of each other.

205. Microfilaments and microtubules form a complex network of fibers within the eukaryotic cell that can be disassembled and reassembled. If this were to occur, what is likely to be the immediate result?

    A. Depolarization
    B. Protein synthesis
    C. Absorption
    D. Change in cell shape

206. The semiconservative hypothesis of replication refers to:

    A. the process of transcription.
    B. the formation of chromatids.
    C. one aspect of protein formation.
    D. the activity of lysogenic viruses.

207. In general, each cell synthesizes its own macromolecules and does not receive them previously formed from other cells. For example, muscle cells make their own glycogen, rather than receiving it intact from the:

    A. pancreas.
    B. kidney.
    C. liver.
    D. small intestine.

208. Which statement is true concerning the sites at which muscles attach to bones?

    A. The origin of a muscle is never on a bone that forms part of a movable joint.
    B. The insertion of a muscle is usually on the same bone as the body of the muscle.
    C. The same bone can serve as the origin for one muscle and the insertion for a different muscle.
    D. No muscles are attached to bones forming immovable joints.

209. In certain insects, juvenile hormone suppresses metamorphosis from larva to adult. Instead, this hormone allows the young organism to grow in size while remaining in the immature larval stage. Eventually, the juvenile hormone decreases, causing metamorphosis to take place. If the corpora allata, the site of juvenile hormone production and release, is surgically re-

moved at an early larval stage, what is expected to happen?

    A. A tiny adult will form.
    B. The larva will continue to grow, and metamorphosis will occur at the normal age.
    C. The larva will no longer grow or undergo metamorphosis.
    D. The larva will continue to grow until it looks like a giant, adult-sized larva.

210. Which statement is most likely to be true concerning obligate anaerobes?

    A. These organisms can use oxygen if it is present in their environment.
    B. These organisms cannot use oxygen as their final electron acceptor.
    C. These organisms carry out fermentation for at least 50 percent of their ATP production.
    D. Most of these organisms are vegetative fungi.

211. A countercurrent mechanism in the kidney helps maintain a high concentration of salt in the interstitial fluid of the medulla, the site adjacent to where the hypotonic filtrate passes before its elimination out of the body. This permits efficient:

    A. secretion of excess salts.
    B. adjustment of filtrate pH.
    C. filtration of venous blood returning to the heart.
    D. reabsorption of water.

212. Point mutations are changes in a single DNA nucleotide base pair. An addition results in an extra base pair, while a deletion results in an omitted base pair along the DNA molecule. In contrast, a substitution results in an incorrect base pair replacing the correct one. Which point mutations have the highest probability of causing drastic results?

    A. Substitutions
    B. Deletions
    C. Additions and deletions
    D. All three have equal chances of causing drastic results.

213. Foods rich in fiber are basically plant materials high in cellulose, a cell wall polysaccharide that we cannot digest. The nutritional benefit(s) provided by such foods result from:

   A. other macromolecules present that can be digested and absorbed.
   B. macromolecules (like cellulose) that are absorbed without digestion and then catabolized inside the cells.
   C. microbes that are the normal symbionts of plant tissues.
   D. All of the above

214. Water and small proteins leak out of capillaries at their arterial ends because hydrostatic pressure (exerted mainly by blood pressure pushing outward against the capillary walls) is greater than colloid osmotic pressure (a fluid-retaining force caused by large solutes in the blood). Most of the fluid returns at the venule end because blood pressure:

   A. increases and large solutes decrease.
   B. decreases and large solutes decrease.
   C. increases and large solutes stay the same.
   D. decreases and large solutes stay the same.

215. The most stable isomer of 1,3-dimethylcyclohexane is:

(A)

(B)

(C)

(D)

216. The dehydration of

$$CH_3-CH_2-\underset{\underset{OH}{|}}{\overset{\overset{CH_3}{|}}{C}}-CH_3$$

yields mostly which of the following?

   A. $CH_2=CH-\underset{\underset{OH}{|}}{\overset{\overset{CH_3}{|}}{C}}-CH_3$

   B. $CH_3-CH=\overset{\overset{CH_3}{|}}{C}-CH_3$

   C. $CH_3-CH_2-\overset{\overset{CH_3}{|}}{C}=CH_2$

   D. $CH_3-CH_2-\overset{\overset{CH_2}{||}}{C}-CH_3$

217. The aldohexoses shown below are examples of which of the following?

   A. Enantiomers
   B. Optically inactive isomers
   C. Anomers
   D. Epimers

218. Which of the following is the oxidation
product of

$$CH_3-CH-CH_2-CH_2OH?$$
$$|$$
$$OH$$

A.
$$O$$
$$\|$$
$$CH_3-CH-CH_2-C-H$$
$$|$$
$$OH$$

B.
$$O$$
$$\|$$
$$CH_3-C-CH_2-C-OH$$
$$\|$$
$$O$$

C.
$$O$$
$$\|$$
$$CH_3-CH-CH_2-C-OH$$
$$|$$
$$OH$$

D.
$$CH_3-CH-CH_2-CH_2OH$$
$$|$$
$$OH$$

219. The following two reactions were carried out.

Reaction I

$$\begin{array}{c} H \\ | \\ C_6H_5-C-CH_2 \end{array} + C_2H_5O^\ominus \xrightarrow{k_I} C_6H_5CH=CH_2 + C_2H_5OH$$
$$\begin{array}{cc} | & | \\ H & Br \end{array} \qquad\qquad +Br^-$$

Reaction II

$$\begin{array}{c} D \\ | \\ C_6H_5-C-CH_2 \end{array} + C_2H_5O^\ominus \xrightarrow{k_{II}} C_6H_5CD=CH_2 + C_2H_5OD$$
$$\begin{array}{cc} | & | \\ D & Br \end{array} \qquad\qquad +Br^-$$

The rate constant k_I was seven times greater than the rate constant k_{II}. Therefore:

A. the rate determining step involves the breaking of a β-carbon-hydrogen bond.
B. the rate determining step involves the breaking of the carbon-bromine bond.
C. the rate of the reaction does not depend on the breaking of a carbon-hydrogen bond.
D. the rate of the reaction does not depend on the breaking of the carbon-bromine bond.

END OF TEST 4.

**IF YOU FINISH BEFORE THE TIME IS UP, YOU MAY
CHECK YOUR WORK ON THIS TEST ONLY.**

PRACTICE EXAM I ANSWER KEY

VERBAL REASONING		PHYSICAL SCIENCES		BIOLOGICAL SCIENCES	
1. B	45. C	66. D	110. C	143. C	187. A
2. B	46. D	67. C	111. A	144. A	188. C
3. B	47. A	68. B	112. B	145. B	189. C
4. B	48. B	69. B	113. D	146. D	190. B
5. C	49. C	70. A	114. A	147. C	191. C
6. B	50. C	71. D	115. C	148. B	192. C
7. B	51. D	72. A	116. B	149. C	193. D
8. A	52. B	73. A	117. A	150. C	194. B
9. B	53. D	74. B	118. A	151. B	195. D
10. C	54. A	75. B	119. A	152. A	196. A
11. B	55. D	76. C	120. D	153. D	197. C
12. D	56. B	77. B	121. A	154. B	198. C
13. D	57. B	78. A	122. C	155. C	199. B
14. B	58. B	79. B	123. C	156. D	200. D
15. D	59. D	80. A	124. A	157. B	201. A
16. A	60. B	81. A	125. B	158. D	202. B
17. D	61. A	82. C	126. A	159. C	203. A
18. A	62. C	83. C	127. D	160. A	204. D
19. C	63. B	84. D	128. B	161. D	205. D
20. B	64. D	85. B	129. D	162. B	206. B
21. D	65. A	86. B	130. C	163. D	207. C
22. B		87. C	131. B	164. B	208. C
23. C		88. A	132. A	165. B	209. A
24. D		89. B	133. C	166. B	210. B
25. C		90. D	134. D	167. C	211. D
26. D		91. B	135. D	168. C	212. C
27. A		92. B	136. B	169. A	213. A
28. D		93. B	137. A	170. B	214. D
29. A		94. C	138. B	171. C	215. B
30. A		95. D	139. A	172. D	216. B
31. B		96. A	140. B	173. D	217. D
32. C		97. B	141. C	174. A	218. B
33. B		98. A	142. C	175. A	219. A
34. A		99. B		176. A	
35. C		100. C		177. A	
36. C		101. B		178. D	
37. B		102. B		179. C	
38. D		103. C		180. C	
39. A		104. A		181. D	
40. C		105. D		182. B	
41. D		106. C		183. D	
42. B		107. A		184. B	
43. C		108. C		185. D	
44. A		109. B		186. C	

PRACTICE EXAM I EXPLANATORY ANSWERS

VERBAL REASONING

1. **B** The answer to this question is based on the following statements made in paragraphs 2 and 3 and on the overall tone of the article. "It is only with respect to those laws which offend the fundamental values of human life that moral defense of civil disobedience can be rationally supported" (paragraph 2). "The assumption that a law is a valid target of civil disobedience is filled with moral and legal responsibility that cannot be taken lightly. To be morally justified in such a stance one must be prepared to submit to legal prosecution for violation of the law and accept the punishment if his attack is unsuccessful" (paragraph 3).

2. **B** The answer to this question is based on the following statement in paragraph 2: "However, disobedience of laws not the subject of dissent, but merely used to dramatize dissent, is regarded as morally as well as legally unacceptable."

3. **B** The answer to this question is based on the following statement in paragraph 2: "It is only with respect to those laws which offend the fundamental values of human life that moral defense of civil disobedience can be rationally supported."

4. **B** The answer to this question is based on the following statement in paragraph 3: "To be morally justified in such a stance, one must be prepared to submit to legal prosecution for violation of the law."

5. **C** The answer to this question is based on the following statement in paragraph 4: "For a just society to exist, the principle of tolerance must be accepted, both by the government in regard to properly expressed individual dissent and by the individual toward legally established majority verdicts."

6. **B** The answer to this question is based on the same statement from paragraph 2 that answers question 3 (refer to the answer for question 3).

7. **B** The answer to this question can be inferred from the statement from paragraph 4 that answers question 5 (refer to the answer for question 5).

8. **A** The answer to this question is based on the following statement in paragraph 3: "One should even demand that the law be enforced and then be willing to acquiesce in the ultimate judgment of the courts."

9. **B** The answer to this question is supported by this statement in the first paragraph: "Sooner or later on the basis of observation and analysis, what astronomers detect finds its way into theory. . ."

10. **C** This answer to this question is based on the following statement in paragraph 5: "Even such indirect observations need elaborate and highly sensitive equipment that wasn't in place until about five years ago."

11. **B** The answer to this question can be inferred from this statement in the last paragraph: "Certain quantities that physicists insist should be the same after an interaction as before—momentum, energy, and angular momentum—could be conserved only if another particle of zero charge and negligible mass were emitted."

12. **D** The answer to this question is based on the following statement in paragraph 4: "Having no charge, it does not interact with the fields around which most particle detection experiments are built; it can be detected only inferentially, by identifying the debris from its rare interaction with matter."

13. **D** The answer to this question is based on the following statement in paragraph 2: "Despite the construction, finally, of a string of elaborate observatories, some buried in the earth from southern India to Utah to South America, the last five years as well have produced not a single, validated observation of an extraterrestrial neutrino."

14. **B** The answer to this question is based on the following statement in paragraph 5: "The goal is worth the effort, however: once detected, extraterrestrial neutrinos will provide solid, first-

hand information on the sources and conditions that spawned them."

15. **D** The answer to this question is based on the statement found in paragraph 7 that is given also as the answer to question 11.

16. **A** The answer to this question is based on the statement in paragraph 7 that is given in the answer to question 11.

17. **D** The answer to this question is based on the following statement in paragraph 1: ". . . cannot overlook the absence of common sense and impartiality. . ."

18. **A** The answer to this question is based on the following statement in paragraph 1: "Many persons who appreciate and admire Mr. Swinburne's genius cannot help regretting that he should ever have descended from the serene heights of poetry into the arena of criticism."

19. **C** The answer to this question is based on the following statement in paragraph 3: "A careful comparison of *Essays and Studies* with another volume published about eleven years later, under the title of *Miscellanies,* shows that their author has either deliberately or unconsciously contradicted many of the opinions he had previously expressed . . . ."

20. **B** The answer to this question is based on the following two statements in paragraphs 2 and 5: "Mr. Swinburne's criticism is characterized by an utter want of proportion and aggressive dogmatism which finds vent in offensive and vituperative language quite unsuited to the dignity of literature . . ." (paragraph 2). ". . . he is too one-sided, too extravagant, too unrestrained" (paragraph 5).

21. **D** The answer to this question is based on the statement in paragraph 1, which is quoted in the answer to question 17.

22. **B** This inference is based on the following statement made in paragraph 4: "Indeed, nearly all that he has written about this rather overrated representative of the French romanticist school is little better than hysterical declamation."

23. **C** This assumption can be made based on the following statement in paragraph 5: "This fact, however, remains; his judgments upon books

and their authors are the reverse of impartial, and it is manifest that Nature never intended him for a critic."

24. **D** The last two paragraphs of the article clearly state that Mr. Swinburne was not an impartial, astute, nor perceptive critic.

25. **C** The answer to this question is based on the following statements in paragraph 2: "A prolific photographer, he also took thousands of photographs documenting the daily lives and customs of the peoples he saw. After his death, James's unique pictorial history of the region was donated to the Southwest Museum in Los Angeles . . . founded to preserve and interpret the art, artifacts, and documentary material of the prehistoric and historic cultures of the Americas."

26. **D** The answer to this question is based on the following statement in paragraph 8: "The more than eleven thousand nitrate-based negatives in the museum's collection 'are still in good condition . . . ' but experts have already detected . . . signals of deterioration."

27. **A** The answer to this question is based on the following statements in paragraph 5: ". . . James and many other photographers of the early 1900s often used a nitrate-based film . . . Within decades, however, the nitrate-based film begins to deteriorate . . . the early photographers . . . 'just didn't realize it would deteriorate so quickly.'"

28. **D** The answer to this question is based on the following statement in paragraph 1: "A proper, English-born minister, George Wharton James seemed out of his element when he arrived in the still-wild West in 1881."

29. **A** The answer to this question is based on the following statements in paragraph 8: ". . . experts have already detected early warning signals of deterioration. 'The negatives could turn to powder before we know it,' she [Moneta] notes, adding the museum's anxiety over the film has increased greatly in the past five years."

30. **A** The answer to this question is based on the following statement in paragraph 2: "After his death, James's unique pictorial history of the region was donated to the Southwestern Museum in Los Angeles . . . founded . . . to pre-

serve . . . the art, artifacts, and documentary material of the prehistoric and historic cultures of the Americas."

31. **B** The answer to this question can be inferred from the following statements in paragraphs 4 and 6: "There is very little documentation of that period remaining . . ." (paragraph 4). "The photo library is a treasure house for researchers—particularly those living in the West—since it contains vintage prints which show . . . the daily life of the native Americans" (paragraph 6).

32. **C** The answer to this question is based on the following statement in the passage: "But . . . his strength lies in a dramatic insight which goes far toward the making of a master of the playwright's art . . . ."

33. **B** The answer to this question is based on the following statement in the passage: ". . . of all the Elizabethan playwrights he is one of the most unwearied . . . ."

34. **A** The answer to this question can be inferred from the following statements in the passage: "It would grieve me to seem unjust toward a writer to whom I have long felt very specially attracted . . . ." and ". . . his strength lies in a dramatic insight which goes far toward the making of a master of the playwright's art . . . ."

35. **C** The answer to this question is based on the following statement in the passage: ". . . his strength lies in a dramatic insight which goes far toward the making of a master playwright's art . . . ."

36. **C** The answer to this question is found in the article as a whole as it discusses almost nothing else but Heywood's creative ability. The following two statements are an example of this focus. The first statement says, "His creative power was, however, of that secondary order which is content with accommodating itself to conditions imposed by the prevailing tastes of the day." The second states ". . . his practiced inventiveness displays with the utmost abundance; of all the Elizabethan playwrights he is one of the most unwearied . . . ."

37. **B** This inference could be based on many statements in the article, but the following two statements give the best basis for the inference: "Yet

the highest praise which it seems right to bestow upon Thomas Heywood is that which was happily expressed by Tieck when he described him as the 'model of the light and rapid talent'" is the first statement, and the second is "His creative power was, however, of that secondary order which is content with accommodating itself to conditions imposed by the prevailing tastes of the day."

38. **D** The answer to this question is based on the following statement in paragraph 1: "During the past four decades the fishery scientists of the West have studied the dynamics of fish populations with the objective of determining the relationship between the amount of fishing and the sustainable catch."

39. **A** The answer to this question is based on the following statement in paragraph 3: "The rate of growth of individuals, the time of sexual maturity, and the accumulation of reserves vary according to the food supply."

40. **C** The answer to this question is based on the following statement in paragraph 2: "Much of it (theory) is based on the Darwinian concept of a constant overpopulation of young that is reduced by density-dependent mortality resulting from intraspecific competition."

41. **D** The answer to this question is based on the following statement in paragraph 3: "He argues that Darwin's concept of constant overpopulation has led to the neglect of the problem of protecting spawners and young fish."

42. **B** The answer to this question is based on the following statement in paragraph 1: "During the past four decades the fishery scientists of the West have studied the dynamics of fish populations with the objective of determining the relationship between the amount of fishing and the sustainable catch."

43. **C** The answer to this question is based on the following statement in paragraph 3: "Nikolskii considers the main laws of population dynamics to be concerned with the succession of generations; their birth, growth, and death."

44. **A** This inference is based on the following statements in paragraphs 2 and 3. In paragraph 2, the Darwinian point of view and food supply are not mentioned. "Much of it [the theory] is

based on the Darwinian concept of a constant overpopulation of young that is reduced by density-dependent mortality resulting from intraspecific competition." In paragraph 3, part of the explanation of the non-Darwinian point of view of G. V. Nikolskii is stated: "The mass and age structure of a population are the result of adaptation to the food supply. The rate of growth of individuals, the time of sexual maturity, and the accumulation of reserves vary according to the food supply."

45. **C** The answer to this question is based on the following statement in paragraph 3: "The mass and age structure of a population are the result of adaptation to the food supply." The answer is also listed above as part of the answer to question 44.

46. **D** The answer to this question is based on the following statement in paragraph 5: "The real question concerns, rather, the responsibility of criticism to defend the integrity of art against all encroachments. . . ."

47. **A** The answer to this question is based on the following statement in paragraph 5: "By concentrating in the most disinterested way on its traditional tasks of elucidation and evaluation, criticism will make its necessary contribution to the life of art and the freedom of the spirit."

48. **B** The answer to this question is based on the following statement in paragraph 3: "Therefore, so as not to conceal this admixture of description and judgment, critical evaluation is best performed as honestly as possible with reasoned arguments and detailed examples."

49. **C** The answer is based on the following statement: " . . . when all the institutions of society—the museums, the media, the universities, the galleries, the collectors, and all government agencies . . . —are prejudiced in favor of whatever is deemed on any grounds new and innovative in the arts, the challenge to criticism is monumental."

50. **C** The answer to this question is based on the following statement in paragraph 3: "The first task of the critic is to see the work of art and describe its qualities . . . This is the task of elucidation, and it is fundamental to all criticism worthy of the name."

51. **D** The answer to this question is based on a number of statements, but the following statement in paragraph 5 best sums up the answer: "The question in a democratic society is not whether criticism has a role to play; that is taken for granted."

52. **B** The answer to this question can be inferred from the following statements in paragraph 2: The "message" in Muir's quote "first found institutional expression on a global scale in the 1972 United Nations Conference on the Human Environment . . . " "There 130 nations . . . acknowledged a mutual obligation in maintaining a livable global environment."

53. **D** The answer to this question is found in the following statement in paragraph 4: "Although Americans tend to bask in the notion that we are environmentally progressive, in truth the United States is in many ways a mirror of global environmental problems—a story of too little and too late . . ."

54. **A** The answer to this question can be inferred in the following statement in paragraph 5: "The United States did move quickly, as the Environmental Revolution dawned in the late 1960s, to enact constructive measures: the epochal National Environmental Policy Act; laws to abate air and water pollution and even noise; laws to deal with solid waste, to protect wildlife, to save coasts from degradation; and more."

55. **D** The answer is based on the following statement: "The United States exemplifies the worldwide conflict . . . between professed desires for environmental quality versus addiction to lifestyles that are environmentally destructive in every aspect. . . ."

56. **B** The answer to this question can be inferred from the following statement in paragraph 7: "Greens have been elected to legislative bodies in West Germany, France, Italy, Austria, Luxembourg, Switzerland, Belgium, Finland, and Portugal."

57. **B** This answer is based on the following statements in paragraph 10: " . . . it seems only a matter of time . . . until it brings significant changes in national lifestyles that are conspicuously inimical to environmental quality. Such conspicuous habits include demands for gas-guzzling cars, a voracious pattern of energy

consumption, throwaway consumerism, recreational vehicles designed to ravage deserts, the equation of growth with good, and all the rest."

58. **B** The answer to this question is based on the following statement in paragraph 5: "Although we have been spending roughly $85 billion a year—$340 per capita—on pollution controls, we are still far short of our goals of clean air and water."

59. **D** The answer to this question is based on the following statement in paragraph 2: "It is thus necessary that, if action needs to be taken, it should be taken on a global scale with the participation of as many countries as possible for a sustained period of time."

60. **B** The answer is based on the process of eliminating choices A, C, and D, which are supported by statements in the article. Choice B is the remaining possible answer as it is not supported by any statement in the article. Choice A is supported by the following statements in paragraph 6: " . . . the United States and other countries should begin to think of ways to reduce greenhouse gas emissions . . . The source of these reductions would be different for every country." Choice C is inferred by several statements in paragraph 6 and supported directly by a statement in paragraph 7. "The source of these reductions would be different for every country. For one, it may be changing land-use patterns to reduce tropical deforestation. For another, it may be improving energy efficiency" (paragraph 6). "Since greenhouse gas emissions have already increased, some amount of adaptation may be necessary even if we limited emissions today" (paragraph 7). Choice D is supported by the following statements in paragraph 7. "Moreover, if concerted action on an international level is to be undertaken, then a consensus must emerge on the seriousness of the climate change problem. Only through internationally coordinated research on the impacts of climate change can this be accomplished."

61. **A** The answer to this question is based on the following statement in paragraph 3: "If we wait until we can actually measure warming before we take action, then we may have to live with warmings for many generations, since it takes many years before emission reductions could have an impact on atmospheric concentrations and the climate system."

62. **C** The answer to this question is based on a number of statements in paragraph 1: "The way we live is profoundly affected by our climate. When and where we farm, how much we heat and cool our homes, how we obtain our water—all depend on the climate we experience. Climate determines whether we have a bumper crop or a shortage." There is no mention of climate and clothing.

63. **B** The answer to this question is found in several statements in paragraph 6: "Yet, we do not have the luxury of sitting on our hands while a scientific consensus emerges. Rather, the United States and other countries should begin to think of ways to reduce greenhouse gas emissions, in the event that it ultimately proves necessary to do so."

64. **D** The correct answer is based on summarization of paragraphs 5 and 7.

65. **A** The answer to this question can be found in several statements in paragraph 2: "No one country dominates in the emission of greenhouse gases, and any country that takes action to control emissions will achieve only limited success if other countries do not follow suit. It is thus necessary that, if action needs to be taken, it should be taken on a global scale with the participation of as many countries as possible for a sustained period of time."

PHYSICAL SCIENCES

66. **D** $6.6 \times 10^{-7} \text{m} / 3.89 \times 10^{-7} \text{ m} = 1.7$

67. **C** $389 \times 10^{-9} \text{ m} = 3.89 \times 10^{-7} \text{ m}$

68. **B** Higher energy differences correspond to higher frequencies and thus shorter wavelengths.

69. **B** $E = h\nu = hc/\lambda$

70. **A** No spectral line occurs at 610 nm; to Scientist 1, this fact means no corresponding transition exists.

71. **D** Scientist 2 believes hydrogen to have a broad range of emissions, only a few of which pass through the glass in the measuring instrument.

72. **A** If other atoms showed the same spectra in the same spectrometer, there would be proof that

the device, not the atoms, was the source of the spectral lines.

73. **A** Evidently, the spectrometer *will* pass a broad spectrum of wavelengths. Thus, Scientist 2's objection to Scientist 1's position is refuted.

74. **B** PbS has the smaller K_{sp}, so the tendency for its separate ions to combine is greater.

75. **B** The sulfide concentration is maintained at 0.1 so A is incorrect, and the powers of 2 are not needed as in C and D.

76. **C** $(1 \times 10^{-20} M/\text{L})(6 \times 10^{23} \text{ ions/mol}) (10^{-3} \text{ L/cc}) = 6 \text{ ions/cc}$

77. **B** If pH is low, $[H^+]$ is high, and $[S^{2-}]$ is low.

78. **A** $[S^{2-}] = (1 \times 10^{-23})/(10^{-2})^2 = 1 \times 10^{-19} M$

79. **B** $[H^+] = ((10^{-23})/10^{-20})^{\frac{1}{2}} = 0.032 M$

80. **A** The solubility in this case is equal to the number of moles per liter of magnesium ion liberated by a dissociation. Note that K_{sp} is *not* wanted.

81. **A** Since hydroxide is a product in the equilibrium, adding more of it will drive the equilibrium to the left, with the result that less of the salt will dissociate.

82. **C** The student needs to insert "0.1" as the concentration of hydroxide, then square it, since there are 2 OH⁻'s in the solubility equation. It is not correct to double the concentration of hydroxide before squaring, as in D.

83. **C** A solution buffered to pH 5.0 is weakly acidic. The H^+ ions will remove OH⁻ ions from the solution, shifting the equilibrium to the right and increasing the solubility.

84. **D** Here $[OH^-] = K_w/[H^+] = 1 \times 10^{-14}$

85. **B** Solubility is surely pH-dependent, but K_{sp} is not. Since other magnesium salts would not necessarily have hydroxides in their formulas, these concerns need not apply to them.

86. **B** $n = PV/RT$, so n decreases as T increases.

87. **C** Note pressure is in atm, temperature is in K.

88. **A** Note, molar mass = mass/number of moles

89. **B** Use MW = g/n = gRT/PV. All answers except B give an error in the wrong direction.

90. **D** There would be fewer of the aggregated

molecules than there would be if the molecules did not bind to each other. Since the aggregates would be more massive, they would move more slowly.

91. **B** Since the measured MW is about three times the correct MW, on average three molecules must bind together.

92. **B** Concentrations of reactants, not products, determine rate in both theories, according to the text.

93. **B** Here you must have understood the relation of numbers of reactants in the overall equation to exponents in the rate law.

94. **C** The theories differ in that the first calls for the use of the coefficients in the *overall* reaction as exponents in the rate law, while the second asks that the coefficients from the *slow step* be employed. In a single-step reaction, the theories predict the same thing.

95. **D** The product concentration doesn't affect the rate.

96. **A** The slow stage controls the overall rate, according to Theory 2.

97. **B** Be sure to use column 3, not column 4. The value for PbS is clearly the lowest in the column; it takes more examination to see that the value for BaF_2 is the highest.

98. **A** You need to find the ratio of the column 3 value to the column 1 value; this ratio is 10, not $\frac{1}{10}$.

99. **B** This considerable difference in solubility is found for all rows of the table.

100. **C** Each value in column 4 is 10 times greater than the corresponding value in column 2; answer C reflects this fact.

101. **B** Use column 2, and divide K_{sp} for PbS by K_{sp} for $CaSO_4$.

102. **B** Here you can look for the greatest pure-water solubility, i.e., the greatest value in column 3 among the three lead salts.

103. **C** The chart shows the pure-water solubility of BaF_2 to be greater than that when $.1\ M\ Ba^{2+}$ is present. Therefore, as $Ba(NO_3)_2$ is added, solid BaF_2 precipitates.

104. **A** Since K_{sp} is smaller for $BaSO_4$ than for $CaSO_4$, $BaSO_4$ will precipitate. Only if the Ba^{2+} in solution is effectively used up will Ca^{2+} precipitate. As an alternative solution, examine the solubilities in Column 4, to see that the solubility of $BaSO_4$ is much lower than that of $CaSO_4$.

105. **D** Weight is the product of mass and the acceleration of gravity.

$$F_{gravity} = Wgt = mg = (100\ kg)\ (9.8\ m/s^2)$$
$$Wgt = 980\ kg\ m\ s^{-2} = 980\ N$$

106. **C** The entire 200 N force was used to overcome the frictional force. The applied force of 200 N is parallel to the direction of motion of the block. Therefore, none of the applied force was used to overcome gravity. Since the velocity is constant, none of the force was used to accelerate the block.

107. **A** Work is force times distance in the same direction of force. The applied force and the direction of motion are both horizontal so the work performed is

$$W = Fd = (200\ N)\ (8\ m) = 1600\ N\text{-}m = 1600\ J$$

108. **C** $v^2 = v_0^2 + 2ax = 0 + 2\ (9.8\ m/s^2)\ (8\ m)\ v = 12.5\ m/s$

109. **B** $E = \frac{1}{2}\ mv^2 = \frac{1}{2}\ (100\ kg)\ (12.5\ m/s)^2\ E = 7840\ J$

110. **C** $P_2 = I_2^2 R_2 = (2\ A)^2\ (60\ \Omega) = 240\ W$

111. **A** Energy is the product of power and time: $E = Pt = I^2Rt = 240\ W\ (3\ s) = 720\ W\text{-}s = 720\ J$

112. **B** Since R_1 and R_2 are connected in parallel, the voltage drop across each must be identical: $V_1 = V_2 = I_2R_2 = (2\ A)\ (60\ \Omega) = 120\ V$

113. **D** The parallel resistors R_1 and R_2 can be replaced by a single resistance, R_{eq}, which will be in series with R_3. The current in R_{eq} must equal the sum of the currents in R_1 and R_2. Once this current is found, the voltage of R_{eq} can be computed. The voltage of the source is the sum of the voltages for R_3 and R_{eq}.

$V_1 = V_2 = I_1R_1 = I_2R_2$, therefore
$$I_1 = \frac{I_2R_2}{R_1} = \frac{(2\ A)\ (60\Omega)}{30\ \Omega} = 4\ A$$
$$I_{eq} = I_1 + I_2 = 4\ A + 2\ A = 6\ A$$

Since R_3 and R_{eq} are in series, the same current must flow through both resistors, so that $I_{tot} = 6\ A$

The total resistance of the circuit is given by

$$R_{tot} = R_3 + R_{eq}$$

We can either stop and calculate R_{eq} so we can get R_{tot}, or we can use the value of I_3 and R_3 to find V_3, then find

$$V_{tot} = V_3 + V_{eq}$$
$$V_3 = I_3R_3 = (6\ A)\ (40\ \Omega) = 240\ V$$
$$V_{tot} = V_3 + V_{eq} = 240\ V + 120\ V = 360\ V$$

114. **A** The terminal voltage is the voltage when the source is connected in a closed circuit. The terminal voltage equals the emf minus Ir, produced by current flowing through the source. For the circuit shown, I_{tot} was 6 A so Ir = (6 A) (4 Ω) = 24 V

And the emf is found from:

$$\text{terminal voltage} = \text{emf} - \text{Ir}$$

so emf = term. volt. + Ir = 360 V + 24 V = 384 V

115. **C** Since all of the walls of the apparatus that the ray passes through are parallel, and since the ray exits into the same medium it originally entered from (air), the path of the ray as it exits must be parallel to its path when it entered from the air into chamber 1. This angle is given as 45° to the normal of the first wall. Therefore, the ray should exit into the air with an angle of 45° to the normal of the outside wall. Trace F looks closest to 45°.

116. **B** By definition, the refractive index is the ratio of the speed of light in a vacuum to its speed in the medium of interest, water. Therefore,

$$v = c/n$$
$$v = (3.00 \times 10^8\ m/s)/1.33 = 2.26 \times 10^8\ m/s$$

Choices C and D are easily eliminated because they are too large. We don't expect light to travel as fast in a physical medium as it does in a vacuum, so that eliminates C. And, nothing travels faster than the speed of light in a vacuum, so that eliminates choice D. The product of n and v equals c. This eliminates choice A as too small. Since $n \sim 1$, we expect v to be fairly close to C.

117. **A** Choices C and D can be eliminated because the angle of the beam in air is $45°$. The liquid has a greater optical density than air; therefore, it will slow the light down more than air does. The incident angle will be shifted toward the normal and will be less than that in the air. The ratio of the sine of the angle of incidence, $\sin x$, to the sine of the angle of refraction, $\sin 45$, where the beam exits into the air, is equal to the ratio of the index of refraction for medium 2 to the index of refraction for air, which is 1.

$\sin x = (1/2)\sin 45 = 0.35,$

which is less than $30°$

118. **A** The sine of the critical angle is the reciprocal of the refractive index: $\sin 0_{crit} = 1/2.00 = 0.500$

119. **A** Stress $= F/A$ where F is the tension on the wire and A is the cross-sectional area of the wire:

$A = \pi r^2 = \pi (2.00 \ 10^{-3} m / 2)^2$

$= 3.14 \ 10^{-6} m^2$ stress $= F/A$

$= 628 N/3.14 \ 10^{-6} m^2 = 2.00 \ 10^8 N/m^2$

Choice D can be eliminated because it has no units, which fits the property of strain. Similarly, choice B can also be eliminated because it has the wrong units for stress.

120. **D** Strain is the fractional change in length to the original length:

strain $= \Delta \ell / \ell = 0.24 m/240 m = 1.0 \times 10^{-3}$

Choices A and B can be eliminated because strain has no units.

121. **A** Any modulus is the ratio of stress to strain $= 2.0 \times 10^{11} N/m^2$

122. **C** The elastic modulus being described is for a change in length, which is given by Young's modulus. By definition, Young's modulus is the

ratio of the tensile stress to the tensile strain:

$$Y = (F/A)/(\Delta \ell / \ell)$$

123. **C** The ability of a substance to return to its original shape once a deforming force is removed is called elasticity.

124. **A** The shortest pipe length will be associated with the wavelength for the fundamental tone. For a closed-end pipe this is: $\lambda = 4 \ell$. The wavelength is the ratio of the speed to the frequency: $\lambda = v/v$. Therefore, the shortest length is:

$$\ell = v/4v = \frac{360 \ m/s}{4 \ (450 \ s^{-1})} = 0.20 \ m = 20 \ cm$$

125. **B** Acceleration is the change in velocity; therefore,

$$a = \frac{\Delta v}{\Delta t} = \frac{100 \ m/s - 80 \ m/s}{2 \ s} = 10 \ m/s^2$$

Choice C can be eliminated immediately because the units meter per second is for velocity, not acceleration.

126. **A** $v = v_0 + at$. Estimate the acceleration due to gravity using $a = -g = -9.8 \ m/s^2 \sim -10 \ m/s^2$. The velocity is approximately

$v = 40.0 \ m/s - 10 \ m/s^2 (2 \ s)$

$= 40 \ m/s - 20 \ m/s = 20 \ m/s$

The closest choice to 20 m/s is A.

$v = 40.0 \ m/s - 9.80 \ m/s^2 (2.00 \ s) = 20.4 \ m/s$

127. **D** From Newton's second law, $F = ma$, so the acceleration is

$$a = F/m = \frac{10 \ N}{2.0 \ kg.} = \frac{10 \ kg \ m \ s^{-2}}{2.0 \ kg} = 5.0 \ m/s^2$$

The velocity is $v = v_0 + at$ where $v_0 = 0$ so that

$$v = at = \frac{(5.0 \ m)}{s^2} 5.0 \ s = 25 \ m/s$$

128. **B** This expression gives the number of moles of $NiCl_2$ (and therefore of Ni). It must equal the number of moles of product, which has 1 Ni per molecule. There is no need to work with the MW of the product, since its weight is not requested.

129. **D** Only D shows each of the oxygens surrounded by an octet as well as showing the required 14 electrons.

130. **C** This solution is a buffer, for which

$$[H^+] = K_a [HFor]/[For–] = K_a$$
$$pH = -\log (1.8 \times 10^{-4}) = 3.7$$

131. **B** Heat lost by graphite = heat gained by water: (1.0 mol) (heat cap. for graphite) (temperature drop for graphite) = (1.0 mol) (heat cap. for water) (temp gain for water)

132. **A** A 0th order reaction proceeds with a constant rate, so the time to go from one-half to one-quarter of the original amount will be only half the time needed to go from all of the reactants to one-half of them. (Had the reaction been first-order, the answer would have been 5 minutes.)

133. **C** Since the egg is cooked in water, it can't be heated above the boiling temperature of the liquid. The boiling temperature is lower at high altitudes, where the external pressure is lower and molecules can more easily escape from the liquid phase into the vapor.

134. **D** The "n" quantum number is used as the beginning of the orbital's name: "4." The value of "*l*" is translated into the second designation; when "*l*" = 2, the orbital is called "*d*." Hence "4*d*."

135. **D** Spontaneity of a reaction is determined by the free energy, $\Delta G = \Delta H - T\Delta S$.

136. **B** The force of interaction between two charges is:

$F = \dfrac{kq_1 q_2}{r^2}$. Since the charges are alike, the force is repulsive (positive sign). This eliminates choice D immediately.

$$F = (9 \quad 10^9 \frac{Nm^2}{C^2}) = \frac{(10 \quad 10^{-6} C)(10 \quad 10^{-6} C)}{(10 \quad 10^{-2} m)^2} =$$

$$\frac{(9 \quad 10^9)(10 \quad 10^{-12})}{(10 \quad 10^{-4})} N = 9 \quad 10^9 \quad 10^{-11} \quad 10^3 N =$$

$$9 \quad 10^1 \ N = 90 \ N$$

137. **A** Power can be expressed as $P = V^2/R$. Solving for R gives:

$$R = \frac{V^2}{P} = \frac{120 \ V}{1200 \ W} = \frac{(120 \ V)(120 \ V)}{1200 \ W} = \frac{120 \ V^2}{10 \ W} = 12 \ \Omega$$

138. **B** Intensity, power and radial distance between source and observer are related by:

$$I = \frac{P}{4\pi r^2}$$

Since the source doesn't change, the power is constant; therefore, the ratio of the two intensities becomes

$$\frac{I_{6 \ feet}}{I_{3 \ feet}} = \frac{P / (4\pi (6 \ ft)^2)}{P / (4\pi (3 \ ft)^2)} = \frac{(6 \ ft)^2}{(3 \ ft)^2} = \frac{36 \ ft^2}{9 \ ft^2} = 4$$

Choices C and D can be eliminated immediately because the brightness must increase, not decrease, as the source is brought closer to the observer.

139. **A** Conservation of mass means you get $_{2}^{4}x$, which corresponds to an alpha particle being emitted.

140. **B** Because the resistors are in series, the same current must flow through both resistors. Apply Ohm's law to find the voltage across the 40 Ω-resistor.

$$V = IR = (2.0 \ A) (40 \ \Omega) = 80 \ V$$

141. **C** Conservation of mass and charge means that the sum of mass numbers on the reactant side must add up to 235 + 1 = 236. Since 144 + 89 + x = 236, x must equal 3. There are 3 neutrons emitted.

142. **C** Choices A and D are immediately eliminated because they represent the difference and the

sum of the two vectors and only occur if they are both colinear. The resultant is equivalent to the hypotenuse of a right triangle with the adjacent legs of 6 N and 8 N. This is an example of a 3-4-5 right triangle where each side is multiplied by the constant 2. The resultant is $2 \times 5 = 10$ N.

BIOLOGICAL SCIENCES

143. **C** A basic knowledge of digestive processes is required, i.e., the stomach is a highly acidic environment, whereas the small intestine is slightly alkaline. The lower part of the graph shows that Enzyme X works best at a pH close to 2, while Enzyme Y works best at a pH closer to 8.

144. **A** Because the two enzymes have two different, non-overlapping pH ranges, they could not be at work in the same place at the same time. In addition, the graph does not refer to the temperature ranges of X and Y (only A and B). Although Enzyme X generally works more slowly than Enzyme Y, neither enzyme works at all at pH:4.5.

145. **B** The key to this question is the temperature range at which the two enzymes work. Only Enzyme A has a temperature range encompassing human body temperature ($37°C$). An enzyme whose peak activity is close to $75°C–80°C$ (Enzyme B) is unlikely to be found in the human body.

146. **D** Both enzymes overlap between $40°C$ and $50°C$. Choices A and B are too broad, and each includes a range of temperatures beyond which one of the enzymes cannot work.

147. **C** When an enzyme is not active in a particular environment, it may be because that environment affects its conformation. The only possible answer, therefore, is C. For choices B and D, no information is provided in the graph.

148. **B** Some knowledge about factors that affect enzyme activity is needed here. Within an enzyme's normal range of activity, a clear indication that all enzyme molecules are saturated with substrate is a leveling off of the rate of reaction curve (an increase in enzyme concentration would help increase activity again).

149. **C** When enzymes are at work, they help bring their substrate(s) to the "transition state," at which time bonds can break and the reaction can proceed. To be able to do this, the enzyme must be in an environment compatible with its range of activity. A pH below 5.5 is not within the activity range of Enzyme Y. Therefore, it would be unable to bring its substrate(s) to the transition state.

150. **C** The understanding that each single bacterial cell can give rise to an entire colony is helpful. The passage states that the presence of fewer colonies is indicative of cells dying, while smaller colonies suggests that growth has been inhibited. Side 1 (the UV radiated side) has *fewer and smaller colonies* compared to the unradiated side, as well as compared to the dish irradiated with green light.

151. **B** Only Side 1 was exposed to UV light. Therefore, ten colonies grew compared to 30 on the unexposed side (1/3).

152. **A** The observation that the number and size of colonies exposed to green light (Dish B/Side 1) is about the same as the number and size of colonies not exposed to anything (Dish A/Side 2; Dish B/Side 2) demonstrates that green light has no effects. What should also be clear is that in both experiments, cultures were only incubated in the dark (exposure to light in Experiment 2 took place *before* incubation).

153. **D** In both experiments, Side 2 was always treated identically to Side 1 *except* for the variable being tested—the type of radiation.

154. **B** In *both* experiments, Dish A/Side 1 was exposed to *UV radiation*. In Experiment 2, exposure to incandescent light took place *after* UV. Therefore, any change (in this case, a restorative effect) was due to the incandescent light. This effect is referred to as photoreactivation. (Neither experiment compared exposure to UV light versus exposure to incandescent light.)

155. **C** The passage states that UV radiation is absorbed by purines and pyrimidines. Since these bases are part of nucleotide structure in the DNA, answer C is correct.

156. **D** The only difference in procedure between the new experiment and Experiment 1 is the presence of the glass lid prior to UV radiation. Since the number and size of colonies on the UV-exposed side (in the new experiment) were

equivalent to those on the unexposed side, one must conclude that the glass lid protected the bacterial cells (glass *does* absorb UV—that's why we can't get a sunburn through a window!).

157. **B** If each of these structures has endocrine functions, the secretions must enter the blood. The hypothalamus only regulates the activity of the pituitary gland.

158. **D** The question states that an increase in blood volume will increase blood pressure. When reabsorption of sodium occurs, reabsorption of water usually follows (increasing blood volume). Therefore, without knowing anything about ANF, choice D is the only possible answer.

159. **C** Knowledge about the role of bicarbonate ion (here, in the form of sodium bicarbonate) as an alkaline secretion that helps neutralize acidity is helpful. The arrival of acidic chyme signals the small intestine to release secretin ("proximate" reason). The fact that pancreatic enzymes are most active in the slightly alkaline pH of the small intestine (they require a slightly alkaline environment to function properly) is the "ultimate" reason.

160. **A** When cells in a noncyclic environment (darkness) display a cyclic pattern of response, an "internal" cyclic rhythm is suggested. Choices B and C do not apply to the conditions described in the question. There is no relevant basis for selecting choice D.

161. **D** The passage states that thymosin only influences the differentiation of T-lymphocytes. Choices A, B and C are each specific roles of lymphocytes (either T- or B-lymphocytes).

162. **B** Knowledge of the source and function of bile is important. The liver produces bile, while the gall bladder stores and concentrates bile. The role of bile is to emulsify fats so that they can be efficiently digested by pancreatic lipase. Without the gall bladder, bile can still be sent to the small intestine via the liver directly.

163. **D** According to the figure, the peak secondary response to antigen A (day 40) came approximately 30 days after the peak primary response (day 9–10). The peak primary response to antigen B appears to occur on day 40. Therefore, day 70 is the appropriate answer for this question.

164. **B** Initial exposure to antigen A occurs prior to day 2, while peak primary response is approximately at day 9–10. Similarly, the initial exposure to antigen B occurs at day 28, while peak primary response is approximately at day 37–38. Thus, choice B is the correct answer.

165. **B** The peak primary response is approximately 20 units. The peak secondary response is somewhat less than 10,000 units. Therefore, it is between 100 and 1000 times as great.

166. **B** Since macrophages ". . . digest the antigen-bearing agent . . .," it should immediately be recognized that they carry out phagocytosis. Neither red blood cells nor platelets take part in this process. The macrophages are most likely neutrophils or monocytes (granular and non-granular white blood cells, respectively).

167. **C** Initial contact with a dead or weakened form of the antigen in the form of a vaccine provides effective immunity when the "real" organism makes contact the second time.

168. **C** Careful referral to the passage reveals that T-cells play important roles during both stages of the immune response.

169. **A** The ability to draw inferences from previous information is important here. If the primary immune response (response to initial treatment) to penicillin causes an allergic response, the secondary immune response (response to the drug the next time it is administered) may be much more severe and extremely dangerous (as shown earlier, the secondary response can produce between 100 and 1000 times as many antibodies).

170. **B** When acetylcholine is released by motor neurons, it initiates depolarization of the sarcolemma. Calcium returns to the sarcoplasmic reticulum only *after* depolarization has occurred. Additionally, neurons of the sympathetic nervous system would never be on the "receiving" side of a neuromuscular junction.

171. **C** Basic knowledge of the organization of the nervous system is needed. Motor neurons, by definition, carry impulses *from* the CNS *to* the effectors. Only choice C is a plausible answer.

172. **D** Each answer is a reasonable option. ATP is needed for a variety of processes involved in

muscle relaxation (repolarization of the sarco-lemma, return of calcium to the SR, events at the neuromuscular junction, etc.). Interrupted blood flow can prevent efficient delivery of oxygen needed for ATP production during cellular respiration. Salt imbalances (sodium, potassium, calcium) can also prevent normal muscle function.

173. **D** Knowledge about neuromuscular junctions is required. The motor end plate is the site directly under the axon terminals of the motor neuron (where the motor neuron and muscle cell membrane meet).

174. **A** To answer this question correctly, knowledge that the CNS consists of the brain and spinal cord, and that myelin sheaths are found on axons is necessary.

175. **A** Understanding the inheritance pattern of sex-linked traits is essential. Males always inherit sex-linked traits (on the X-chromosome) from their mothers. In addition, sex-linked traits are much more commonly expressed in males since they only have one X-chromosome.

176. **A** The more soluble a substance is, the further it will be carried in solution. Additionally, the passage states that adsorption is the tendency of substances in a mixture to adhere to the material over which they are passed. Thus, the greater the adsorptive tendency, the *sooner* they will leave the mixture (and the *lower* they will be on the paper).

177. **A** Since chromatography is designed to separate substances from a mixture, the three colored bands most likely represent three separate pigments ("Substances with color can easily be detected on the paper.") found in leaves.

178. **D** A careful reading of the graph reveals that this is the only correct answer. Answer B is incorrect because substance A has a broad range of low absorbance (high transmittance). Although the three substances each have two major absorbance peaks, the second peak of substance B (in the red range) does not reach 40 percent absorbance.

179. **C** The passage states that unless light is absorbed, its energy cannot be put to use. Substance A has absorbance peaks in the red and violet-blue range. These are the wavelengths used by this pigment (chlorophyll a) to run the light reactions of photosynthesis.

180. **C** Green wavelengths are among the *least* absorbed by the plant pigments, especially substances A and B (chlorophylls a and b, respectively). The appearance of the leaves is due to those wavelengths of light that are *reflected* and thus, visible to the eye. Substance C (a carotenoid pigment) mostly reflects the yellows, oranges and reds, thereby contributing to the color changes seen in autumn when the chlorophylls are no longer present.

181. **D** If different pigments absorb different wavelengths, more of the light energy reaching the plant can be harnessed at the same time. The light absorbed for photosynthesis has nothing to do with heat dissipation. Similarly, making different pigments would probably be energetically more expensive since a different synthetic pathway would also require the anabolism of different enzymes and different "machinery" for dealing with new metabolites, etc.

182. **B** This question is about a typical Mendelian cross. Having "at least one normal allele" is simply another way of referring to the probability of a child having the normal phenotype (3:1 ratio).

183. **D** The probability of one child being a carrier is 1/2 or 50% (the child has a two in four chance of receiving the Pp genotype). Each subsequent child will have the same chances. However, it should be understood that the probability of two children being carriers (considering the two events together), is the *product* of the two events happening separately ($1/2 \times 1/2 = 1/4$).

184. **B** Amino acids do cross the placenta into the embryo's circulation (that is how the baby gets the building blocks for synthesizing its own proteins!). However, since the mother cannot make the enzyme to metabolize phenylalanine (remember, she has PKU), she must be careful with her diet. Otherwise, the high levels of the amino acid again in her blood can pass to the baby's blood (regardless of the baby's genotype) and cause the same situation that confronts PKU children.

185. **D** It must be understood that any individual with one allele (it is a dominant trait) for polydactyly will express the trait.

186. **C** A basic knowledge of human sex-determination and the general characteristics of the sex-chromosomes is required. Only males have a Y-chromosome. Therefore, only males can express holandric traits. Similarly, since the Y-chromosome is not homologous to the X-chromosome, every trait will be expressed (as are all X-linked traits carried by a male).

187. **A** An affected individual must be homozygous recessive. If the parents are heterozygotes, one in four offspring can be homozygous dominant (all offspring do not have to be heterozygous).

188. **C** $H\!-\!C\!\equiv\!C\!-\!H + HOH \rightarrow H_2C\!=\!C\!-\!H \rightleftarrows H_3C\!-\!C\!=\!O$

                                           OH   H

                                  enol form   keto form

189. **C** The weaker acid holds on more tightly to its proton than the stronger acid, which will release its proton more readily. As a result, the concentration of the weaker acid will increase over the stronger acid.

190. **B** The aromatic structure is lost in the keto form so that the enol structure is favored.

191. **C**

                         H

                      |

$-C\!=\!C\!-\!N\!-\!R' \rightleftarrows \left[-C\!=\!C\!-\!N\!-\!R'\ \underset{\Theta}{}\ \updownarrow\ -\underset{\Theta}{C}\!-\!C\!=\!N\!-\!R' \right] + H^+ \rightleftarrows -\overset{|}{C}\!-\!\overset{|}{C}\!=\!N\!-\!R'$

192. **C** The imine is the chief product.

193. **D** There is no hydrogen joined to N.

194. **B** There are two equivalence points (or full neutralization points) ii and iv indicating two acidic protons.

195. **D** When the amino acid is acidified its structure is

$$\overset{\oplus}{H_3N}\!-\!\underset{\underset{R}{|}}{CH}\!-\!COOH$$

It therefore behaves like a diprotic acid with two acid dissociation constants, K_{a1} and K_{a2}. The pK_a values are

$$pK_{a1} = -\log K_{a1}$$

$$pK_{a2} = -\log K_{a2}$$

Each amino acid has its characteristic pK_a values at each 1/2 neutralization or equivalence point (after adding 0.50 mol and 1.50 mol of NaOH pH = pK_a). Therefore, by measuring the pH after addition of 0.50 mol of NaOH you have the value of pK_{a1}. After the addition of 1.50 mol of NaOH, pH = pK_{a2}.

196. **A** $pI = \dfrac{pK_{a1} + pK_{a2}}{2}$ at this pH the amino acid is a zwitterion

$$\overset{\oplus}{H_3N}-CH-COO^{\ominus}$$
$$|$$
$$R$$

$$pI = \frac{2.40 + 9.80}{2} = 6.10$$

197. **C** At this point in the titration the first 1/2 equivalence point has been passed. At the first 1/2 equivalence point one-half of the diprotic acid

$$\overset{\oplus}{H_3N}-CH-COOH$$
$$|$$
$$R$$

has been converted into its conjugate base

$$\overset{\oplus}{H_3N}-CH-COO^{\ominus}$$
$$|$$
$$R$$

$$\overset{\oplus}{H_3N}-CH-COOH + OH^{\ominus} \rightarrow \overset{\oplus}{H_3N}-CH-COO^{\ominus}$$
$$|\qquad\qquad\qquad\qquad\qquad |$$
$$R\qquad\qquad\qquad\qquad\qquad R$$

Therefore, at the first 1/2 equivalence point

$$[\overset{\oplus}{H_3N}-CH-COOH]=[\overset{\oplus}{H_3N}-CH-COO^{\ominus}]$$
$$|\qquad\qquad\qquad\qquad\qquad |$$
$$R\qquad\qquad\qquad\qquad\qquad R$$

As you add more NaOH you increase

$$[\overset{\oplus}{H_3N}-CH-COO^{\ominus}]$$
$$|\qquad\qquad\text{so that it exceeds the}$$
$$R$$

concentration of the diprotic form.

198. **C**

199. **B** After the addition of 1.5 mol of NaOH

$$[\overset{\oplus}{H_3N}-CH-COO^{\ominus}]=[H_2N-CH-COO^{\ominus}]$$
$$|\qquad\qquad\qquad\qquad\qquad |$$
$$R\qquad\qquad\qquad\qquad\qquad R$$
$$\text{acid}\qquad\qquad\qquad\text{conjugate base}$$

A buffer solution contains similar concentrations of an acid and its conjugate base (or a base and conjugate acid).

200. **D**
$$CH_3$$
$$|$$
$$CH_3-C-CH_2Br$$
$$|$$
$$Br$$

There are two kinds of protons in this molecule: the six methyl protons and the two —CH_2— protons. Splitting is not observed because these non-equivalent protons are not on adjacent carbons. Hence, two NMR signals are observed in a 3:1 ratio.

201. **A** There are four non-equivalent protons: methyl protons (a), —CH$_2$— protons (d), and the two vinyl protons (a) and (b). The vinyl protons are non-equivalent because of their different chemical environments.

Consequently, 4 NMR signals will be observed.

202. **B** A deuteron gives no signal in a proton NMR spectrum because it absorbs at a much higher field. Consequently, by replacing H with D, signals are removed from the spectrum so that only two NMR signals will appear in a 3:2 peak ratio. No splitting will occur because the non-equivalent hydrogens are not attached to adjacent carbon atoms.

203. **A** The Br atom withdraws negative charge via an inductive effect deshielding the proton and causing a downfield shift.

204. **D** Nuclei of some elements generate a magnetic moment. When such nuclei are exposed to a magnetic field, their magnetic moment can be aligned with *or* against the field. The magnetic moment of the nucleus is aligned with the field in the more stable state. Energy can be absorbed to excite the nucleus into a higher energy state in which the magnetic moment of the nucleus is aligned against the field. An NMR spectrum records these absorptions. Some examples of nuclei which generate a magnetic field include protons, ^{13}C, and ^{19}F.

205. **D** Familiarity with the parts of a eukaryotic cell is required. The microtubules and microfilaments make up part of the cell's cytoskeleton. A change in their arrangement can lead to cell movement or a change in cell shape.

206. **B** It should be known that the semiconservative hypothesis refers to the accepted model of how DNA replication occurs. This takes place at the onset of mitosis or meiosis—when chromatids are synthesized.

207. **C** Knowledge about the roles of the liver is required. In addition, it should be understood that the liver first catabolizes its stored glycogen back to glucose. The monosaccharides enter the bloodstream, not the entire insoluble polysaccharide.

208. **C** Basic knowledge about muscle and joint anatomy is required. The origin of a muscle is the end which attaches to a site (bone) that usually does not move when the muscle contracts. In contrast, the insertion is the end that usually does move when the muscle contracts. The same bone can serve as the origin (site) for one muscle while serving as the insertion (site) for a different muscle.

209. **A** No previous knowledge about insects, hormones, or metamorphosis is necessary. The ability to logically apply the given information is required. If juvenile hormone inhibits metamorphosis, removal of the hormone (and its source) should cause metamorphosis to occur.

210. **B** An understanding of the role of oxygen in cellular respiration is needed, as is familiarity with microbiology terminology. Obligate anaerobes can survive only in the absence of oxygen.

211. **D** A basic understanding of kidney function and osmotic interactions is required. If a hypotonic filtrate (less solute, more water) passes a hypertonic tissue (more solute, less water), water will move from filtrate to surrounding tissue.

212. **C** Substitutions affect only one codon, and as a result, only one amino acid. Both additions and deletions affect the codons in which they occur, and every codon thereafter (frameshift mutations).

213. **A** An understanding of the relationship between

digestion and absorption is helpful. Except for the associated beneficial effects of maintaining normal digestive function and regularity, fiber itself provides little or no nutrition. The foods containing fiber, however, have other nutritional substances that we are able to digest and absorb.

214. **D** A basic knowledge about the major osmotic components of blood plasma is important, as is an understanding of the relationship between blood pressure and blood vessel distance from the heart. The major osmotic blood proteins (such as albumin) are too large to leave the capillaries. Thus, colloid osmotic pressure (COP) normally remains the same at both ends of the capillary. However, blood pressure decreases in vessels as distance from the heart increases, resulting in hydrostatic pressure being lower than COP at the venule end.

215. **B** In this isomer the bulky methyl groups are in equatorial positions where they have more room.

216. **B** The most substituted alkene is favored in elimination reactions.

217. **D** Epimers are diastereomeric aldoses that differ only in their configuration about carbon-2.

218. **B**

219. **A** A bond to deuterium is broken more slowly than a bond to protium (H). Observation of such a primary hydrogen isotope effect elucidates the rate determining step in a reaction.

PRACTICE EXAM II

	Time
Verbal Reasoning Questions 1–65	85 minutes
Physical Sciences Questions 66–142	100 minutes
Writing Sample 2 Essays	60 minutes
Biological Sciences Questions 143–219	100 minutes

ANSWER SHEET
PRACTICE EXAM II

VERBAL REASONING

1. Ⓐ Ⓑ Ⓒ Ⓓ
2. Ⓐ Ⓑ Ⓒ Ⓓ
3. Ⓐ Ⓑ Ⓒ Ⓓ
4. Ⓐ Ⓑ Ⓒ Ⓓ
5. Ⓐ Ⓑ Ⓒ Ⓓ
6. Ⓐ Ⓑ Ⓒ Ⓓ
7. Ⓐ Ⓑ Ⓒ Ⓓ
8. Ⓐ Ⓑ Ⓒ Ⓓ
9. Ⓐ Ⓑ Ⓒ Ⓓ
10. Ⓐ Ⓑ Ⓒ Ⓓ
11. Ⓐ Ⓑ Ⓒ Ⓓ
12. Ⓐ Ⓑ Ⓒ Ⓓ
13. Ⓐ Ⓑ Ⓒ Ⓓ
14. Ⓐ Ⓑ Ⓒ Ⓓ
15. Ⓐ Ⓑ Ⓒ Ⓓ
16. Ⓐ Ⓑ Ⓒ Ⓓ
17. Ⓐ Ⓑ Ⓒ Ⓓ
18. Ⓐ Ⓑ Ⓒ Ⓓ
19. Ⓐ Ⓑ Ⓒ Ⓓ
20. Ⓐ Ⓑ Ⓒ Ⓓ
21. Ⓐ Ⓑ Ⓒ Ⓓ
22. Ⓐ Ⓑ Ⓒ Ⓓ
23. Ⓐ Ⓑ Ⓒ Ⓓ
24. Ⓐ Ⓑ Ⓒ Ⓓ
25. Ⓐ Ⓑ Ⓒ Ⓓ
26. Ⓐ Ⓑ Ⓒ Ⓓ
27. Ⓐ Ⓑ Ⓒ Ⓓ
28. Ⓐ Ⓑ Ⓒ Ⓓ
29. Ⓐ Ⓑ Ⓒ Ⓓ
30. Ⓐ Ⓑ Ⓒ Ⓓ
31. Ⓐ Ⓑ Ⓒ Ⓓ
32. Ⓐ Ⓑ Ⓒ Ⓓ
33. Ⓐ Ⓑ Ⓒ Ⓓ
34. Ⓐ Ⓑ Ⓒ Ⓓ
35. Ⓐ Ⓑ Ⓒ Ⓓ
36. Ⓐ Ⓑ Ⓒ Ⓓ
37. Ⓐ Ⓑ Ⓒ Ⓓ
38. Ⓐ Ⓑ Ⓒ Ⓓ
39. Ⓐ Ⓑ Ⓒ Ⓓ
40. Ⓐ Ⓑ Ⓒ Ⓓ
41. Ⓐ Ⓑ Ⓒ Ⓓ
42. Ⓐ Ⓑ Ⓒ Ⓓ

43. Ⓐ Ⓑ Ⓒ Ⓓ
44. Ⓐ Ⓑ Ⓒ Ⓓ
45. Ⓐ Ⓑ Ⓒ Ⓓ
46. Ⓐ Ⓑ Ⓒ Ⓓ
47. Ⓐ Ⓑ Ⓒ Ⓓ
48. Ⓐ Ⓑ Ⓒ Ⓓ
49. Ⓐ Ⓑ Ⓒ Ⓓ
50. Ⓐ Ⓑ Ⓒ Ⓓ
51. Ⓐ Ⓑ Ⓒ Ⓓ
52. Ⓐ Ⓑ Ⓒ Ⓓ
53. Ⓐ Ⓑ Ⓒ Ⓓ
54. Ⓐ Ⓑ Ⓒ Ⓓ
55. Ⓐ Ⓑ Ⓒ Ⓓ
56. Ⓐ Ⓑ Ⓒ Ⓓ
57. Ⓐ Ⓑ Ⓒ Ⓓ
58. Ⓐ Ⓑ Ⓒ Ⓓ
59. Ⓐ Ⓑ Ⓒ Ⓓ
60. Ⓐ Ⓑ Ⓒ Ⓓ
61. Ⓐ Ⓑ Ⓒ Ⓓ
62. Ⓐ Ⓑ Ⓒ Ⓓ
63. Ⓐ Ⓑ Ⓒ Ⓓ
64. Ⓐ Ⓑ Ⓒ Ⓓ
65. Ⓐ Ⓑ Ⓒ Ⓓ

PHYSICAL SCIENCES

66. Ⓐ Ⓑ Ⓒ Ⓓ
67. Ⓐ Ⓑ Ⓒ Ⓓ
68. Ⓐ Ⓑ Ⓒ Ⓓ
69. Ⓐ Ⓑ Ⓒ Ⓓ
70. Ⓐ Ⓑ Ⓒ Ⓓ
71. Ⓐ Ⓑ Ⓒ Ⓓ
72. Ⓐ Ⓑ Ⓒ Ⓓ
73. Ⓐ Ⓑ Ⓒ Ⓓ
74. Ⓐ Ⓑ Ⓒ Ⓓ
75. Ⓐ Ⓑ Ⓒ Ⓓ
76. Ⓐ Ⓑ Ⓒ Ⓓ
77. Ⓐ Ⓑ Ⓒ Ⓓ
78. Ⓐ Ⓑ Ⓒ Ⓓ
79. Ⓐ Ⓑ Ⓒ Ⓓ
80. Ⓐ Ⓑ Ⓒ Ⓓ
81. Ⓐ Ⓑ Ⓒ Ⓓ
82. Ⓐ Ⓑ Ⓒ Ⓓ
83. Ⓐ Ⓑ Ⓒ Ⓓ
84. Ⓐ Ⓑ Ⓒ Ⓓ
85. Ⓐ Ⓑ Ⓒ Ⓓ
86. Ⓐ Ⓑ Ⓒ Ⓓ
87. Ⓐ Ⓑ Ⓒ Ⓓ
88. Ⓐ Ⓑ Ⓒ Ⓓ
89. Ⓐ Ⓑ Ⓒ Ⓓ
90. Ⓐ Ⓑ Ⓒ Ⓓ
91. Ⓐ Ⓑ Ⓒ Ⓓ
92. Ⓐ Ⓑ Ⓒ Ⓓ
93. Ⓐ Ⓑ Ⓒ Ⓓ
94. Ⓐ Ⓑ Ⓒ Ⓓ
95. Ⓐ Ⓑ Ⓒ Ⓓ
96. Ⓐ Ⓑ Ⓒ Ⓓ
97. Ⓐ Ⓑ Ⓒ Ⓓ
98. Ⓐ Ⓑ Ⓒ Ⓓ
99. Ⓐ Ⓑ Ⓒ Ⓓ
100. Ⓐ Ⓑ Ⓒ Ⓓ
101. Ⓐ Ⓑ Ⓒ Ⓓ
102. Ⓐ Ⓑ Ⓒ Ⓓ
103. Ⓐ Ⓑ Ⓒ Ⓓ
104. Ⓐ Ⓑ Ⓒ Ⓓ
105. Ⓐ Ⓑ Ⓒ Ⓓ
106. Ⓐ Ⓑ Ⓒ Ⓓ
107. Ⓐ Ⓑ Ⓒ Ⓓ

BIOLOGICAL SCIENCES

108. Ⓐ Ⓑ Ⓒ Ⓓ	143. Ⓐ Ⓑ Ⓒ Ⓓ	192. Ⓐ Ⓑ Ⓒ Ⓓ
109. Ⓐ Ⓑ Ⓒ Ⓓ	144. Ⓐ Ⓑ Ⓒ Ⓓ	193. Ⓐ Ⓑ Ⓒ Ⓓ
110. Ⓐ Ⓑ Ⓒ Ⓓ	145. Ⓐ Ⓑ Ⓒ Ⓓ	194. Ⓐ Ⓑ Ⓒ Ⓓ
111. Ⓐ Ⓑ Ⓒ Ⓓ	146. Ⓐ Ⓑ Ⓒ Ⓓ	195. Ⓐ Ⓑ Ⓒ Ⓓ
112. Ⓐ Ⓑ Ⓒ Ⓓ	147. Ⓐ Ⓑ Ⓒ Ⓓ	196. Ⓐ Ⓑ Ⓒ Ⓓ
113. Ⓐ Ⓑ Ⓒ Ⓓ	148. Ⓐ Ⓑ Ⓒ Ⓓ	197. Ⓐ Ⓑ Ⓒ Ⓓ
114. Ⓐ Ⓑ Ⓒ Ⓓ	149. Ⓐ Ⓑ Ⓒ Ⓓ	198. Ⓐ Ⓑ Ⓒ Ⓓ
115. Ⓐ Ⓑ Ⓒ Ⓓ	150. Ⓐ Ⓑ Ⓒ Ⓓ	199. Ⓐ Ⓑ Ⓒ Ⓓ
116. Ⓐ Ⓑ Ⓒ Ⓓ	151. Ⓐ Ⓑ Ⓒ Ⓓ	200. Ⓐ Ⓑ Ⓒ Ⓓ
117. Ⓐ Ⓑ Ⓒ Ⓓ	152. Ⓐ Ⓑ Ⓒ Ⓓ	201. Ⓐ Ⓑ Ⓒ Ⓓ
118. Ⓐ Ⓑ Ⓒ Ⓓ	153. Ⓐ Ⓑ Ⓒ Ⓓ	202. Ⓐ Ⓑ Ⓒ Ⓓ
119. Ⓐ Ⓑ Ⓒ Ⓓ	154. Ⓐ Ⓑ Ⓒ Ⓓ	203. Ⓐ Ⓑ Ⓒ Ⓓ
120. Ⓐ Ⓑ Ⓒ Ⓓ	155. Ⓐ Ⓑ Ⓒ Ⓓ	204. Ⓐ Ⓑ Ⓒ Ⓓ
121. Ⓐ Ⓑ Ⓒ Ⓓ	156. Ⓐ Ⓑ Ⓒ Ⓓ	205. Ⓐ Ⓑ Ⓒ Ⓓ
122. Ⓐ Ⓑ Ⓒ Ⓓ	157. Ⓐ Ⓑ Ⓒ Ⓓ	206. Ⓐ Ⓑ Ⓒ Ⓓ
123. Ⓐ Ⓑ Ⓒ Ⓓ	158. Ⓐ Ⓑ Ⓒ Ⓓ	207. Ⓐ Ⓑ Ⓒ Ⓓ
124. Ⓐ Ⓑ Ⓒ Ⓓ	159. Ⓐ Ⓑ Ⓒ Ⓓ	208. Ⓐ Ⓑ Ⓒ Ⓓ
125. Ⓐ Ⓑ Ⓒ Ⓓ	160. Ⓐ Ⓑ Ⓒ Ⓓ	209. Ⓐ Ⓑ Ⓒ Ⓓ
126. Ⓐ Ⓑ Ⓒ Ⓓ	161. Ⓐ Ⓑ Ⓒ Ⓓ	210. Ⓐ Ⓑ Ⓒ Ⓓ
127. Ⓐ Ⓑ Ⓒ Ⓓ	162. Ⓐ Ⓑ Ⓒ Ⓓ	211. Ⓐ Ⓑ Ⓒ Ⓓ
128. Ⓐ Ⓑ Ⓒ Ⓓ	163. Ⓐ Ⓑ Ⓒ Ⓓ	212. Ⓐ Ⓑ Ⓒ Ⓓ
129. Ⓐ Ⓑ Ⓒ Ⓓ	164. Ⓐ Ⓑ Ⓒ Ⓓ	213. Ⓐ Ⓑ Ⓒ Ⓓ
130. Ⓐ Ⓑ Ⓒ Ⓓ	165. Ⓐ Ⓑ Ⓒ Ⓓ	214. Ⓐ Ⓑ Ⓒ Ⓓ
131. Ⓐ Ⓑ Ⓒ Ⓓ	166. Ⓐ Ⓑ Ⓒ Ⓓ	215. Ⓐ Ⓑ Ⓒ Ⓓ
132. Ⓐ Ⓑ Ⓒ Ⓓ	167. Ⓐ Ⓑ Ⓒ Ⓓ	216. Ⓐ Ⓑ Ⓒ Ⓓ
133. Ⓐ Ⓑ Ⓒ Ⓓ	168. Ⓐ Ⓑ Ⓒ Ⓓ	217. Ⓐ Ⓑ Ⓒ Ⓓ
134. Ⓐ Ⓑ Ⓒ Ⓓ	169. Ⓐ Ⓑ Ⓒ Ⓓ	218. Ⓐ Ⓑ Ⓒ Ⓓ
135. Ⓐ Ⓑ Ⓒ Ⓓ	170. Ⓐ Ⓑ Ⓒ Ⓓ	219. Ⓐ Ⓑ Ⓒ Ⓓ
136. Ⓐ Ⓑ Ⓒ Ⓓ	171. Ⓐ Ⓑ Ⓒ Ⓓ	
137. Ⓐ Ⓑ Ⓒ Ⓓ	172. Ⓐ Ⓑ Ⓒ Ⓓ	
138. Ⓐ Ⓑ Ⓒ Ⓓ	173. Ⓐ Ⓑ Ⓒ Ⓓ	
139. Ⓐ Ⓑ Ⓒ Ⓓ	174. Ⓐ Ⓑ Ⓒ Ⓓ	
140. Ⓐ Ⓑ Ⓒ Ⓓ	175. Ⓐ Ⓑ Ⓒ Ⓓ	
141. Ⓐ Ⓑ Ⓒ Ⓓ	176. Ⓐ Ⓑ Ⓒ Ⓓ	
142. Ⓐ Ⓑ Ⓒ Ⓓ	177. Ⓐ Ⓑ Ⓒ Ⓓ	
	178. Ⓐ Ⓑ Ⓒ Ⓓ	
	179. Ⓐ Ⓑ Ⓒ Ⓓ	
	180. Ⓐ Ⓑ Ⓒ Ⓓ	
	181. Ⓐ Ⓑ Ⓒ Ⓓ	
	182. Ⓐ Ⓑ Ⓒ Ⓓ	
	183. Ⓐ Ⓑ Ⓒ Ⓓ	
	184. Ⓐ Ⓑ Ⓒ Ⓓ	
	185. Ⓐ Ⓑ Ⓒ Ⓓ	
	186. Ⓐ Ⓑ Ⓒ Ⓓ	
	187. Ⓐ Ⓑ Ⓒ Ⓓ	
	188. Ⓐ Ⓑ Ⓒ Ⓓ	
	189. Ⓐ Ⓑ Ⓒ Ⓓ	
	190. Ⓐ Ⓑ Ⓒ Ⓓ	
	191. Ⓐ Ⓑ Ⓒ Ⓓ	

Writing Sample 1

_____

_____

_____

_____

_____

_____

_____

_____

_____

_____

_____

_____

_____

_____

_____

_____

_____

_____

_____

_____

_____

_____

_____

_____

_____

_____

_____

_____

_____

_____

END OF PART 1

Writing Sample 2

_____

_____

_____

_____

_____

_____

_____

_____

_____

_____

_____

_____

_____

_____

_____

_____

_____

_____

_____

_____

_____

END OF PART 1

VERBAL REASONING

Time: 85 Minutes
Questions 1–65

Directions: There are nine passages in this test. Each passage is followed by questions based on its content. After reading a passage, choose the one best answer to each question and indicate your selection by blackening the corresponding space on your answer sheet.

Passage I (Questions 1–6)

If the world experiences significant temperature increases due to the Greenhouse Effect, both people and nature will have to adapt. One way people will need to adapt is in the way they use energy.

(5) For example, everyone uses energy in ways that are affected directly by weather conditions. Heating, cooking, refrigerating, and water heating are important uses of energy that are affected directly by temperature, humidity, and other weather conditions. One con-
(10) sequence of higher temperatures caused by global warming would be lowered demand for energy used for heating in the winter and increased demand for energy used for cooling in the summer. Under the Greenhouse Effect, the changing seasonal patterns in energy
(15) use—less energy needed in winter and more consumed in summer—and the overall impact on total energy demand could have important implications for energy planning and ultimately on the cost of energy for individuals and businesses.

(20) While climate change could affect a wide range of energy sources and uses, the implications for the demand for electricity are particularly significant. This is because the primary weather-sensitive energy uses—space heating and cooling, water heating, and refriger-
(25) ating—make up a significant portion of total electricity sales for public utilities. These "end-uses" can account for as much as one-third of a power company's total sales and even more during daily and seasonal peak-usage periods.

(30) Also, because of the large investments by utilities in long-lived capital-intensive power plants, the industry must focus on long-term planning. In other words, utilities must begin planning their investments now to meet their power generation needs into the next
(35) century.

To address these issues, the Environmental Protection Agency (EPA) and ICF Incorporated, an environmental and energy consulting firm, have assessed the potential impacts of the Greenhouse Effect on the
(40) demand for electricity and the consequences of these impacts for utility planning. Based on this study, preliminary regional and natural estimates were developed for a period from the present to the middle of the next century (2055).

(45) By the year 2055, the Greenhouse Effect could measurably change regional demands for electricity in the United States. A principal factor in generating capacity requirements is the peak (highest hourly) demand the utility must meet. For most utilities in the United
(50) States, this occurs on a day during a summer hot spell. Peak electricity demands are driven largely by peak use of air conditioning. Because the Greenhouse Effect is expected to have a significant influence on air conditioning and other summertime uses of electricity, higher
(55) temperatures in the future could lead to significant increases in the capacity needed to satisfy those uses.

Capacity requirements would not increase in all states, however. Because of greater demands for heating than cooling in colder regions, some utilities expe-
(60) rience peak demands in the winter. In these cases, warmer winter temperatures caused by the Greenhouse Effect could reduce the amount of generating capacity required. Such reductions in new capacity requirements induced by the Greenhouse Effect are restricted to a
(65) few states in the Northeast (Maine, New Hampshire, and Vermont) and in the Northwest (Washington, Oregon, Montana, and Wyoming).

The EPA-ICF study estimated that the investment in new power plants necessitated by the Greenhouse
(70) Effect could total several hundred billion dollars (not including any increase in costs due to inflation) over the next seventy years. In addition, increased fuel and operating and maintenance costs to generate electricity with these plants could reach several billion dollars per
(75) year by 2055. Much of these costs would undoubtedly be reflected in higher electric bills for consumers.

Of course, it is difficult, if not impossible, to predict the future. The extent and rate of climate change that will occur are very uncertain. Nonetheless, the pic-
(80) ture painted by the study results is a very real possibility. The findings suggest that a substantial amount of our resources could be devoted to planning for and adapting to the Greenhouse Effect in this one sector alone. There are a number of other ways the Green-
(85) house Effect could make an impact on electric utilities (for example, reductions in the availability of water in rivers used to generate hydropower), and there are many other sectors of the world economy and environment that will feel the effects of climate change.
(90) Designing and implementing strategies that will help to mitigate the Greenhouse Effect and to adapt to climate changes that do occur are the challenges facing policy makers and planners today.

1. The passage states that in some parts of the country, peak demand for electricity might decrease under the Greenhouse Effect because:

   A. these regions use more electricity for heating than for cooling and the need to heat would be reduced.
   B. conservation efforts might eliminate the need for more electricity.
   C. increases in rainfall might increase the number of cloudy days and reduce temperatures.
   D. we might switch from electric power to solar power.

2. The passage indicates that electricity demands caused by the Greenhouse Effect:

   A. will not be felt for seventy years.
   B. may result in greater dependence on hydropower.
   C. are most likely to increase in the Northeast and Northwest.
   D. could be significantly changed by the year 2055.

3. It would be reasonable to take the writer's argument further and assume that the writer:

   A. would advocate planning for the greenhouse effect in other areas of our society.
   B. believes that the only aspect of our society that will be affected by the greenhouse effect is the use of electricity.

   C. does not believe the greenhouse effect is going to occur.
   D. believes adjustment to the greenhouse effect will not cause major disruption in our society.

4. If the Greenhouse Effect takes place, the author believes that peak demand for electricity will decrease in the Northeast United States during the:

   I. winter.
   II. summer.
   III. spring.

   A. I only
   B. II only
   C. I and II only
   D. II and III only

5. It can be assumed from the article that the author:

   A. thinks the Greenhouse Effect is a near certainty.
   B. believes we should stop the Greenhouse Effect before it is too late.
   C. believes utilities have not planned enough in the past and need to do a better job in the future.
   D. believes that nonelectrical sources of energy need to be found to reduce the demand for electricity.

6. According to the article, long-range planning is important to utilities because:

   A. without it, they would run out of electricity.
   B. huge capital investments will be needed to build new generating facilities.
   C. the government needs to know well in advance if there are going to be any shortfalls in power generation.
   D. of the time it takes to build generating facilities.

Passage II (Questions 7–15)

As a child of the frontier, it was natural for George Caleb Bingham (1811–79), the "Missouri painter," to paint the fur trappers, flatboatmen, country politicians, and squatters he knew so well. He portrayed them as
(5) rugged and self-reliant Americans, emblems of the frontier spirit.

Bingham came of age in the Golden Age of American painting (1830–60), when the work of American artists was, for the first time, appreciated and pur-
(10) chased not only by the wealthy—whose taste tended toward European works and artists—but also by an emerging and increasingly affluent middle class with an appetite for art that reflected the American spirit.

Today, Bingham ranks among the best of the
(15) nineteenth-century American narrative painters. "He was a powerful figure who broke new ground in illustrating the simple joys of American life and who prepared the way for the giants—Winslow Homer and Thomas Eakins—to follow," says E. Maurice Bloch,
(20) emeritus professor of art history at the University of California at Los Angeles. Bloch is author of *The Paintings of George Caleb Bingham: A Catalogue Raisonné*, published by the University of Missouri Press.

Bloch's *catalogue raisonné* places Bingham's life
(25) and work in the context of the social, artistic, and political climate of nineteenth-century America. The catalogue also reflects on Bingham's philosophy of art and examines the issue of patronage and national support for artists.

(30) To his foes, Bingham was volatile, irascible, and pugnacious—with a colorful vocabulary to match. "He never attempted to mitigate the combative part of his personality," says Bloch. To his close friends, though, he was fiercely loyal and often charming, witty, and
(35) even affectionate.

Like many American artists, Bingham was largely self-taught and "he was proud of it," according to Bloch. Inspired by an itinerant painter, Bingham started out as a journeyman portraitist, traveling from town to town
(40) through Missouri and Mississippi. The stiffness of his early work began to soften after he studied for several months at the Philadelphia Academy of Art. He was also exposed to other artists while he worked as a portraitist for several years in Washington, D.C.

(45) Bingham gained a national reputation through the American Art Union, an important corporate patron that encouraged artists to paint works appealing to patriotic feeling. The Art Union bought such works and distributed them by lottery to its members. The Art Union
(50) bought nineteen of Bingham's paintings between 1845 and 1851, exhibited them for long periods, promoted his work in its magazine, and engraved *The Jolly Flatboatman* in an edition of 10,000.

Despite national recognition, Bingham never
(55) achieved federal patronage. He sought, but did not win, a commission "to paint a western subject by a western artist" for a new extension to the Capitol in Washington, D.C. Although he has always been well known in Missouri, his national reputation began to fade even
(60) before his death in 1879. Not until 1935, after an exhibition of American realists at the Museum of Modern Art, did contemporary scholars become interested in Bingham's work.

Having studied Bingham's life and work for more
(65) than forty years, Bloch notes, "It would have been possible to write an excellent book on Bingham by noting only a narrow circle of authentic works. But the much greater mass of questionable works and copies acted as a magnet and a challenge." The catalogue raisonné,
(70) which supersedes an earlier version written by Bloch, includes one hundred works discovered in recent years. In addition, the attribution of twenty works previously thought to be by Bingham has been changed.

Because most of Bingham's paintings are held in
(75) private collections, this catalogue raisonné with its 370 black-and-white and 34 color illustrations may become indispensable to students and scholars.

7. According to the passage, the golden age of American painting:

 A. lasted for most of the nineteenth century.
 B. was the period from 1830 to 1860.
 C. was over before George Caleb Bingham came of age.
 D. benefited from the patronage of the Philadelphia Academy of Art.

8. Based on reading the article, it would be reasonable to say that Bloch believes Bingham was:

 I. an artist whose works varied enormously in quality.
 II. a very important early American artist.
 III. worth remembering as a historic figure in the art movement but not as an artist.

 A. I only
 B. II only
 C. I and II only
 D. I and III only

9. Bloch describes Bingham as:

   A. nice, social, dedicated, and kind.
   B. calm, diligent, sensitive, and distant.
   C. aggressive, talented, cultured, and caustic.
   D. loyal, charming, witty, and affectionate.

10. Bingham's training as an artist was reflective of most American artists of the time in that he was:

    A. largely self-taught.
    B. trained by itinerant artists.
    C. molded by the art schools dominant in the East.
    D. commissioned by wealthy patrons.

11. The article states that Bingham gained his national reputation:

    A. through the American Art Union.
    B. by getting a commission from the federal government to paint western scenes.
    C. by studying at the Philadelphia Academy of Art.
    D. by traveling and painting scenes all over the United States.

12. It can be inferred from the article that Bingham did much of his painting in:

    A. Texas and New Mexico.
    B. Missouri and Kansas.
    C. Missouri and Mississippi.
    D. Mississippi and Texas.

13. According to the article, E. Maurice Bloch:

    A. dubbed Bingham the "Missouri painter."
    B. studied the work of Winslow Homer and Thomas Eakins.
    C. taught art history at the University of Missouri.
    D. studied Bingham's life and work for over forty years.

14. The recognition of Bingham's reputation as one of the U.S.'s leading nineteenth-century narrative painters is a testament to Bingham's:

    A. ability to depict in his art the spirit of American individualism and self-reliance.
    B. ability to incorporate patriotic themes in his art, thereby promoting a sense of vibrant nationalism.
    C. ability to create an appreciation of American artistic talent.
    D. creative artistic drive, which coincided with the American public's gradual preference for American over European art.

15. According to the article, Bingham's paintings were highly reflective of the:

    A. nineteenth-century American middle class.
    B. early nineteenth-century American city dweller.
    C. frontier-American pioneer spirit.
    D. mid-nineteenth-century mercantile class.

Passage III (Questions 16–21)

Throughout the nation, the current focus in education is on excellence. Recommendations from four independent national panels call for increased emphasis on: the five new basics (English, mathematics, sci-
(5) ence, social studies, and computer science), increased graduation requirements, a longer school day and school year, performance-based pay, incentives for outstanding teacher achievement, and alternate career ladders.

A master teacher plan is one of several proce-
(10) dures recommended to improve the quality of teachers and instruction in the classroom and to raise the achievement of students. A master teacher plan would provide a reward system for excellent teaching and make the profession more attractive to bright, talented college
(15) students seeking a professional career. It would also aid in retaining outstanding tenured teachers.

In response to the recommendations of the President's Commission on Excellence in Education, the Department of Defense Dependents School has
(20) implemented several educational reforms, one of which is a Master Teacher Pilot Program. In the development of the pilot program in the Department of Defense Dependents School's Panama Region, 374 classroom teachers and special area teachers responded to a
(25) 25-item questionnaire on issues related to the Master Teacher Pilot Program. The survey revealed:

- The professional community is uncertain about its readiness for a master teacher program.

- Elementary teachers are more receptive to the
(30) concept of a master teacher plan than are secondary teachers.

- Almost 75 percent of the teachers believe an alternate career path is needed in the teaching profession.

(35) • The ultimate professional goal for 50 percent of the teachers is to remain classroom teachers.

• Fewer than 10 percent of all teachers aspire to be administrators.

• Fifty percent of the teachers believe that a master
(40) teacher program could provide for professional growth.

• The majority of teachers believe that a master teacher program is likely to create tension, jealousy, favoritism, competition, and low morale.

(45) • About two-thirds of the teachers believe the major problem in the development of a master teacher program is the construction of accurate, impartial, and fair evaluation instruments.

• Measurement and selection issues were the biggest
(50) concerns reported by the teachers.

• About one-third of the teachers would like to be considered for a master teacher position.

• Approximately 70 percent of the teachers prefer to have their building principal perform the
(55) observation and evaluation for the selection of master teachers.

• The majority of teachers believe that at least half the master teacher's time should be spent in the classroom.

(60) Teachers in the Panama Region then responded to a second survey about the criteria to be used in selecting master teachers.

What is to be the profile of a master teacher? First and foremost, the master teacher would have compre-
(65) hensive knowledge about his or her subject. The master teacher would be highly skilled in managing and instructing a class of students. Management of the total class as well as individual student behavior was deemed important. The master teacher would also excel in or-
(70) ganizational planning, use of class time, and knowledge and use of instructional materials.

The most significant instructional skill of a master teacher would be the application and adaptation of major educational concepts and theories to provide for
(75) individual student differences, when designing lessons and in using instructional strategies to implement lessons. Students of master teachers would learn content as measured by teacher-developed tests. The master teacher would demonstrate clarity in both verbal and
(80) written expression. The master teacher would work well with students, would show consideration for others, and would have a commitment to professional growth and to the school program. The master teacher would frequently initiate and complete educational tasks and
(85) would show support for other group members. He or

she would be well informed of recent developments in education.

The Department of Defense Dependents School has accepted the challenge for educational reform; the Master
(90) Teacher Program is one small step in an overall plan for excellence. In this endeavor, active teacher participation is vital to the success of a master teacher program.

16. Recommendations from four independent national panels call for increased emphasis on all of the following subjects **EXCEPT**:

   A. science.
   B. computer science.
   C. mathematics.
   D. foreign language study.

17. According to the author, a master teacher plan would provide:

   I. a reward for excellence.
   II. professional development for new teachers.
   III. specialized teachers for the elementary schools.

   A. I only
   B. I and II only
   C. II only
   D. II and III only

18. Based on the article, it would be reasonable to assume that the author:

   A. is strongly opposed to the concept of a master teacher.
   B. is mildly critical of the master teacher concept.
   C. believes that the master teacher idea is good, but disagrees with the way it is being used by the armed forces.
   D. believes that the master teacher concept is a positive step toward improving education.

19. According to the author, which one of the following is the most important attribute of the master teacher?

   A. The ability to train other teachers
   B. Skill in classroom management
   C. The ability to communicate well with students
   D. Comprehensive knowledge of the subject areas taught

20. Which of the following was **NOT** one of the findings of the Panama Region survey?

    A. High school teachers were not as receptive to the master teacher concept as were elementary school teachers.

    B. Development of fair and impartial evaluation instruments is a major problem in implementing a master teacher program.

    C. The majority of teachers aspire to be administrators.

    D. More than 50 percent of all the teachers surveyed believe a master teacher program will result in low morale.

21. According to the article, the ideal master teacher would be highly skilled in:

    I. managing and instructing a class of students.
    II. providing for individual students' needs.
    III. verbal and written expression.
    IV. administrative techniques.

    A. I and II only
    B. I, II, and III only
    C. I, II, and IV only
    D. III only

Passage IV (Questions 22–29)

Consider for a moment these chemicals: safrole, hydrazine, tannin, and ethyl carbamate. We ingest them every day when we consume pepper, mushrooms, tea, and bread. Now consider this: each of these chemicals
(5) is a naturally occurring carcinogen. Do they jeopardize human health? Should this information lead to a movement to eliminate tea, outlaw mushrooms, condemn pepper, and banish bread from our tables?

Of course not. Yet that's where a manipulation
(10) of the numbers, and a misinterpretation of the facts, can take us. The numbers can be made to show that a substance is killing us—even when there isn't the remotest possibility. How, then, can a mother be sure that her food purchases will nourish her family and not con-
(15) tribute to its morbidity?

If you listen to every restrictive environmental report that has received media attention, you know that in addition to apples, you shouldn't eat most other fruits, not to mention meats, fish, fowl, vegetables, eggs, or
(20) milk products. You shouldn't even drink the water. This begs the question, how can we make intelligent choices about risk?

Determining levels of safety in the environment, which is broadly defined to include lifestyle, must start
(25) with some basic premises. The first is that public health means preventing premature disease and death. The second is that public health policy should ensure safety, not harass industry or needlessly terrify the public.

What Americans suffer from is not a lack of data.
(30) It's something else entirely. The malady that needs immediate attention is called nosophobia. It's akin to hypochondria, but different.

Hypochondriacs think they are sick. Nosophobics think they will be sick in the future because of lurking
(35) factors in their diet and general environment. They fixate on an array of allegedly health-threatening gremlins. Due to this phobia, they believe that living—and eating and drinking—in America is inherently hazardous to their health. They are sure there is a death-dealing
(40) carcinogen on every plate, a life-sapping toxin under every pillow. They see salvation only in ever-increasing federal regulations and bans.

The nosophobics' fears of Alar and other agricultural chemicals used in the United States are obvi-
(45) ously purely emotional. These are fears of "invisible hazards," which have always played a special role in the mass psychology of paranoia, according to Park Elliott Dietz, Professor of Law and Psychiatry at the University of Virginia. Yesterday's invisible hazards
(50) give rise to monster legends, claims of witchcraft, and vampire myths. Today, notes Dr. Dietz, we see the same phenomenon among those who exaggerate the hazards of radiation, chemicals, toxic waste, and food additives.

The most deadly public health issues that threaten
(55) our lives have been obscured in the face of trumped-up charges against the food we eat, the water we drink, and the air we breathe. They fall under the category of hazardous lifestyles. And the data detailing the toll they take on human lives—not the lives of laboratory rats
(60) and mice—are compelling and truly frightening.

Cigarette smoking claims 1200 lives a day. In just one year, over 400,000 will perish because they'd rather die than switch. Another obvious example of a hazardous lifestyle habit is excessive or abusive alcohol con-
(65) sumption, which claims 100,000 lives annually. Add to this the use of addictive substances, such as heroin, cocaine, and crack, which claim some 50,000 lives each year.

These numbers are in. They aren't hypothetical.
(70) They aren't based on probability theories that require one to suspend disbelief. These data detail a real loss of life. Clearly, our focus should be on environmental lifestyle issues that, left unchecked, are systematically and prematurely killing our population. As a society,
(75) however, we seem more willing to assume the enormous and deadly risks of smoking or not wearing seatbelts—risks that are within our power to prevent.

Ironically, what we appear to be unwilling to tolerate are the minute, infinitesimal risks we perceive to be (80) outside our control. Today's prime example is the risk the public perceives when chemicals are married to food.

What most don't understand is that food is 100-percent chemicals. Even the foods on our holiday (85) dinner tables—from mushroom soup to roasted turkey to apple pie—contain naturally occurring chemicals that are toxic when taken in high doses. Undoubtedly, there are some who may think we should start worrying about levels of allyl isothiocyanate in broccoli, because this (90) naturally produced chemical is, in high doses, an animal carcinogen. Where does it end? Worrying about more numbers to focus more attention on non-issues accomplishes absolutely nothing.

22. According to the article, public health policy should not:

    A. needlessly harass industry or terrify the public.
    B. avoid controversial issues just to protect industry.
    C. hide dangers in eating certain foods from the public simply to keep the public from becoming fearful.
    D. try to change people's lifestyles.

23. According to the author, which of the following foods naturally contain toxic chemicals?

    I. Grains and dairy products
    II. Mushrooms and bread
    III. Salmon and trout

    A. I only
    B. II only
    C. III only
    D. II and III only

24. The article defines nosophobics as those who are:

    A. environmentally conscious.
    B. committed to improving the quality of life.
    C. overly concerned about their lifestyle.
    D. fearful of future illness due to current hazards in their food or environment.

25. It would be reasonable to infer from this article that the author thinks we should:

    A. spend more time regulating carcinogens that occur naturally in food.

    B. spend more time worrying about the quality of our air than worrying about additives in food.
    C. not worry so much about the potential effects of what we add to food.
    D. more closely regulate what we allow to be added to food.

26. The author implies that our current fear of chemicals in the food and the environment is similar to which of the following?

    A. The fear of technology exhibited in the seventeenth and eighteenth centuries
    B. The fear of the study of science throughout the European Renaissance period
    C. The fear of witchcraft and vampires in past centuries
    D. The fear of the unknown

27. The author believes that one of the most important steps we can take to lengthen our lives is to:

    A. eat only organic produce.
    B. change our lifestyles by avoiding smoking, drinking, and other drug-taking.
    C. pay more attention to the fat content of the food we eat.
    D. pay more attention to exercise.

28. One possible explanation of the fear of chemicals in food and the environment can be interpreted as:

    A. a legitimate public concern.
    B. a symptom of a paranoia among an isolated segment of the population.
    C. a public-oriented fear substantiated by reliable studies performed by consumer food organizations.
    D. a hoax perpetuated by a disgruntled few.

29. According to the author, cigarette smoking kills:

    A. 1200 people a year.
    B. 50,000 people a year.
    C. 100,000 people a year.
    D. 400,000 people a year.

Passage V (Questions 30–36)

How can a society's economic system produce the greatest good for the largest number of its members? Can the Aristotelian idea of the "good life" be conceived independently of the ability to acquire (5) wealth? What is the happiness that Americans believe they have the right to pursue? The people of Seattle are confronting questions like these in an adult education program created by the Metrocenter YMCA in conjunction with the continuing education program at the Uni- (10) versity of Washington.

In 1981, during a City Fair program sponsored by the YMCA, some of the citizens of Seattle examined the hard economic questions facing their city. "People felt that decisions about economic growth in- (15) volved more than statistics," says Richard Conlin, a project director for Metrocenter YMCA. They discovered that economic questions are not only technical and political, but ethical and religious as well. "People wanted to talk about the economy in terms of values," (20) Conlin says. "Yet when they began to discuss the economy, they felt they lacked the ability to understand and articulate the philosophical issues that lie at the heart of the social contract."

To make the readings more accessible, the schol- (25) ars included commentaries that place them in social and historical contexts. "When Plato and Aristotle examined the question, 'What is the good life?' they were living in an age of anxiety. The city-state of Athens was in decline. Their best hopes were a society that (30) could ensure a reasonable quality of life for individuals despite a political environment threatening chaos," says Heyne. "When Aristotle asserted that 'man is by nature a political animal,' he meant that man, who is neither beast nor god, does not live in isolation," says (35) Heyne, "but in a community." Thus, according to Aristotle, the pursuit of material wealth should be a means to strengthen the community, the *polis*. People who pursue material wealth for its own sake, Aristotle wrote, "are intent upon living only and not living well."

(40) "Adam Smith, on the other hand, did not believe that the desire for wealth was in any way unnatural or a threat to the well-being of the society," says Heyne. Increasing wealth was a universal urge, Smith wrote in his classic treatise of 1776, *The Wealth of Nations*. (45) People want to "better their condition, . . . a desire that comes with us from the womb and never leaves us till we fall into the grave." "But Smith knew something that Aristotle couldn't consider," says Heyne. "Smith had observed the process of economic growth visible (50) in Europe in the sixteenth and seventeenth centuries. He had seen how a society could increase the production power over time, expanding the supply of 'necessities and conveniences of life.' This was not unnatural

or a threat to the well being of future generations. 'Capi- (55) tal has been silently and gradually accumulated by the private frugality . . . of individuals to better their own condition. . . . This effort, protected by law and allowed by liberty . . . has maintained the progress of England toward opulence and improvement . . . ,' Smith wrote."

(60) "We won't find simple answers for our age in the writing of these philosophers," says Heyne. "Their worlds differed so much from ours. But those differences can be instructive. If we can understand why Aristotle opposed economic growth and why Adam (65) Smith extolled it, it will prompt us to think about how decisions are actually made in modern democracies."

Arlis Steward, director of Metrocenter YMCA's community development programs, says that "the challenge of this project was to select an anthology that (70) people would not only read but would reflect upon before coming to get things done. Our economic system, as Adam Smith noted, depends basically upon self-interested behavior. Could a system based on nobler obligations be as effective in coordinating the ev- (75) eryday details of a highly specialized economic system?"

30. The article implies that a basic reason for setting up the program was to:

   A. develop an adult education program that discussed philosophy.
   B. develop a program that would help the public to be better informed on social questions.
   C. help adults better understand economic questions particularly as they concerned the city of Seattle.
   D. allow the University of Washington to effectively reach out to the adult community.

31. The inclusion by the YMCA's community adult education programs of the works of philosophers of diverse thinking and historical periods, such as Aristotle and Adam Smith, was a reflection of:

   A. an effort to instruct the public's general understanding of contemporary economic issues through analysis of different philosophical approaches.
   B. a realization that philosophers offered solutions to economic problems that apply today.

C. a commitment to reintroducing classical writers no longer read by the general public.

D. an effort to help the general public accept the growing policy of harsh economic reforms occurring in Seattle.

32. According to Richard Conlin, people in Seattle found that economic questions were not only technical and political but also:

A. cultural and social.

B. philosophical and historical.

C. were based on knowledge of the past, present, and future.

D. ethical and religious.

33. According to the article, which of the following correctly reflects the views of Adam Smith and Aristotle toward economic growth?

A. Adam Smith opposed economic growth and Aristotle extolled it.

B. Both Aristotle and Adam Smith extolled economic growth, but for different reasons.

C. Both Aristotle and Adam Smith opposed economic growth, but for different reasons.

D. Aristotle opposed economic growth while Adam Smith extolled it.

34. One can infer from the article that we can better understand our modern day society by exploring the works of philosophers of the past because these works offer:

I. viable solutions to contemporary problems.

II. ways of viewing variable approaches to contemporary decision-making.

III. idealized answers applicable to today's realistic situations.

A. I only

B. II only

C. I and II only

D. II and III only

35. Based on the article, it would be reasonable to assume that the author:

A. supports the program that the YMCA created.

B. opposes the kind of program the YMCA created.

C. supports the concept of the program, but is not satisfied with the program as implemented.

D. believes that programs such as the one that the YMCA developed should be developed by universities instead of YMCAs.

36. Which of the following expresses one of the basic differences between the philosophies of Adam Smith and Aristotle?

A. Adam Smith felt that wealth should be accumulated for the good of society if it was to have any real value, and Aristotle believed that the accumulation of wealth was of value in itself.

B. Aristotle thought that wealth had value only when it was accumulated for the good of society, and Adam Smith felt the accumulation of wealth was of value in its own right.

C. Aristotle was more philosophical and Adam Smith was more pragmatic.

D. Adam Smith was more interested in money than Aristotle.

Passage VI (Questions 37–44)

One hallmark of the Southern literary tradition has been the varied ways that writers have drawn upon Southerners' almost instinctive relationship to their surroundings. Working within a land-oriented cultural
(5) ethos, Southern writers have evoked a familiar, often haunting sense of place that gives the South a distinctive regional identity. Writers as well as artists have variously envisioned the land as a nostalgic emblem of the past, a source of goodness or a reflection of the
(10) divine, a product of decay, an exemplar of the bizarre, and a symbol of the human condition. Their portrayals range from the mythic and romantic to the factual and realistic.

"What is distinctive about the South," says Robert
(15) C. Stewart, executive director of the Alabama Humanities Foundation, "and about the Southerners' response to it, is that it remained primarily agricultural well into the twentieth century, long after the rest of the nation had become urbanized. This has kept much of the South poor
(20) economically, though not poor in spirit. Memories of defeat in the Civil War and of poverty during the Reconstruction and Depression eras have sometimes figured predominantly in the Southern consciousness. Consequently, Southerners have had mixed feelings about the
(25) land rather than purely idealized reactions, with pastoral myths often giving way to hard reality."

To help Alabamians examine their traditional relation to the land, Stewart directed the development of "In View of Home: Twentieth-Century Visions of the
(30) Alabama Landscape," a public program that combines a traveling photography exhibition with a seven-week series of reading and discussion programs, continuing through May at eight public libraries across the state . . . The program introduces participants to some of the ma-
(35) jor works of twentieth-century Southern literature and to a renewed sense of their roots in the land and its continuing vitality.

In selected readings, Stewart worked with Kieran Quinlan, an assistant professor of English at the Uni-
(40) versity of Alabama at Birmingham. Southern literature, Quinlan says, is a particularly effective tool for grappling with a sense of regional identity: "Southern literature came into its own after the First World War, when Southern writers stopped blaming the Northeast
(45) for the South's problems and instead turned a critical eye on themselves."

What these writers found in the South, however, makes today's Southerner uncomfortable. "There is a tendency to deny what Faulkner or Agee found to be
(50) quintessentially Southern," Quinlan says. "The progressive South is uncomfortable with its rural heritage. Our program is an attempt to look squarely at its complicated past."

Participants are learning that Southern writers do
(55) not present a uniform view of "home." Among the works being read is William Faulkner's *The Bear* (1942), which depicts a mythic landscape and treats the theme of humanity's withdrawal from civilization. Jean Toomer's *Cane* (1923) portrays the spiritual land-
(60) scape and the folk rhythms of black life in rural Georgia. And the Agrarians, represented by John Crowe Ransom's essay "Reconstructed but Unregenerate" (1930) and Andrew Lytle's short story "Jericho, Jericho, Jericho" (1984), who present the rural South as
(65) the philosophic preserve of the Jeffersonian values that first formed this nation.

"With Walker Percy's *The Last Gentleman* (1966) and Mary Ward Brown's *Tongues of Flame* (1986), Southern literature reaches the point at which it ceases
(70) to be distinctively Southern and becomes broadly American," says Quinlan.

As chronicled in the works of these and other contemporary Southern writers, the South is moving inexorably into the urban, industrial mainstream. With
(75) fewer people living close to the land, the experiences that in many ways made Southerners "Southern" are becoming alien. "This program enables participants to think about some crucial cultural issues now that the great majority of Alabamians are living in urban ar-
(80) eas," says Stewart. "As we move farther from the land of our parents and grandparents, we need to reflect on their special relationship with the land, whether we will have it today, and what will become of it as we move into the 1990s."

(85) "In View of Home" is part of Alabama Reunion, a year-long, state-wide celebration.

37. According to the article, which of the following is true?

   A. The South became industrial before the North.

   B. The South has never become industrialized.

   C. The South remained agricultural long after the North had become largely urban.

   D. The South is still predominately agricultural while the rest of the country is predominately urban.

38. The article states that Southern writing has slowly evolved since World War-I from a tendency to criticize the North for the South's problems to a self-assessment of the South's virtues and faults. The implication is that contemporary Southern writers:

    A. are no longer concerned with the South's regional identity and urge moving away from Southern literary tradition.
    B. acknowledge the South's rural literary past as their writings become more mainstream.
    C. have disavowed their regional heritage in a gradual effort to become more "American."
    D. have become prolific in writings that renew their literary ties to a nostalgic and romantic view of the past.

39. According to the author, which two books mark the point at which Southern literature stops being regional and becomes broadly national?

    A. *Cane* and *The Bear*
    B. *Their Eyes Were Watching God* and *Mules and Men*
    C. *Tobacco Road* and *God's Little Acre*
    D. *The Last Gentleman* and *Tongues of Flame*

40. The author suggests that today's progressive South:

    A. is uncomfortable with the process of urbanization that has taken place during this century.
    B. is uncomfortable with its rural past.
    C. would prefer to forget its history of slavery and segregation.
    D. feels that remembering past literary history is important to understanding the present.

41. Based on the article, it would be reasonable to assume that the author believes that what made Southerners quintessentially Southerners was:

    I. the segregation of black and white society.
    II. the South's antagonism to the North.
    III. the predominately rural culture that dominated through the early part of the twentieth century.

A. I only
B. III only
C. I and II only
D. II and III only

42. As shown through "In View of Home," Southern writers offered a:

    A. romantic view of an antebellum aristocratic society that dominated the region.
    B. picture of a homespun, frolicking, spirited rural society.
    C. variety of images of the South that reflected its wide diversity.
    D. view of a society still tormented by its historical support of slavery.

43. According to the article, the work of contemporary Southern writers is a reflection of the South's:

    A. moving into the urban, industrial mainstream.
    B. moving further into the nationalistic mainstream of literature.
    C. re-evaluating its rural beginnings.
    D. losing its vital, regional character.

44. Based on what the author stated, which of the following is most likely to occur?

    A. Southern literature will remain distinctive from Northern literature.
    B. In the future there will be no distinctive Southern literature and Southern writers will be largely indistinguishable from Northern writers.
    C. In the future, the basic difference in writing styles will be between rural and urban writers rather than between Southern and Northern writers.
    D. While there has been much talk about the historic difference between Southern writers and Northern writers, realistically there has been very little difference.

Passage VII (Questions 45–51)

Since 1977, Richard D. Brown, a professor of history at the University of Connecticut, has been reading through diaries from the various social strata. Most of these diaries have been used by historians only to gauge reac-
(5) tions to a specific event—how the scholar-clergyman William Bentley felt about Shays' Rebellion, for example—and few have been studied closely. Brown's perspective is much wider. Among the eleven chapters from his work, *The Diffusion of Information in Early America,*
(10) *1700-1865,* there are discussions of declining isolation among Yankee farmers, the development of the legal profession as seen through the careers of John Adams and Robert Treat Paine, and the flow of information among merchants and mariners in port cities.

(15) Diaries are the best sources of this type of inquiry, according to Brown, because they enable one "to see a person whole, to see how print and oral communication fit together in a person's life, to determine which is more important and exactly how both are
(20) used." Up to this point, scholars of journalism have written the history of communications, and they have tended to focus on particular forms, such as how newspapers developed from a primitive state to the present.

Brown finds long diaries like that kept by Boston
(25) judge Samuel Sewall from 1685 until 1729 especially valuable because they provide a constant against which changing mores can be examined over time. "For the first part of Sewall's diary," Brown says, "there are no newspapers in America. When the first newspaper is
(30) published, he gets one. So you can trace the effect of newspapers in Sewall's life over the next twenty-five years, and you see that they didn't make a whole lot of difference for him. People in Sewall's time did not read newspapers for news. Word of mouth was much faster.
(35) What newspapers did provide was the text of official documents, such as laws or treaties, and the speeches of high officials."

Because keeping a diary was a good deal more common during the eighteenth and nineteenth centu-
(40) ries than at present, Brown had to choose from the multitude available in university libraries and historical societies. The vast majority, being of the line-a-day or weather-report variety, were clearly of little interest. He also avoided the atypical experiences found in battle
(45) or travel diaries and screened out the many diaries concerned chiefly with the writer's spiritual health, concentrating instead on those that offer a reasonably full record of the author's experiences over at least a year. In particular, Brown sought out generic types—ordi-
(50) nary folks, such as farmers, merchants, women, artisans—rather than notables. There were, however, a few major figures—Sewall, Bentley, John Adams, William Byrd II—whose diaries, while frequently studied, were

so revealing about patterns of social intercourse that
(55) they could not be ignored.

Based on a full reading of these diaries, about eighty altogether, Brown has revised some of his preconceptions about the movement of information. "Initially, I thought I would see successive stages in an in-
(60) formation revolution over the period," he recalls. "During much of the eighteenth century, information was a scarce commodity, and its dispersal was hierarchical: a community's leaders controlled important communications and diffused them by word of mouth to other
(65) people. Then, with the Revolution and the explosion of printing in the 1780s and 1790s, came a much more egalitarian flow of information.

"Instead of this rather simple model of one system being supplanted by another, however, I found a
(70) picture of overlap and layering. Things were different in the 1800s not because the old face-to-face ways had been erased but because new developments had multiplied ways of diffusing information. The radical difference between the America of 1700 and 1850 was
(75) the extraordinary abundance of information. People gradually became selectors of information according to their individual temperament, their occupation, their social class. For example, a New England farmer thought that it was far more important to be informed
(80) about the land in his area than about the Constitution. In these farmers' diaries, one can see a tremendous information network that had little to do with print. Every time they left the farm they spoke with all sorts of people about local matters—the marriage market for
(85) their daughters, births and deaths, the availability of land. In short, people acquire the information pertinent to their lives.

"By the nineteenth century a dramatic change had occurred," Brown says. "The ideology of the Revolu-
(90) tion required that the people—that is, all sorts of people, who run the nation in a democracy—be well-informed. It was the beginning of the idea that we should worry if a high percentage of people don't know who their senator is. This notion had many implications: it led to the
(95) public-school movement, the founding of academies, the rise of the lecture circuit, all aimed at upgrading the knowledge of the average citizen."

45. Diaries are a good source for gaining a better understanding of how people lived in the early eighteenth century because:

    A. they are the only written record that remains from that period.

    B. diaries were widely written during this period of time and often captured the day-to-day experiences of the average person.

C. diaries were written by those who were on the bottom of society and books and newspapers were written by those who were on the top.
D. all the decision makers of the period kept diaries, and by reading these diaries we can learn how the important decisions were made.

46. On the basis of the fact that the number of newspapers in America increased dramatically between 1700 and the middle of the eighteenth century, we can reasonably assume all BUT one of the following:

A. more people in America could read in 1850 than in 1700.
B. newspapers became an increasingly important source of information during this period.
C. the quality of writing in newspapers improved during the period in discussion.
D. one of the results of the American Revolution was to encourage people to be better informed; one way to be better informed was to read the newspaper.

47. All but which one of the following are mentioned as means by which Americans selected their own information by the mid-nineteenth century?

A. Individual temperament
B. Occupation
C. Social class
D. Geographical location

48. Although Richard Brown usually read diaries of little-known people, he did study the diaries of a few major figures, including:

A. Alexander Hamilton and Benjamin Franklin.
B. John Adams and Samuel Sewall.
C. Patrick Henry and Thomas Jefferson.
D. George Washington and Henry Clay.

49. In the early 1700s in what is today the United States, people read newspapers to:

A. better understand the views of others.
B. get the official text of treaties and speeches.
C. read the political satire of the time.
D. follow literary events.

50. The idea that the people need to be well informed developed during the:

A. eighteenth century as newspapers became more widely available.
B. eighteenth century because new technologies made information more available.
C. early nineteenth century because of an expanded need for leadership in the United States.
D. early nineteenth century as a product of the American Revolution.

51. According to the article, the primary method of obtaining information in the eighteenth century was:

I.   word of mouth.
II. newspapers.
III. town meetings.

A. I only
B. II only
C. I and II only
D. II and III only

Passage VIII (Questions 52–58)

In order to understand and deal with the acid rain problem, programs that examine possible control measures and increase scientific knowledge have been developed and are being carried out cooperatively by the
(5) United States and Canada.

Initially, sulphur and sulphuric compounds were selected for study because they were known to be capable of causing damage over large areas of eastern North America and because of the prospect for sub-
(10) stantial increases in the atmospheric sulphur load in connection with the United States' plans to increase the use of coal. Scientists in both the United States and Canada are also examining other major pollutants, such as the oxides of nitrogen, heavy metals, hydrocarbons,
(15) and fine particles. Similar studies are being made in Scandinavia.

Results of these early studies enabled the two countries to recognize and clarify the time-sensitive nature and the ultimate irreversibility of the impact of acid rain. A
(20) national program was recently modified to meet two clearly stated objectives, one aimed at short-term efforts and the other at long-term efforts. Elements of this program include emission inventories, the systematic study of precipitation, and the study of the progressive deterio-
(25) ration of the watersheds and fish population.

Long-range transport of air pollution represents a serious environmental problem for Canada. While much scientific work still needs to be carried out, some action must be taken as soon as possible. Such action (30) not only should prevent further increases in emissions but should reduce emissions from their current levels. Action by Canada alone will be insufficient in view of the continental dimension of the problem and the climatic behavior that favors transport of United States' (35) pollutants over Canada.

In recognition of the importance of the task at hand, Canada looks forward to close cooperation with the United States, particularly through the development of a bilateral agreement.

52. According to the article, a planned United States increase in its burning of coal will increase the atmospheric load of:

   A. hydrocarbons.
   B. sulphuric compounds.
   C. fine particles.
   D. sulphur.

53. The article emphasizes the ability of the United States and Canada to work cooperatively on the acid rain program. Which of the following offers the BEST assessment of the advantage of such cooperation?

   A. Neighboring countries can develop and implement mutually beneficial programs that increase understanding and control of environmental problems.
   B. Neighboring countries can reinforce close working relations based on governmental research.
   C. Neighboring countries working together increase and strengthen their nationalistic programs on environmental issues.
   D. Neighboring countries have no choice but to work together to confront mutual environmental concerns.

54. The first compounds that were selected for study were:

   A. sulphur and sulphuric compounds.
   B. ozone and hydrocarbons.
   C. sulphur and hydrochloric acid.
   D. sulphuric compounds and oxides of nitrogen.

55. The article points out that climatic conditions result in transport of pollutants from:

   A. Canada to the United States.
   B. the United States to Canada.
   C. the United States to Sweden.
   D. east to west across the United States.

56. The article states that the damage done by acid rain to ponds and forests is:

   A. irreversible.
   B. reversible over a short period of time.
   C. reversible with bilateral action.
   D. reversible over a long period of time.

57. The article implies that a forceful, aggressive program to resolve problems with acid rain must be undertaken:

   I. with close cooperation between the United States and Canada.
   II. with the United States always taking the initiative.
   III. among governments of the world despite its great cost.

   A. I only
   B. II only
   C. I and II only
   D. I and III only

58. The writer of the article suggests that while more research must be done, the two actions that must be taken are:

   A. a ban on the burning of coal and an increase in the budget for research.
   B. a bilateral action by the United States and Canada to freeze emissions at their current level and to work to reduce those emissions in the future.
   C. a multinational agreement between Sweden, the United States and Canada to freeze emissions at their current level and then to reduce them.
   D. a unilateral commitment to studying watersheds and fish population.

Passage IX (Questions 59–65)

In 1855, when the population of the United States was about one-ninth what it is today, and when nineteen states had yet to join the Union, Thomas Bulfinch's *The Age of Fable; or, Stories of Gods and Heroes* be-
(5) gan its long and influential life. Americans may confuse the author with his architect father, Charles Bulfinch; nevertheless, in the American mind, the name of Bulfinch is indelibly associated with classical mythology.

(10) Without a doubt, *The Age of Fable* formed the image that millions of Americans had of the classical gods and heroes. . . The mythology learned by Americans was Bulfinch's mythology. . . Bulfinch did not . . . simply adapt the myths for contemporary readers . . .
(15) he wrote to instruct by making the material entertaining. "Thus we hope to teach mythology," he explains in his preface, "not as a study, but as a relaxation from study; to give our work the charm of a story-book, yet by means of it to impart a knowledge of an important
(20) branch of education." Bulfinch recreated dozens of myths, discussed their use in modern poetry, and wrote for both adults and young people.

The Age of Fable consists of prose narratives of classical myths, chiefly from Ovid (as well as some sto-
(25) ries from Norse, Oriental, and Egyptian mythologies); information about ancient classical writers and artists; and lists for reference. Intertwined with Bulfinch's narrative are myth-related quotations from poetry, chiefly British. The subject of the book, he emphasizes in his
(30) preface, is not just mythology, but "mythology as connected with literature."

Bulfinch's strong background in classical literature, especially Roman, accounts for his success in adapting Ovid for American readers. Although he in-
(35) cluded material from other ancient authors, notably Homer and Virgil, the majority of the myths in *The Age of Fable* are his own translations from the *Metamorphoses,* the chief source for classical myth in Western literature and art. Bulfinch abridged, bowdlerized,
(40) and rearranged Ovid, and at times he added a tidbit or two from other sources. Yet, his translations of the ancient author's powerfully wrought details of physical description and human behavior convey Ovidian sprightliness and charm.

(45) Having retold Ovid's story, Bulfinch notes in passing that it is an allegory for the seasons, and he then shifts into "poetical citations," as he calls them in his preface, which illustrate the use of the myth of Proserpine by modern poets. Annotating as he quotes,
(50) he cites short passages from Milton (whom he quotes forty times in *The Age of Fable*); Thomas Hood; Coleridge; and, in two separate passages, one of his favorites, the Irish poet Thomas Moore.

Bulfinch drew his 188 "citations" from the work
(55) of forty poets. All were British except for three— Longfellow, Lowell, and Stephen Greenleaf Bulfinch, brother of the author. The shining lights of English literature—Milton, Coleridge, Spenser, Shakespeare, Dryden, Pope, Swift, Wordsworth, Keats, Shelley, and
(60) Tennyson—dominate. Also included, however, are some of the minor poets popular in Bulfinch's time, for example, Erasmus Darwin, Charles Darwin's uncle.

In using poetry as a counterpoint in *The Age of Fable,* Bulfinch was tapping into an interest of the gen-
(65) eral educated public. His criterion for choosing selections, he explains in his preface, was popularity; these are passages which "are most frequently quoted or alluded to in reading or conversation." Many of the poets who appear in *The Age of Fable* are represented in
(70) William Holmes McGuffey's *Eclectic Readers* and also in the "gift books." A phenomenon of Bulfinch's era, those literary annuals containing poetry, stories, and moral maxims were great favorites with middle-class Americans and helped create, in that level of society, a
(75) demand for literature and art.

What led Bulfinch . . . to put together the combination of ancient myth and modern poetry that is *The Age of Fable*? . . . Unquestionably, he was following the altruistic example of his architect father and hop-
(80) ing to serve an American public confronted by enormous societal change. He was responding, in particular, to the rise of science and technology, a decline in classical learning and increasing educational opportunities . . . For the purpose of educating his fellow citi-
(85) zens, Bulfinch directed his book to . . . out-of-school audiences. He imagined *The Age of Fable* not in a classroom, but in the "parlor." His audience was not to be schoolchildren, but "the reader of English literature, of either sex," others "more advanced" who may require
(90) mythological knowledge when they visit museums or "mingle in cultivated society," and also, readers "in advanced life."

The presence of *The Age of Fable* . . . across America for well over a hundred years has assured for
(95) Bulfinch a place as progenitor of the strong American fascination with classical mythology in art and literature. . . . What Bulfinch proves is that in America the poetry and story of our common classical past are not for the few, but for the many.

59. The popularity of *The Age of Fable* during the latter part of the nineteenth century can be interpreted as being due to all BUT one of the following reasons:

    A. the public's acceptance of the combination of classical mythology and modern poetry as devised by Bulfinch.
    B. the growth of an educated public and its interest in and use of references from the book in everyday speech and reading material.
    C. the appeal of the book to an increasingly sophisticated adult audience.
    D. a reflection of the waning influence of classical learning due to the Industrial Revolution.

60. Which of the following was **NOT** one of Bulfinch's intents in writing *The Age of Fable*?

    A. To provide didactic entertainment
    B. To generate interest in translations of a classical work
    C. To reach an audience of adults and young people
    D. To educate schoolchildren in particular

61. One can infer from the article that the predominance of the poets cited by Bulfinch indicates:

    I. a strongly American influence.
    II. a heavily British influence.
    III. a distinctly European influence.

    A. I only
    B. II only
    C. III only
    D. II and III only

62. The widespread appeal of Bulfinch's rewriting of ancient mythology during the nineteenth century does **NOT** reflect which one of the following?

    A. A fairly well-read and well-educated middle class of Americans
    B. A demand for writings reflecting a tradition in classical works

    C. A strong feeling among Americans of the necessity to revamp the educational system
    D. A trend among most Americans to quote or read passages for conversation

63. Using classical literature as his basis, Bulfinch was demonstrating the nineteenth century's educational tendency to:

    A. borrow from the past to explain the present.
    B. look upon a foundation in the classics as a reflection of a proper education.
    C. inculcate a teaching method accessible to the affluent.
    D. generate learning through memorization of ancient works.

64. The author suggests that the enduring popularity of *The Age of Fable* **CANNOT** be attributed to which one of the following?

    A. American interest in and attraction to classical literature
    B. An interplay of interesting narrative stories and poetry
    C. Bulfinch's ability to interpret and translate classical work with skill and intelligence
    D. The inclusion of well-known British writers

65. One can infer from the article that the author believes Bulfinch's legacy to the American public is a work that:

    A. successfully introduced classical mythology interspersed with literature.
    B. was dedicated to preserving a segment of classical mythology in order to educate the American people.
    C. reflected the importance of both classical mythology and mid-nineteenth century British writers.
    D. successfully preserved classical mythology while instructing the educated.

END OF TEST 1.

**IF YOU FINISH BEFORE THE TIME IS UP, YOU MAY
CHECK YOUR WORK ON THIS TEST ONLY.**

PHYSICAL SCIENCES

Time: 100 Minutes
Questions 66–142

Directions: This test contains 77 questions. Most of the questions consist of a descriptive passage followed by a group of questions related to the passage. For these questions, study the passage carefully and then choose the best answer to each question in the group. Some questions in this test stand alone. These questions are independent of any passage and independent of each other. For these questions, too, you must select the one best answer. Indicate all your answers by blackening the corresponding circles on your answer sheet.

A periodic table is provided at the beginning of this book. You may consult it whenever you wish.

Passage I (Questions 66–75)

By tabulating standard thermodynamic functions, we gain the ability to calculate thermodynamic properties for a broad range of reactions. We can calculate not only the basic state functions, but also related quantities such as the equilibrium constant.

The table below lists various thermodynamic properties—standard enthalpies and free energies of formation, absolute entropies, and standard heat capacities—for a range of hydrocarbons and oxygen-containing compounds. All compounds are in the gaseous state at 25° C unless otherwise noted.

Compound	ΔH_f° (kJ/mol)	ΔG_f° (kJ/mol)	S° (J/mol K)	C_p° (J/mol K)
C (gas)	715	67.1	158	20.9
C (graphite)	0	0	57.3	8.4
CO	−110	−137	197	29.2
CO_2	−394	−395	214	37.2
CH_4	−749	−50.6	186	35.1
C_2H_6	−84.5	−32.9	229	52.7
C_2H_4	51.9	68.1	220	43.5
C_3H_8	−103.8	−23	270	73.6
C_6H_6	82.9	130	269	81.6
CH_3OH	−201	162	240	43.9
CH_3Cl	−808	−57.3	234	40.6
CH_2Cl_2	−92.5	−66.1	270	51.0
$CHCl_3$	−103	−70.2	295	65.6
HCHO	−116	−113	219	35.6
H_2	0	0	131	28.9
H_2O	−242	−228	189	33.5
O_2	0	0	205	29.3
O_3	143	163	239	39.3

66. Under standard conditions, how many of the substances listed in the table can be formed spontaneously from their constituent elements?

    A. 6
    B. 9
    C. 10
    D. 11

67. Using the values in the table, what is $\Delta S°$ (in J/mol K) for the following reaction?

    $$2H_2(g) + O_2(g) \rightarrow 2H_2O(g)$$

    A. −89
    B. −147
    C. −484
    D. −456

68. Sufficient heat is aded to a 10-gram sample of gaseous carbon atoms to raise the temperature by 10 K. If the same amount of heat was added to a 10-gram sample of graphite, what would be the value of the temperature increase?

    A. 2K
    B. 4K
    C. 10K
    D. 25K

69. For the data shown in the table, the molar heat capacities of saturated hydrocarbons:

    A. decrease with increasing chain length.
    B. increase with increasing chain length.
    C. do not show a consistent trend.
    D. remain constant with increasing chain length.

70. The value of $\Delta H_f°$ for C_2H_2 (not shown in the table) is considerably higher than that for C_2H_4. The heat capacities for the two compounds are very similar. Therefore, which of the following is (are) likely to be true?

    I. The energy of a double bond differs substantially from that of a triple bond.
    II. If 1.0 J of heat is added to a mixture containing equal moles of each compound, the C_2H_2 will absorb considerably more heat than the C_2H_4.
    III. When each compound is decomposed into its elements at their standard states, more energy is released by C_2H_2.

A. I only
B. II only
C. III only
D. I and III only

71. Among the halogenated hydrocarbons shown in the table, which of the following increases as the number of chlorines increases?

    A. $\Delta H°$ only
    B. $\Delta H°$ and $\Delta G°$ only
    C. $S°$ and $C_p°$ only
    D. All four thermodynamic functions shown

72. What is the change in free energy (in kJ) when 2.000 moles of C_6H_6 are oxidized to CO_2 and H_2O?

    A. −1375
    B. −1442
    C. 2750
    D. −2880

73. The difference in the values of the thermodynamic functions between gas-phase carbon and graphite can be explained by which of the following?

    I. The enthalpy of formation of graphite is lower than that of gas-phase carbon, owing to covalent bonding in the graphite.
    II. The free motion and greater molar volume of the gaseous atoms are reflected in a greater value of the entropy for the gas.
    III. The greater molar volume of the gas leads to a greater ΔG than in graphite.

    A. I only
    B. II only
    C. III only
    D. I and II only

74. Which of the following graphs best illustrates the formation of CH_4 from its elements?

(A)

(B)

(C)

(D)

75. Which of the following expressions can be used to calculate the equilibrium constant for the following reaction?

$$CO(g) + 1/2\ O_2(g) \rightarrow CO_2(g)$$

A. $\ln K = -258/RT$
B. $\ln K = 258/RT$
C. $\ln K = 284/RT$
D. $K = 258/RT$

Passage II (Questions 76–82)

The kinetic theory predicts that gas molecules will move in all directions at a range of speeds. The average kinetic energy of the molecules is $\frac{3}{2}RT$ per mole, where R (the gas constant) = 8.31 J/mol K. Since the kinetic energy is related to speed, we can show that for an ideal gas, the root-mean-square speed (a quantity that is usually very close to the average speed) is given by

$$(3RT/M)^{1/2}$$

where M is the molar mass in g/mol.

In the following graph, the curves show the fraction of molecules having a given speed, for the temperatures of 300K and 600K.

76. Which of the following expresses the ratio of average speeds of a molecule of O_2 to a molecule of H_2 when both are at the same temperature?

A. 1/16
B. 16
C. 1/4
D. 4

77. If the temperature of a mole of gaseous O_2 is raised from 100°C to 200°C, the average speed of the molecules is:

A. lowered by the factor 100/200.
B. raised by the factor 200/100.
C. raised by the factor 473/373.
D. raised by the factor $(473/373)^{1/2}$.

78. Based on the graph, the most probable speed at 600K is closest to which of the following?

   A. 0 m/s
   B. 0.075 m/s
   C. 1,600 m/s
   D. 2,300 m/s

79. Based on the graph, for 600K, what is the approximate fraction of molecules having speeds greater than 1,600 m/s?

   A. 0.10
   B. 0.25
   C. 0.50
   D. 0.75

80. Based on the graph, the curve for 1,200K is most likely to peak at which of the following?

   A. 165 m/s
   B. 1,000 m/s
   C. 1,600 m/s
   D. 3,200 m/s

81. The fact that there are no negative speeds on the graph reflects:

   A. the experimenter's failure to measure negative speeds.
   B. the fact that speed is the magnitude of velocity.
   C. the fact that all molecules in a diatomic gas travel in a positive direction.
   D. the fact that kinetic energy must always be positive or zero.

82. Which of the following may be inferred from the speed distributions shown on the graph?

   I. At higher temperatures, the average speed is higher.
   II. At lower temperatures, the speed distribution is more widely distributed.
   III. The average speed is proportional to the absolute temperature.

   A. I only
   B. II only
   C. III only
   D. I and II only

Passage III (Questions 83-91)

The following graph shows a titration of 100 mL of an unknown weak acid of undetermined concentration with 0.20 M NaOH.

A student is told that the unknown acid is one of those listed in the following table.

Acid	K_a	pK_a
hydrogen sulfate	1.2×10^{-2}	1.92
formic	1.8×10^{-4}	3.74
acetic	1.8×10^{-5}	4.74
dihydrogen phosphate	6.2×10^{-8}	7.21

83. Which of the following is the number of moles of NaOH added at the endpoint of the titration shown in the graph?

   A. 0.0050
   B. 0.010
   C. 0.10
   D. 1.0

84. The data in the graph indicate that the concentration of the unknown acid is which of the following?

   A. 0.010
   B. 0.050
   C. 0.10
   D. 0.40

85. In the titration shown in the graph, as the volume of NaOH added is changed from 8 to 30 mL, the change in $[H^+]$ is approximately:

    A. an increase of about 30 percent.
    B. a decrease of about 30 percent.
    C. an increase of about a factor of 10.
    D. a decrease of about a factor of 10.

86. Based on the graph, the ratio $\Delta V_{OH^-} / \Delta pH$ is smallest when ΔV_{OH^-} equals:

    A. 0 mL.
    B. 5 mL.
    C. 25 mL.
    D. 50 mL.

87. Based on the information given, what is the pH when $\Delta V_{OH^-} = 100$ mL?

    A. 12
    B. 13
    C. 14
    D. Cannot be determined

88. Based on the data in the table and the titration curve shown in the graph, which of the following is the unknown acid?

    A. Hydrogen sulfate
    B. Formic acid
    C. Acetic acid
    D. Dihydrogen phosphate

89. A second sample of the unknown acid is titrated with NaOH of the same concentration, and the endpoint is found to occur at 60 mL. The solution is then titrated with 30 mL of 0.20 M HCl. The resulting pH is closest to which of the following?

    A. 3
    B. 4
    C. 5
    D. 7

90. At the 40-mL point on the graph, the solution most closely resembles which of the following mixtures (where "conjugate acid/base" refers to the unknown acid)?

    A. 4 parts strong base to 1 part strong acid
    B. 4 parts conjugate base to 1 part conjugate acid
    C. 1 part conjugate base to 4 parts conjugate acid
    D. 1 part conjugate base to 5 parts conjugate acid

91. The student wishes to choose an indicator to signal the equivalence point of the titration. Indicators that change color at pH 7.5 or 8.5 are available. Which should she choose?

    A. 7.5 only
    B. 8.5 only
    C. Either 7.5 or 8.5
    D. Neither would be accurate

Passage IV (Questions 92–96)

An investigator studies several properties related to silver and chlorine and to their salt, AgCl:

Experiment 1. The investigator determines the first ionization energy, ΔH_{IE}, of gas-phase Ag:

$$Ag(g) \rightarrow Ag^+ + e- \qquad \Delta H_{IE} = 728 \text{ kJ/mol}$$

Experiment 2. The investigator determines the heat of sublimation of solid silver:

$$Ag(s) \rightarrow Ag(g) \qquad \Delta H_{subl} = 286 \text{ kJ/mol}$$

Experiment 3. Next, the investigator determines the dissociation energy of diatomic chlorine, Cl_2:

$$Cl_2(g) \rightarrow 2Cl(g) \qquad \Delta H_{diss} = 239 \text{ kJ/mol}$$

Experiment 4. The investigator finds the solubility product of solid AgCl in water:

$$AgCl(s) = Ag^+ (aq) + Cl^+(aq) \qquad K_{sp} = 1.8 \times 10^{-10}$$

Experiment 5. Finally, the investigator measures the value of the heat of formation of AgCl:

$$Ag(s) + \tfrac{1}{2} Cl_2 \rightarrow AgCl(s) \ \Delta H_f = -128 \text{ kJ}$$

92. Of the reactions for which ΔH is given, how many can be said with certainty to proceed spontaneously?

    A. 1
    B. 2
    C. 3
    D. Cannot say without further information.

93. Find the energy taken in or given off when 20 moles of gaseous chlorine *atoms* are converted to gaseous Cl_2 molecules.

    A. 2390 kJ given off
    B. 2390 kJ taken in
    C. 4780 kJ given off
    D. 4730 kJ taken in

94. Use the data given to calculate the concentration of silver ion, $[Ag^+ (aq)]$, expected in pure water.

    A. $1.8 \times 10^{-10}M$
    B. $1.3 \times 10^{-10}M$
    C. $1.3 \times 10^{-5}M$
    D. 728 kJ

95. Using the results of the experiments, what en-

ergy would be necessary to produce 0.10 mol of gas-phase silver ion (Ag^+) from metallic silver?

    A. 28.6 kJ
    B. 72.8 kJ
    C. 101.4 kJ
    D. 1014 kJ

96. Find the heat added or given off when 0.5 mol AgCl(s) is converted to gaseous Ag atoms and gaseous Cl atoms.

    A. 139 kJ added
    B. 267 kJ added
    C. 278 kJ given off
    D. 534 kJ added

Passage V (Questions 97–101)

A "phase diagram" is used by chemists to display graphically the different solid, liquid, and gas phases—as well as mixtures of these—that exist in a pure compound or combination of compounds. Depending on the situation, the diagram may show the variation of phases with temperature, pressure, percentage of one component of a mixture, or other variables.

Figure 1 shows a temperature-pressure phase diagram for Substance 1, a pure compound. Figure 2 is a similar diagram for Substance 2. Figure 3 shows the temperature behavior of the phases in a mixture of aluminum which contains a small, variable amount of silicon. Note that this diagram refers to two different solids, labeled "solid 1" and "solid 2." Each of these solids contains a mixture of aluminum and silicon, but they differ in percent composition and in crystal structure.

FIG02

FIG03

97. In Figure 1, which point corresponds to a pressure and temperature at which sublimation is taking place?

A. Point A
B. Point B
C. Point C
D. Point D

98. Consider Figures 1 and 2. Which would best describe water, given that water has the unusual property of expanding as it freezes?

A. Fig. 1, owing to the slope of boundary between solid and liquid.
B. Fig. 1, owing to the slope of boundary between gas and liquid.
C. Fig. 2, owing to the slope of boundary between solid and liquid.
D. Fig. 2, owing to the slope of boundary between solid and gas.

99. Figure 3 displays the phases that result when small amounts of silicon are added to aluminum at different temperatures. One property of these substances that helps to determine the shape of the diagram is the atomic radius. Which of the following best predicts the relationship of the radii of aluminum and silicon?

A. The radius of aluminum is larger since as one moves to the right on the periodic table, there is an increase in nuclear charge which tends to pull the outer electrons more closely toward the nucleus.
B. The radius of silicon is larger since as one moves to the right on the periodic table, there is a decrease in nuclear charge which tends to pull the outer electrons more closely toward the nucleus.
C. The radius of aluminum is larger since as one moves to the right on the periodic table, electrons are added to a new shell, one which puts them farther from the nucleus.
D. The radius of silicon is larger since as one moves to the right on the periodic table, electrons are added to a new shell, one which puts them farther from the nucleus.

100. Referring to Figure 3, determine the phase that will exist in a mixture of aluminum and 1.00% silicon at 550°C.

A. Liquid only
B. Liquid plus solid 1
C. Liquid plus solid 2
D. Solid 1 only

101. Which of the following statements may be inferred from the diagram?

According to the diagram, as the percentage of silicon increases:

 I. The minimum temperature needed for the existence of any solid decreases.
 II. The maximum temperature at which solid 2 appears increases sharply, then levels out.
 III. The minimum temperature at which liquid is found decreases at a roughly constant rate.

A. I only
B. II only
C. III only
D. I and II only

Passage V (Questions 102–108)

The state function entropy measures the increase (or decrease) in "disorder" of a system when it undergoes a change, such as a chemical reaction. Generally, reactions such as gas-phase dissociations proceed with a positive entropy change, since several fragments are created from an initial molecule. (Dissociations in a solvent are not easy to predict, however, as you will see as you work some examples.)

Is a positive entropy change enough to ensure that a reaction will proceed? No. Entropy enters into one of the terms in the expression for the free energy, which determines spontaneity.

The table below shows the entropy changes associated with a number of reactions.

Reaction	ΔS°_{298} (J/mol K)
1. $Cu(s) \rightarrow Cu(g)$	133
2. $H_2(g) \rightarrow 2H(g)$	98.6
3. $NaCl(s) \rightarrow Na^+(aq) + Cl^-(aq)$	43
4. $H_2O(g) \rightarrow H_2O(l)$	−119
5. $HCl(g) \rightarrow H^+(aq) + Cl^-(aq)$	−131
6. $C(diamond) \rightarrow (graphite)$	3.3
7. $MgCl_2(s) \rightarrow Mg^{2+}(aq) + 2Cl^-(aq)$	−97.1
8. $LiCl(s) \rightarrow Li^+(aq) + Cl^-(aq)$	14

102. How many of the reactions in the table are spontaneous?

A. 0
B. 5
C. 8
D. Cannot be determined

103. An investigator who wishes to test the hypothesis that the entropy change is positive for a reaction that results in more product molecules or ions than reactants would find what pattern in the data?

A. Confirming instances: reactions 1,2,3
 Disconfirming instances: reactions 7.8
B. Confirming instances: reactions 2,3,7,8
 Disconfirming instances: 5
C. Confirming instances: reactions 2,3,8
 Disconfirming instances: reaction 5, 7
D. Confirming instances: reactions 2,3
 Disconfirming instances: reactions 7,8

104. An investigator wishing to predict the direction of entropy change as dry ice (solid CO_2) sublimes to its vapor would get the best prediction from which of the following reactions?

A. 1
B. 3
C. 4
D. 6

105. Given the value of ΔS° for reaction 3 and the high solubility of NaCl in water, it can be said that the enthalpy change of NaCl solution:

A. must be negative.
B. must be positive.
C. must be zero.
D. could be negative, zero, or positive.

106. The ΔS for a phase change equals the enthalpy change for the phase change divided by the Kelvin temperature at the phase change. In order to predict the melting temperature of ice, an investigator would need to know:

A. only data given in the table.
B. the data given, plus the enthalpy of fusion of ice at its boiling point.
C. the data given, plus the enthalpy of fusion of ice at its melting point.
D. both the enthalpy and entropy of fusion of ice at its melting point.

107. In order to explain the difference between the S° values given for the two forms of carbon, an investigator might reasonably suggest which of the following?

I. A mole of diamond consists of fewer particles than a mole of graphite.
II. Diamond is a more stable structure than graphite.
III. The structure of diamond is more orderly than that of graphite.

A. I only
B. II only
C. III only
D. I and III only

108. An investigator wishes to account for the difference in $\Delta S°$ between Reactions 7 and 8. Which of the following would **NOT** help to explain the difference?

I. Entropy changes increase as the number of product molecules increase.
II. When Mg^{2+} is dissolved, its large positive charge causes a more orderly arrangement of water molecules around it than in the case of Na^+.
III. The heat of solution is greater for $MgCl_2$ than for NaCl.

A. I only
B. II only
C. III only
D. I and III only

Passage VI (Questions 109–115)

An experiment is performed to examine the nuclear decay reaction associated with a sample of phosphorous-30 isotope. An initial mass of 32.0 grams of the isotope is placed in a shielded reaction chamber. After 10.0 minutes the chamber is opened. Only 2.0 grams of the parent isotope remain. In addition, a different element is found in the chamber. Further examination shows that the new substance is an isotope of silicon. The reaction occurring probably can be summarized by:

$$^{30}_{15}P \rightarrow \, ^{A}_{Z}Si + \, ^{0}_{+1}X$$

109. What is the half-life of $^{30}_{15}P$?

A. 7.5 min
B. 5.0 min
C. 2.5 min
D. 2.0 min

110. A second particle, $^{0}_{1}X$, is emitted along with silicon in the decay process. What is the most likely identity of this second particle?

A. Electron
B. Positron
C. Neutron
D. α – particle

111. What is the mass number for the silicon isotopes?

A. 30
B. 15
C. 14
D. 16

112. How many neutrons are present in the silicon isotope produced?

A. 29
B. 16
C. 15
D. 14

113. What is the atomic number of the silicon?

A. 30
B. 16
C. 15
D. 14

114. The silicon isotope given above falls:

A. above the belt of stability.
B. below the belt of stability.
C. on the belt of stability.
D. None of the above

115. What is the atomic number of a stable phosphorus nucleus?

A. 30
B. 14
C. 15
D. 29

Passage VII (Questions 116–120)

Miguel is taking a high school physics class. His teacher has told him to design and carry out any simple experiment that will allow him to observe an aspect of physics. Miguel goes home feeling quite perplexed because he can't think of an experiment. While sitting in the kitchen he notices his baby sister trying first to pull and then to push a box across the highly polished kitchen floor. The little girl is trying to give a ride to her stuffed bear, which is sitting in the box. Miguel suddenly "sees" his experiment. He decides to follow his sister's progress across the kitchen floor by plotting the estimated velocity of the box versus time.

In his report, Miguel notes that he is assuming that the kitchen floor is perfectly horizontal and frictionless. When his sister is through playing, Miguel measures the combined mass of the box and stuffed bear and finds that the total is 4.0 kg. The graph of his observed velocity *vs.* time is shown below.

116. What is the best estimate of the distance the box moved during the last two recorded minutes?

   A. 1.0 m
   B. 2.0 m
   C. 3.0 m
   D. 4.0 m

117. Over which of the following time intervals was the kinetic energy of the box greatest?

   A. Minutes 0 to 1
   B. Minutes 2 to 3
   C. Minutes 5 to 6
   D. Minutes 7 to 8

118. What was the net force acting on the box over the interval of 1.5 minutes to 4 minutes?

   A. 0 N
   B. 0.5 N
   C. 2 N
   D. 8 N

119. What was the momentum of the box over the interval of 1.5 minutes to 4 minutes?

   A. 0 kg m/min
   B. 4 kg m/min
   C. 8 kg m/min
   D. 16 kg m/min

120. During which of the following intervals was **NO** work being done on the box?

   A. Minutes 1 to 2
   B. Minutes 2 to 3
   C. Minutes 4 to 5
   D. Minutes 7 to 8

Passage VIII (Questions 121–127)

An instructor in an introductory physics course makes up a set of five simple graphs with unlabeled axes to represent various functions. The graphs are shown below. She then asks her students to answer the following questions.

(A)

(B)

(C)

(D)

(E)

121. If the *x* and *y* axes are volts and amperes, respectively, which graph best represents Ohm's law?

A. A
B. B
C. C
D. D

122. Which graph gives the closest approximation of the relationship between the force of gravity and the radial distance from the center of the Earth?

A. B
B. C
C. D
D. E

123. If the *x* and *y* axes are time and velocity, respectively, which graph describes the behavior of a ball thrown vertically upward?

A. B
B. C
C. D
D. E

124. For Einstein's mass-energy equation $E = mc^2$, which graph provides the best representation of the relationship between energy and mass?

A. A
B. B
C. C
D. D

125. For a body in dynamic equilibrium, which graph gives the expected relationship between velocity and time?

A. A
B. B
C. C
D. D

126. Which graph shows the relationship between pressure and volume of a gas at constant temperature?

A. B
B. E
C. D
D. C

127. Which graph shows the increase in pressure as increasing force pushes water through a hose?

A. A
B. B
C. C
D. E

Questions 128 through 142 are independent of any passage and independent of each other.

128. What is the maximum number of electrons in an atom that can have quantum numbers of $n = 5$ and $l = 2$?

A. 5
B. 8
C. 10
D. 15

129. Which of the following are arranged in decreasing order of expected dipole moment?

A. F_2, Cl_2, Br_2
B. H_2, HBr, HF
C. HF, HBr, H_2
D. K, Na, Li

130. The solubility product for $BaSO_4$ is 1.5×10^{-9}. Which of the following is correct?

I. The solubility of $BaSO_4$ in pure water is greater than the solubility in $0.1\ M$ $Ba(NO_3)_2$.
II. The solubility product of $BaSO_4$ in pure water is greater than the solubility product in $0.1\ M$ $Ba(NO_3)_2$.
III. The reaction of Ba^{2+} with SO_4^{2-} has an equilibrium constant greater than 1.0.

A. I only
B. II only
C. III only
D. I and III only

131. A student finds that $MgCO_3$ is more soluble in HNO_3 than in plain water. Which of the following is a likely explanation for this effect?

A. The NO_3^- ion attaches preferentially to the Mg^{2+}.
B. Mg^{2+} is a strong base and reacts completely with the H^+ from the nitric acid, causing the magnesium salt to dissociate.
C. Carbonate is a weak base and reacts with the H^+ from the strong acid, causing the barium salt to dissociate.
D. The HNO_3 reduces the Mg^{2+} to magnesium metal.

132. For the reaction $E + 2F \rightarrow G$, it is found that doubling the concentration of E quadruples the rate, while doubling the concentration of F has no effect. The rate law is which of the following?

A. rate $= k[E]$
B. rate $= k[E]^2$
C. rate $= k[E]^2[F]$
D. rate $= k[E][F]^2$

133. An electron in a p_z orbital is least likely to be found:

A. in the positive lobe.
B. in the xy plane.
C. in the negative lobe.
D. in the same side of the xy plane as another electron.

134. The pH of a solution of $0.1\ M$ HNO_3 is closest to which of the following?

A. 0.1
B. 1
C. 7
D. 13

135. A gas mixture containing 1 mole of H_2 and 3 moles of N_2 has a total pressure of P atm. Which of the following are the partial pressures of each gas?

A. N_2: 3 atm; $\quad$ H_2: 1 atm
B. N_2: $(2P/3)$ atm; $\quad$ H_2: $(P/3)$ atm
C. N_2: $(P/3)$ atm; $\quad$ H_2: $(2P/3)$ atm
D. N_2: $(3P/4)$ atm; $\quad$ H_2: $(P/4)$ atm

136. Four media are separated from each other by horizontal surfaces. The path of a ray of light passing through the media system is illustrated below. In which medium is the speed of light greatest?

A. I
B. II
C. III
D. IV

137. Ball A is thrown horizontally from the roof of a building. At the same time, ball B, which weighs half as much as ball A, is dropped from the roof. Air resistance is negligible. Since both balls start at the same height and time, which statement is most accurate?

A. A and B will hit the ground simultaneously.
B. Ball A will hit the ground first.
C. Ball B will hit the ground first.
D. There is not enough information to determine which ball will hit the ground first.

138. Which of the following units **CANNOT** be used to represent energy?

A. Joule
B. Kilowatt-hour
C. Kilogram meter per second squared
D. Newton-meter

139. How far can light travel in a vacuum during the same time it takes sound to travel 660 meters in air?

A. 1.0×10^8 m
B. 1.5×10^8 m
C. 3.0×10^8 m
D. 6.0×10^8 m

140. What is the average power output of a 70-kg woman who runs up an incline to a height of 2 meters in 2 seconds?

A. 343 W
B. 686 W
C. 1,372 W
D. 1,715 W

141. Assume that a pole vaulter can convert all of his kinetic energy into potential energy. If a 70.0-kg pole vaulter approaches the vault with a velocity of 9.80 m/s, about how high can he vault?

A. 2.45 m
B. 4.90 m
C. 9.80 m
D. 19.6 m

142. A car drives around a circular track at a constant speed of 20 m/s. If the track is flat and has a radius of 200 m, what is the acceleration of the car?

A. 2.0 m/s^2
B. 10 m/s^2
C. 2.0 m/s^2
D. 0.10 m/s^2

END OF TEST 2.

**IF YOU FINISH BEFORE THE TIME IS UP, YOU MAY
CHECK YOUR WORK ON THIS TEST ONLY.**

WRITING SAMPLE

Time: 60 Minutes
2 Essays

Directions: This test consists of two parts. You will have 30 minutes to complete each part. During the first 30 minutes you may work on Part 1 only. During the second 30 minutes, you may work on Part 2 only. You will have 3 pages for each essay answer, but you do not have to fill all 3 pages. Be sure to write legibly; illegible essays will not be scored.

Part 1

Consider this statement:

Most bad habits are tools to help us through life.

Write a unified essay in which you perform the following tasks. Explain what you think the above statement means. Describe a specific situation in which most bad habits are *not* tools that help individuals through life. Discuss what you think determines whether such habits become useful in assisting individuals through life.

DO NOT START THE NEXT TOPIC UNTIL THE TIME IS UP.

Part 2

Consider this statement:

If you don't learn, you will always find someone else to do it for you.

Write a unified essay in which you perform the following tasks. Explain what you think the above statement means. Describe a specific situation in which one learns on his or her own without relying on another individual to do it. Discuss what you think determines whether learning on one's own enables someone to avoid relying on others.

END OF SECTION 3.

DO NOT RETURN TO PART 1.

BIOLOGICAL SCIENCES

Time: 100 Minutes
Questions 143–219

Directions: This test contains 77 questions. Most of the questions consist of a descriptive passage followed by a group of questions related to the passage. For these questions, study the passage carefully and then choose the best answer to each question in the group. Some questions in this test stand alone. These questions are independent of any passage and independent of each other. For these questions, too, you must select the one best answer. Indicate all your answers by blackening the corresponding circles on your answer sheet.

A periodic table is provided at the beginning of the book. You may consult it whenever you wish.

Passage I (Questions 143–148)

Carbohydrates, fats, and proteins can all be utilized as sources of material for making ATP in cellular respiration. The figure below shows how each of these food molecules can enter the respiratory pathway.

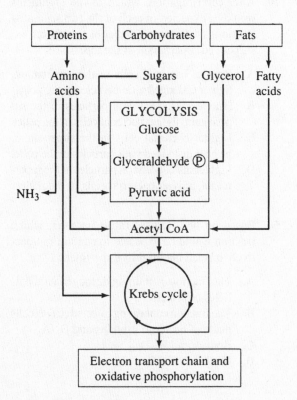

143. Beta oxidation is the process in which fatty acids are converted to a substance that feeds into the respiratory pathway. What is the name of this substance?

   A. Glycerol
   B. Glyceraldehyde phosphate (PGAL)
   C. Acetyl CoA
   D. Glucose

144. One reason fatty acids are an excellent source of fuel is that, gram for gram, they are richer in hydrogens than in glucose. Which of the following is the best estimate of how many ATP molecules a 6-carbon fatty acid would yield if it were completely metabolized in cellular respiration?

   A. Between 2 and 18
   B. Between 18 and 24
   C. Between 24 and 36
   D. More than 36

145. When utilized in cellular respiration, amino acids are deaminated before being metabolized further. After deamination, alanine becomes pyruvic acid, glutamate is converted to alpha-ketoglutarate, and aspartate yields oxaloacetate. Based on information in the figure, alpha-ketoglutarate and oxaloacetate are probably:

A. acetyl CoA.
B. hydrogen acceptors in the electron transport chain.
C. Krebs cycle intermediates.
D. None of the above

146. In the human body, what happens to the ammonia (NH_3) that results from the deamination of amino acids?

A. Most is converted to uric acid before being eliminated in the urine.
B. Most is converted to urea before being eliminated in the urine.
C. Most is converted to creatinine before being eliminated in the urine.
D. Most is eliminated in the urine without further conversion.

147. According to information in the figure, where in the cell does glycerol enter the respiratory pathway?

A. In the cytoplasm
B. Inside the mitochondrial matrix
C. Along the inner mitochondrial membranes (cristae)
D. In the intermembranous space of the mitochondria

148. If the same molecule forms as an intermediate in more than one catabolic pathway, it can often be used in the conversion of one type of substance to another. Therefore, acetyl CoA should enable the body to convert:

A. amino acids to fat.
B. glucose to fat.
C. starch to fat.
D. All of the above

Passage II (Questions 149–154)

A number of historic experiments were designed to identify characteristics of the genetic material. In 1928, Frederick Griffith showed that genetic information could be transferred from dead bacteria (heat-killed) to living bacteria of a different strain. It was not until years later that this genetic material was finally confirmed to be DNA.

Experiments 1 and 2

In 1952, Hershey and Chase examined how the bacteriophage, T2, infects the intestinal bacterium, *E. coli*. They knew that viruses were composed of proteins and DNA, and they used radioactive isotopes of phosphorus and sulfur to label the viral components. After previously labeled phage was mixed in a test tube with bacterial cells long enough to ensure infection, the mixture was agitated in a blender in order to dislodge all viral components that had not entered the bacterial cell. The mixture was then centrifuged at high speed, separating the dislodged viral fraction and bacterial fraction from each other. Two similar experiments were carried out separately. In Experiment 1, only radioactive sulfur was used. In Experiment 2, only radioactive phosphorus was used.

149. After centrifugation, which of the organisms would be expected in each of the two separated fractions (sedimentary pellet at the bottom vs. suspended supernatant at the top)?

A. Heavier bacterial cells in the supernatant, lighter dislodged viral particles in the pellet
B. Heavier dislodged viral particles in the supernatant, lighter bacterial cells in the pellet
C. Lighter bacterial cells in the supernatant, heavier dislodged viral particles in the pellet
D. Lighter dislodged viral particles in the supernatant, heavier bacterial cells in the pellet

150. Based on how viruses infect bacteria, which fraction would be expected to contain radioactively labeled material in Experiment 1?

A. The fraction containing dislodged viral particles of protein
B. The fraction containing infected *E. coli* cells made of bacterial proteins and DNA
C. Both A and B
D. Neither A nor B

151. In Experiment 2, only the fraction containing infected bacterial cells should be labeled. Which of the following best explains this expectation?

A. Viral DNA and proteins were labeled and both are inside the bacteria.

B. Viral and bacterial DNA were labeled and both are inside the bacteria.

C. Only viral DNA was labeled and it is now inside the bacteria.

D. Viral and bacterial proteins were labeled and are both being synthesized by the bacteria.

152. If the infected *E. coli* was returned to a normal, unlabeled culture medium so that the infection had additional time to run its course, the bacterial cells (after growing for many generations) would lyse and many new phages would be released. Which hypothesis is most reasonable?

A. All released phages would contain labeled DNA.

B. No released phages would contain labeled DNA.

C. Most released phages would contain labeled DNA.

D. Most released phages would contain unlabeled DNA.

153. In the 1940s, Beadle and Tatum, working with the red bread mold *Neurospora,* used irradiation to cause mutations in various biosynthetic pathways. When one of the mutant strains could grow on *complete medium* (all essential nutritional ingredients included), but not on *minimal medium* (various nutrients missing that the organism can normally synthesize on its own), a mutation in such a synthetic pathway was suggested. To identify the specific nutrient no longer being synthesized by the organism, an experimenter might:

A. try to grow samples of different strains (each with a different biosynthetic mutation) together on the same minimal medium.

B. try to grow samples of one strain on different minimal media (each medium having one different nutrient added).

C. try to grow samples of different strains (each with a different biosynthetic mutation) together on the same complete medium.

D. try to grow samples of one strain on different media with different combinations of nutrients.

154. In their experiments, Beadle and Tatum occasionally observed *different* mutant strains that could not synthesize the exact same nutrient. Since such biosynthetic pathways were known to involve many steps, these observations provided evidence suggesting that:

A. different mutations affect different synthetic pathways.

B. different mutations affect different enzymes involved in the same pathway.

C. different nutrients are synthesized in different pathways.

D. All of the above

Passage III (Questions 155–161)

Imagine a species of plant with two varieties: dark flowers (due to the dominant allele A) and light flowers (due to the recessive allele a). If the two purebred varieties were pollinated in a typical monohybrid cross, dark flowers would be expected to outnumber light flowers 3:1 in the F_2 generation. It would seem reasonable, therefore, that after a number of generations, the dominant allele would become increasingly prevalent at the expense of the recessive allele. According to the Hardy-Weinberg Equilibrium, however, unless "evolutionary" factors are at work, the two allele frequencies in the breeding population should not change from generation to generation.

Since A and a are the only alleles present in the population for flower shade (algebraically represented by p and q respectively), the sum of these two allele frequencies, regardless of the genotypes in which they are found, must be 100% ($p + q = 1$). All individuals in this population must have one of these genotypes: AA, Aa, or aa. A homozygous dominant (AA) individual can only come about at fertilization if both gametes carry the A allele. The probability of this occurring is $p \times p = p^2$. Similarly, the probability of an individual being homozygous recessive is $q \times q = q^2$. A heterozygote (Aa) can result from both an $A \times a$ cross or an $a \times A$ cross. Thus, the probability of either of these combinations occurring is $(q \times p) + (p \times q) = 2pq$. The sum of all genotypes in the population is:

$$p^2 + 2pq + q^2 = 1$$

155. In a population of 1000 plants in which 910 have dark flowers, there can only be 90 with light flowers. What are the frequencies of each allele?

   A. $p = .7$; $q = .3$
   B. $p = .3$; $q = .7$
   C. $p = .9$; $q = .1$
   D. $p = .1$; $q = .9$

156. Referring to the plant population described in Question 155, how many plants are homozygous dominant?

   A. .49
   B. .81
   C. 490
   D. 810

157. In the plant population described in Question 155, what proportion of individuals will be heterozygotes?

   A. .18
   B. .09
   C. .50
   D. .42

158. Which of the following would have **NO** effect on the allele frequencies observed in the next generation of the plant population described in Question 155?

   A. Predatory caterpillars that preferred the dark-flowered variety
   B. Insect pollinators that could see the light flowers more easily
   C. The dark-flowered variety's pollen grains, which are dispersed more easily by winds
   D. None of the above

159. If approximately one in every 2,500 white individuals in the United States is affected by the autosomal recessive disease cystic fibrosis, what are the frequencies of both the dominant and recessive alleles in the population?

   A. $p = 2499$; $q = 1$
   B. $p = .9996$; $q = .0004$
   C. $p = .98$; $q = .02$
   D. $p = .96$; $q = .04$

160. Based on the information in Question 159, how many white Americans (out of 2500) are carriers for cystic fibrosis?

   A. Approximately 1
   B. Approximately 4
   C. Approximately 10
   D. Approximately 100

161. The cystic fibrosis allele originated as a result of:

   A. genetic drift.
   B. mutation.
   C. nonrandom mating.
   D. gene migration.

Passage IV (Questions 162–167)

The evolutionary origin of viruses remains a mystery.

Hypothesis A

One hypothesis is that the ancestors of modern viruses were free-living heterotrophs that evolved in the early seas and fed on the organic molecules around them. By the time these nutrients became depleted, other heterotrophic and autotrophic forms may have begun to appear, and viruses adapted to a parasitic life-style.

Hypothesis B

A second hypothesis favors the idea that viruses evolved from a cellular form and subsequently became highly specialized parasites. So specialized were they, that they "lost" almost all of their cellular components except the nuclear (genetic) material.

Hypothesis C

A third hypothesis is that viruses arose from bits of nucleic acid that escaped from cellular organisms. They may have survived at first without any form of outer covering before evolving their specialized coats. Various viruses may have arisen this way from different kinds of organisms.

162. Which hypothesis views viruses as having evolved independently from prokaryotes and eukaryotes?

   A. Hypothesis A
   B. Hypothesis B
   C. Hypothesis C
   D. None of the above

163. Which of the following questions would be especially difficult to answer for a proponent of the view that viruses predate cells?

   A. Why are viruses so much smaller than cellular forms?
   B. How could viruses reproduce before cells evolved?
   C. From what precursor molecules could viral DNA and viral proteins have formed?
   D. From what source could viruses have obtained nourishment?

164. Which piece of evidence would strongly support only Hypothesis C?

   A. Viral genetic material is usually made of the same type of nucleic acid as that of the viruses' hosts.
   B. Sometimes, viral genes are virtually identical to host-cell genes.
   C. Viruses are well adapted as parasites to their host cells.
   D. Viruses are all very similar in their genetic makeup.

165. Which hypothesis views cells as having evolved *before* viruses?

   A. Hypothesis A
   B. Hypothesis B
   C. Hypothesis C
   D. Hypotheses B and C

166. Which hypothesis appears strongest in view of the frequent observation today that there is greater genetic similarity between viruses and their hosts than between types of viruses?

   A. Hypothesis A
   B. Hypothesis B
   C. Hypothesis C
   D. Hypotheses B and C

167. Which of the following is **NOT** implied by Hypothesis A?

   A. Photosynthetic organisms evolved after viruses.
   B. Viral ancestors could absorb.
   C. Viral ancestors required host cells to reproduce.
   D. Viral ancestors could metabolize food on their own.

Passage V (Questions 168–174)

A survivorship curve is a representation of the age structure of a population. It shows the number of individuals still alive at each age. The pattern exhibited by a survivorship curve can provide valuable information about an organism's life history characteristics. By examining these curves, we can deduce information concerning a population's average life expectancy, mortality rate, proportion surviving at each age, number dying at each age, potential for growth, and vulnerable periods within the life cycle. The following figure shows three generalized types of survivorship curves, each representing organisms with different combinations of life history characteristics. Each type of organism successfully mates, reproduces, and leaves adequate numbers of offspring to maintain species continuity in its environment.

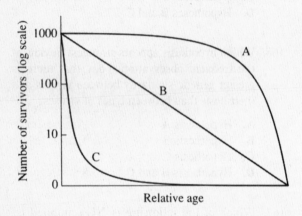

168. Which curve represents a species in which most individuals die before reaching reproductive age?

    A. Curve A
    B. Curve B
    C. Curve C
    D. Curves B and C

169. Which of the following life history characteristics would assure the survival of a species in which most individuals die before reaching reproductive age?

    A. Individuals mate and produce few offspring at a late age.
    B. Individuals produce high numbers of offspring with each mating episode.

    C. Individuals have long courtship periods before carefully choosing mates.
    D. Breeding pairs have few mating episodes but pairs are well distributed across the breeding grounds.

170. Which survivorship curve suggests that mortality occurs as a result of relatively random events with little age bias?

    A. Curve A
    B. Curve B
    C. Curve C
    D. None of the above

171. According to the figure, the highest mortality rate appears to be associated with:

    A. curve A—late in life.
    B. curve B—from midlife to late in life.
    C. curve C—early in life.
    D. Both A and C

172. Which of the following combinations of environmental and life history characteristics is likely to be associated with survivorship curve A?

    A. Late reproductive age, severe predation of young
    B. Few offspring, extensive parental care
    C. Many offspring, limited resources
    D. Limited parental care, severe predation of young

173. "Individuals alive halfway through the average maximum lifespan can expect little or no increase in their probability of dying." For which survivorship curves is this statement correct?

    A. Curves A and B
    B. Curves A and C
    C. Curves B and C
    D. Curves A, B, and C

174. Which of the survivorship curves represents the longest maximum lifespan?

    A. Curve A
    B. Curve B
    C. Curve C
    D. Maximum life spans are the same

Passage VI (Questions 175–181)

A number of experiments have been performed to examine possible mechanisms of development.

Experiment 1

In amphibians, the first cleavage division produces two blastomeres that equally divide the gray crescent, a region near the equator of the egg. When the two blastomeres are separated, each can develop into a normal tadpole. If the zygote is manipulated so that the first cleavage division does not pass through the gray crescent, and these two blastomeres are separated as before, only the one containing the gray crescent develops normally.

Experiment 2

Skin cells from a spotted frog were grown in tissue culture. The nuclei from the cells were transplanted into unfertilized eggs of an unspotted frog whose nuclei had been removed. When grown in the proper environment, a small percentage of these eggs subsequently formed blastulas and eventually developed into tadpoles and adults.

Experiment 3

In the 1920s it was found that the dorsal lip of the blastopore acts as an organizer of early amphibian development in such a way that surrounding cells eventually form the notocord, neural plate, and neural tube. Later in development, the neural tube gives rise to the brain and spinal cord. When dorsal lip cells from one embryo were transplanted to another embryo (into a region where these cells are not usually found), a second brain and spinal cord often developed. In some cases, a second head could be seen growing out of the belly!

175. Which of the following is one conclusion that can be drawn from Experiment 1?

   A. Under normal circumstances, the fate of embryonic cells is determined by the first division of the zygote.
   B. Materials outside cells can have profound effect on the fate of cells.
   C. After the first division, cells normally retain the potential to form all parts of the organism (totipotency).
   D. The directional plane of the first cleavage division plays no role in determining the developmental fate of cells.

176. Experiment 1 also clearly demonstrates that:

   A. cytoplasmic contents are not important at this stage of development.
   B. totipotency can be transferred from one cell to another.
   C. the absence of nuclear material does not limit the developmental potential of a blastomere.
   D. cytoplasmic contents affect the developmental fate of cells at this stage.

177. In Experiment 2, what is the expected appearance of frogs that successfully completed development?

   A. All should be unspotted.
   B. 50% spotted, 50% unspotted (1:1 ratio)
   C. 75% spotted, 25% unspotted (3:1 ratio)
   D. All should be spotted.

178. Were any findings from Experiment 1 also demonstrated by Experiment 2?

   A. Yes, cells can retain their totipotency (even after development has been completed).
   B. Yes, different cytoplasmic ingredients in the enucleated cells clearly affected the fates of the developing cells.
   C. No, too many of the enucleated eggs did not successfully develop.
   D. No, nuclei from spotted frogs were no longer affected by their own normal cellular environment.

179. Results from Experiment 3 demonstrate that:

   A. cytoplasmic factors are of major importance in determining the developmental fate of cells.
   B. nuclear material is secondary to environmental cues in development.
   C. tissue induction takes place in development.
   D. totipotency can be nullified by environmental factors.

180. The organizing effects of the dorsal lip cells can normally be observed:

   A. during cleavage.
   B. in the early blastula.
   C. during early gastrulation.
   D. during early organogenesis.

181. Experiments 1–3 indicate that although cells can retain the genetic potential to form all parts of the organism during development:

    A. environmental factors inside and outside the cell influence the expression of that potential.

    B. interaction between genes and cytoplasmic factors occurs.

    C. interaction between genes and other tissues occurs.

    D. All of the above

Passage VII (Questions 182–187)

Animals move in a variety of ways. Each method of movement results in an energy cost to the organism that is dependent, in part, on the size of the organism. Some organisms are specialized for aquatic movement, others for terrestrial movement, still others for flight. The following figure shows the energy costs of different methods of locomotion for animals of different size.

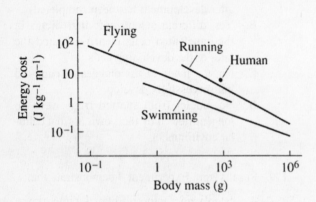

182. Based on the figure, what seems to be the most efficient mode of locomotion, pound for pound?

    A. Running

    B. Flying

    C. Swimming

    D. Flying and swimming (both activities have similar slopes)

183. In J/kg/m (log scale), what is the energy cost of flying for a 1-g (log scale) beast?

    A. 10^2

    B. 10

    C. 1

    D. Less than 1

184. According to the figure, which is the more efficient mode of locomotion for a human?

    A. Running

    B. Swimming

    C. Both are equally efficient

    D. Cannot be determined

185. Based on the figure, which statement is correct?

    A. If two individuals use the same method of movement, the smaller individual is usually more efficient.

    B. If two individuals use the same method of movement, the larger individual is always more efficient.

    C. Body mass is directly proportional to energy cost.

    D. Neither A, B, nor C is correct for all methods of movement.

186. Which of the following would be expected to move with the greatest energy cost (J/kg/m)?

    A. A running human

    B. A 1-g flyer

    C. A 10^3-g swimmer

    D. A 10^6-g runner

187. Which of the following would be expected to move with the least energy cost (J/kg/m)?

    A. A mosquito

    B. A horse

    C. A blue whale

    D. A cheetah

Passage VIII (Questions 188–193)

A heterocylic compound contains a ring with more than one kind of atom. The ring of heterocyclic amines contains carbon and nitrogen. They are a very important kind of amino compound; for example, the bases of DNA are heterocyclic amines. The most important property of heterocyclic amines is their basicity due to the presence of nitrogen. Some examples are shown below.

Pyrrole Pyridine Pyrimidine

188. Pyrrole, pyridine, and pyrimidine all have abnormally low heats of combustion and tend to undergo reactions in which their ring is retained, i.e., substitution reactions. These properties are consistent with:

   A. conjugated dienes.
   B. aromatic compounds.
   C. bases.
   D. alkenes.

189. Which of the following statements is true about the extra pair of electrons in pyrrole and pyridine?

   A. In pyrrole, an sp^2 orbital contains the pair of electrons, while in pyridine, they are involved in the π cloud.
   B. In both pyrrole and pyridine, an sp^2 orbital contains the pair of electrons.
   C. In both pyrrole and pyridine, they are involved in the π cloud.
   D. In pyrrole, they are involved in the π cloud, while in pyridine, an sp^2 orbital contains the pair of electrons.

190. Pyridine is a much stronger base than pyrrole because:

   A. pyrrole will lose its aromatic character if nitrogen accepts H^+.
   B. pyridine has a pair of electrons in an sp^2 orbital that is available for sharing.
   C. the extra pair of electrons on nitrogen in pyrrole is involved in the π cloud and therefore less available for sharing.
   D. All of the above

191. Pyrrole undergoes electrophilic substitution at position 2 because:

   A. the carbocation intermediate has more resonance structures than the intermediate formed when the electrophile attacks position 3.
   B. the inductive effect of N is greater.
   C. the aromatic ring is maintained in the carbocation.
   D. resonance structures cannot be drawn for the carbocation intermediate formed by the attack at position 3.

192. Pyridine undergoes nucleophilic substitution more readily than electrophilic substitution. Which of the following is a reasonable explanation?

   A. The N atom can better stabilize the carbanion intermediate than the carbocation intermediate.
   B. No resonance structures can be drawn for the intermediate formed by the attack of an electrophile.
   C. Nitrogen cannot expand its octet.
   D. The nitrogen atom repels electrophiles.

193. Piperidine ⬡ is formed by the catalytic reduction of pyridine. It is found in some alkaloids, such as nicotine and cocaine. One would expect the basicity of piperidine to be similar to that of:

   A. pyridine.
   B. pyrrole.
   C. dimethylamine.
   D. aniline.

Passage IX (Questions 194–199)

These experiments were performed to study esterification reactions.

Experiment 1

Labeled $CH_3{}^{18}OH$ reacted with acetic acid to form methyl acetate enriched in ^{18}O:

$$CH_3-\overset{\overset{\displaystyle O}{\|}}{C}-OH + CH_3{}^{18}OH \underset{}{\overset{H^+}{\rightleftharpoons}} CH_3-\overset{\overset{\displaystyle O}{\|}}{C}-{}^{18}OCH_3 + H_2O$$

Experiment 2

Acetic acid was reacted with several alcohols. The rate of esterification increased according to

$$CH_3-\overset{\overset{\displaystyle CH_3}{|}}{\underset{\underset{\displaystyle OH}{|}}{C}}-CH_3 < CH_3-\overset{\overset{\displaystyle CH_3}{|}}{CH}-OH < CH_3CH_2OH < CH_3OH$$

Experiment 3

Ethanol was reacted with several carboxylic acids. The rate of esterification increased according to $(CH_3)_3CCOOH < (CH_3)_2CHCOOH < CH_3CH_2COOH < CH_3COOH$

194. The results of Experiment 1 indicate that in esterification the bond that is cleaved in the carboxylic acid, $R-\overset{\overset{\displaystyle O}{\|}}{C}-OH$, is which of the following?

    A. C$\cancel{-}$OH
    B. R$\cancel{-}$C
    C. CO$\cancel{-}$H
    D. $\overset{\cancel{\|}}{C}$

195. The mechanism for the acid-catalyzed hydrolysis of ester $R-\overset{\overset{\displaystyle O}{\|}}{C}-OR'$ involves the breaking of which of the following bonds?

    A. R$\cancel{-}$C
    B. C$\cancel{-}$OR'
    C. CO$\cancel{-}$R'
    D. $\overset{\cancel{\|}}{C}$

196. Strong acids catalyze both esterification and hydrolysis because:

    A. they add to the carbonyl carbon.
    B. they protonate the alcoholic oxygen.
    C. the carbonyl carbon is made more susceptible to attack by a nucleophile when the carbonyl oxygen is protonated.
    D. they remove OH– ions.

197. The results of Experiments 2 and 3 support which of the following statements?

    A. The presence of bulky groups near the site of the reaction slows both esterification and hydrolysis reactions.
    B. The presence of bulky groups on only the alcohol slows both esterification and hydrolysis reactions.
    C. The presence of bulky groups near the site of the reaction slows esterification with no effect on hydrolysis.
    D. The presence of bulky groups near the site of the reaction slows hydrolysis with no effect on esterification.

198. Basic hydrolysis of esters involves attack of OH– and is essentially irreversible.

$$R-\overset{\overset{\displaystyle O}{\|}}{C}-OR' + OH^- \rightarrow R-\overset{\overset{\displaystyle O}{\|}}{C}-O^\ominus + R'OH$$

A basic hydrolysis reaction is carried out using a labeled ester:

$$CH_3-\overset{\overset{\displaystyle O}{\|}}{C}-{}^{18}OC_2H_5 + OH^- \rightarrow CH_3-\overset{\overset{\displaystyle O}{\|}}{C}-O^\ominus + C_2H_5{}^{18}OH$$

Therefore, in basic hydrolysis of an ester, cleavage occurs between:

A. oxygen and the alkyl group of the alcohol.
B. the carbonyl carbon and the alkyl group of the acid.
C. the carbonyl carbon and the carbonyl oxygen.
D. oxygen and the acyl group.

199. Esterification and both acidic and basic hydrolysis reactions can be described as attack of:

A. a nucleophile on the carbonyl carbon.
B. a nucleophile on an alkyl carbon.
C. an electrophile on the carbonyl carbon.
D. an electrophile on an alkyl carbon.

Passage X (Questions 200–204)

The infrared spectrum of an organic compound composed of carbon, oxygen, and hydrogen shows strong absorptions at about 3350 cm^{-1}; 1000 cm^{-1}; and 675–870 cm^{-1}. The absorption at 3350 cm^{-1} is both strong and broad. The compound also exhibits strong absorption bonds in the ultraviolet region.

Infrared Absorption by Some Oxygen-containing Compounds

Compound	O—H	C—O	C=O
Alcohols	3200–3600 cm^{-1}	1000–1200 cm^{-1}	—
Phenols	3200–3600	1140–1230	—
Ethers, aliphatic	—	1060–1150	—
Ethers, aromatic	—	1200–1275	—
	1020–1075		
Aldehydes, ketones	—	—	1675–1725 cm^{-1}
Carboxylic acids	2500–3000	1250	1680–1725
Esters	—	1050–1300 (*two bands*)	1715–1740
Acid chlorides	—	—	1750–1810
Amides (RCONH$_2$)	(N—H 3050–3550)	—	1650–1690

200. Based on the table, the infrared spectrum indicates which of the following oxygen-containing functional groups is(are) present?

A. Carbonyl and hydroxyl
B. Hydroxyl and ether
C. Carboxyl group
D. Hydroxyl group

201. Absorption in the ultraviolet region indicates the presence of:

A. a conjugated structure or aromatic group.
B. an alkyl group.
C. one double bond.
D. an ether group.

202. The NMR spectrum contains several signals, one of which exhibits splitting only when a dry, pure sample is used. The splitting disappears on the addition of a trace acid or base. This same signal is absent in the NMR spectrum of the product formed by reaction with a carboxylic acid. The functional group that can account for this behavior is which of the following?

   A.

$$H-\overset{\overset{\displaystyle O}{\|}}{C}-$$

   B.

$$-\overset{\overset{\displaystyle O}{\|}}{C}-OH$$

   C.

$$-\overset{|}{\underset{|}{C}}-OH$$

   D.

$$-\overset{|}{\underset{|}{C}}-O-\overset{\overset{\displaystyle H}{|}}{\underset{|}{C}}-$$

203. The infrared spectrum of the compound also contains moderate and weak bands associated with a mono-substituted benzene. Which of the following is the most likely structure of the compound?

   A. ⬡—COOH

   B. ⬡—CH_2OH

   C. ⬡—O—CH_3

   D. ⬡—CH_3

204. Which of the following spectroscopic techniques should be used to establish the presence of a carbonyl group in an organic molecule?

   A. NMR
   B. Ultraviolet spectroscopy
   C. Infrared spectroscopy
   D. Mass spectrometry

Questions 205–219 are independent of any passage and independent of each other.

205. Eukaryotic chromosomes consist of DNA in association with histone proteins. This association enables the genetic material to remain either tightly coiled, condensed, and visible as distinct chromosomes (only during mitosis) or loose and unwound as chromatin (during the rest of the cell cycle). DNA remains *uncoiled* during most of a cell's life so that:

   A. exposed nucleotides can efficiently provide phosphate groups for ATP production.
   B. the larger surface area covered by the chromatin acts as a more efficient osmotic attractant.
   C. transcription can take place when necessary.
   D. ER channels cannot penetrate the nucleus.

206. During respiratory ventilation, impulses along the phrenic nerves stimulate the diaphragm, causing it to contract and move downward. When this occurs, which of the following takes place in the thoracic cavity and lungs?

   A. Volume increases, pressure increases, and air moves out.
   B. Volume decreases, pressure decreases, and air moves out.
   C. Volume increases, pressure decreases, and air moves in.
   D. Volume decreases, pressure increases, and air moves in.

207. Blood pressure is a function of cardiac output (heart rate × stroke volume), as well as peripheral resistance (a measure of friction between the blood and the blood vessel walls). Factors that can increase peripheral resistance include:

   A. vasoconstriction and low blood viscosity.
   B. vasoconstriction and high blood viscosity.
   C. vasodilation and low blood viscosity.
   D. vasodilation and high blood viscosity.

208. Cerebrospinal fluid (CSF) is produced by special capillary networks in the brain called *choroid plexuses*. CSF circulates through the hollow regions of the brain and spinal cord and around the central nervous system, within its protective coverings. Areas that are part of the CSF pathway include:

A. the ventricles, spinal canal, and cranial nerves.
B. the ventricles, spinal canal, and meninges.
C. the ventricles, spinal canal, and spinal nerves.
D. the meninges, spinal canal, and cranial nerves.

209. The pedigree in the following diagram represents the inheritance of deafmutism over three generations within a family. (An arrow on a circle is a male, and a cross below a circle is a female; affected individuals have blackened circles). What kind of trait is deafmutism?

A. Autosomal dominant
B. Autosomal recessive
C. Sex-linked dominant
D. Sex-linked recessive

210. The human body has various ways to protect itself against pathogens, including specific and nonspecific defense mechanisms. The nonspecific defenses do not distinguish one pathogen from another. Which of the following would **NOT** be considered a component of the nonspecific defenses?

A. Macrophages
B. Inflammation
C. Antibodies
D. Interferon

211. The following diagram represents a major role played by enzymes in living systems. Which statement best describes this role?

A. Enzymes lower the barrier of activation energy.
B. Enzymes allow metabolic reactions to be exergonic.
C. Enzymes act as energy producers.
D. Enzymes act as catalysts to slow down reactions.

212. Parkinsonism is a degeneration of the cerebrum's basal ganglia, which help regulate contractions of skeletal muscles through the release of the neurotransmitter dopamine. Symptoms can include tremor and/or rigidity, wide-eyed staring, and drooling. Intelligence, vision, and hearing remain unaffected by this disorder, which suggests that Parkinsonism does not attack:

A. the medulla oblongata.
B. the diencephalon (thalamus and hypothalamus).
C. the dorsal root ganglia.
D. the cerebral cortex.

213. Individuals with Turner's Syndrome have 45 chromosomes (one sex chromosome is missing in the cells of these "XO" individuals). This usually is caused by meiotic nondisjunction during gametogenesis. Which statement is **NOT** correct concerning people with this disorder?

    A. They are genetic females.
    B. They are subject to sex-linked disorders at frequencies similar to those predicted for normal females.
    C. The nondisjunction event could have occurred during meiosis in either the male or female parent.
    D. If meiosis occurs in Turner's Syndrome individuals, one daughter cell resulting from the first meiotic division will have no sex chromosome.

214. Rigor mortis, a condition in which skeletal muscles temporarily remain in a rigid state of partial contraction due to the absence of ATP, occurs a few hours after death. Which of the following steps is **NOT** necessary for muscle relaxation?

    A. Repolarization of the sarcolemma
    B. The return of calcium to the sarcoplasmic reticulum
    C. The detachment of the troponin-tropomyosin complex from actin
    D. The decomposition of acetylcholine by cholinesterase

215. In the presence of a base, two molecules of an aldehyde or a ketone can combine to form a β-hydroxyaldehyde or β-hydroxyketone in an aldol condensation. Which of the following compounds will not react in an aldol condensation?

    A.

$$CH_3-\underset{\underset{\displaystyle O}{\|}}{C}-CH_3$$

    B.

$$CH_3-\underset{\underset{\displaystyle O}{\|}}{C}-CH_2-\underset{\underset{\displaystyle O}{\|}}{C}-H$$

    C.

$$CH_3-\underset{\underset{\displaystyle CH_3}{|}}{\overset{\overset{\displaystyle CH_3}{|}}{C}}-\overset{\overset{\displaystyle O}{\|}}{C}-H$$

    D.

$$CH_3-\underset{\underset{\displaystyle H}{|}}{\overset{\overset{\displaystyle CH_3O}{|}}{C}}-\overset{\overset{\displaystyle O}{\|}}{C}-H$$

216. How many amide linkages are in Ala-Gly-Phe?

    A. 1
    B. 3
    C. 0
    D. 2

217. The alcohol produced upon basic or acidic hydrolysis of a fat is which of the following?

    A.

$$\underset{\underset{\displaystyle OH}{|}}{CH_2}-\underset{\underset{\displaystyle OH}{|}}{CH_2}$$

    B. $CH_3-CH_2CH_2OH$

    C.

$$CH_3-\underset{\underset{\displaystyle OH}{|}}{CH}-\underset{\underset{\displaystyle OH}{|}}{CH_2}$$

    D.

$$\underset{\underset{\displaystyle OH}{|}}{CH_2}-\underset{\underset{\displaystyle OH}{|}}{CH}-\underset{\underset{\displaystyle OH}{|}}{CH_2}$$

218. Ortho-nitrophenol has a low boiling point and aqueous solubility due to:

    A. intermolecular H-bonding.
    B. intramolecular H-bonding.
    C. van der Waals forces.
    D. London dispersion forces.

219. In the rod cells of the retina of a mammal, the conjugated protein rhodopsin is present. The prosthetic group of rhodopsin is 11-cis-retinal:

When light impinges on the retina, 11-cis-retinal is transformed into 11-trans-retinal:

Energy is then required to convert the trans isomer back into the less stable cis isomer. The difference in stability of the two isomers is due to:

A. an inductive effect.
B. a resonance effect.
C. an isotope effect.
D. steric hindrance.

END OF TEST 4.

**IF YOU FINISH BEFORE THE TIME IS UP, YOU MAY
CHECK YOUR WORK ON THIS TEST ONLY.**

PRACTICE EXAM II ANSWER KEY

VERBAL REASONING		PHYSICAL SCIENCES		BIOLOGICAL SCIENCES	
1. A	45. B	66. C	110. B	143. C	187. C
2. D	46. C	67. A	111. A	144. D	188. B
3. A	47. D	68. D	112. B	145. C	189. D
4. A	48. B	69. B	113. D	146. B	190. D
5. A	49. B	70. D	114. B	147. A	191. A
6. B	50. D	71. C	115. C	148. D	192. A
7. B	51. A	72. D	116. B	149. D	193. C
8. B	52. D	73. D	117. B	150. A	194. A
9. D	53. D	74. C	118. A	151. C	195. B
10. A	54. A	75. B	119. D	152. D	196. C
11. A	55. B	76. C	120. B	153. B	197. A
12. C	56. A	77. D	121. B	154. B	198. D
13. D	57. A	78. D	122. D	155. A	199. A
14. A	58. B	79. D	123. B	156. C	200. D
15. C	59. D	80. D	124. B	157. D	201. A
16. D	60. D	81. B	125. A	158. D	202. C
17. A	61. B	82. A	126. B	159. C	203. B
18. D	62. C	83. B	127. B	160. D	204. C
19. D	63. B	84. C	128. C	161. B	205. C
20. C	64. D	85. D	129. C	162. A	206. C
21. B	65. D	86. D	130. D	163. B	207. B
22. A		87. B	131. C	164. B	208. B
23. B		88. B	132. B	165. D	209. B
24. D		89. B	133. B	166. C	210. C
25. C		90. B	134. B	167. C	211. A
26. C		91. C	135. D	168. C	212. D
27. B		92. D	136. A	169. B	213. B
28. B		93. A	137. A	170. B	214. C
29. D		94. C	138. C	171. D	215. C
30. C		95. C	139. D	172. B	216. D
31. A		96. B	140. B	173. C	217. D
32. D		97. A	141. B	174. D	218. B
33. D		98. C	142. A	175. C	219. D
34. B		99. A		176. D	
35. A		100. D		177. D	
36. B		101. D		178. A	
37. C		102. D		179. C	
38. B		103. C		180. D	
39. D		104. A		181. D	
40. B		105. D		182. C	
41. B		106. D		183. B	
42. C		107. C		184. B	
43. A		108. D		185. B	
44. B		109. C		186. B	

PRACTICE EXAM II EXPLANATORY ANSWERS

VERBAL REASONING

1. **A** The answer to this question is found in the following statement in paragraph 7: "Because of greater demands for heating rather than cooling in colder regions, some utilities experience peak demands in the winter. In these cases, warmer winter temperatures caused by the Greenhouse Effect could reduce the amount of generating capacity required."

2. **D** The answer to this question is found in the following statement in paragraph 6: "By the year 2055, the Greenhouse Effect could measurably change regional demands for electricity in the United States."

3. **A** It is unreasonable to assume that someone so aware of one consequence of the greenhouse effect would be completely unaware of its other effects. The writer specifically mentions possible reduction of the flow of rivers.

4. **A** The answer to this question is found in the following statement in paragraph 7: "Such reductions in new capacity requirements induced by the Greenhouse Effect are restricted to a few states in the Northeast . . . and in the Northwest. . . ."

5. **A** The answer to this question is based on two things: the fact that the author does not question the assumption anywhere in the article, and the following statement in paragraph 6: "Because the Greenhouse Effect is expected to have a significant influence on air conditioning and other summertime uses of electricity, higher temperatures in the future could lead to significant increases in the capacity needed to satisfy those uses." Notice that this statement assumes higher temperatures in the future and only questions how much electricity will be needed to supply the needs of the population in the warmer environment.

6. **B** The answer to this question is based on the following statement in paragraph 4: "Also, because of the large investments by utilities in long-lived capital-intensive power plants, the industry must focus on long-term planning."

7. **B** The answer to this question is based on the following statement in paragraph 2: "Bingham came of age in the Golden Age of American painting (1830-60), when the work of American artists was, for the first time, appreciated. . ."

8. **B** The answer to this question is based on several statements in paragraph 3: "Today, Bingham ranks among the best of the nineteenth-century American narrative painters. 'He was a powerful figure who broke new ground in illustrating the simple joys of American life and who prepared the way for the giants—Winslow Homer and Thomas Eakins—to follow,' says E. Maurice Bloch. . . ."

9. **D** The answer to this question is based on the following statement in paragraph 5: "To his close friends, though, he was fiercely loyal and often charming, witty, and even affectionate."

10. **A** The answer to this question is in paragraph 6: "Like many American artists, Bingham was largely self-taught and 'he was proud of it,' according to Bloch."

11. **A** The answer to this question is based on the following statement in paragraph 7: "Bingham gained a national reputation through the American Art Union, an important corporate patron that encouraged artists to paint works appealing to patriotic feeling."

12. **C** The answer to this question is based on a number of statements. In paragraph 1, Bingham is called the "Missouri painter," and in paragraph 8 ". . . he has always been well known in Missouri. . . ." But the statement that best answers this question is in paragraph 6: ". . . Bingham started out as a journeyman portraitist, traveling from town to town through Missouri and Mississippi."

13. **D** The answer to this question is based on the following statement in paragraph 9: "Having studied Bingham's life and work for more than forty years, Bloch notes, 'It would have been possible to write an excellent book on Bingham by noting only a narrow circle of authentic works.'"

14. **A** Paragraph 1 supplies the answer: "He portrayed them as rugged and self-reliant Americans, emblems of the frontier spirit."

15. **C** The answer to this question is implied in several statements in paragraph 1: "As a child of the frontier, it was natural for George Caleb Bingham . . . to paint the fur trappers, flatboatmen, country politicians, and squatters he knew so well. He portrayed them as rugged and self-reliant Americans, emblems of the frontier spirit."

16. **D** The answer to this question is based on the following statement in paragraph 1: "Recommendations from four independent national panels call for increased emphasis on: the five new basics (English, mathematics, science, social studies, and computer science). . . ."

17. **A** The answer to this question is based on the following statement in paragraph 2: "A master teacher plan would provide a reward system for excellent teaching and make the profession more attractive to bright, talented college students seeking a professional career."

18. **D** The answer to this question is implied by the following statements in paragraphs 2 and 7: "A master teacher plan would provide a reward system for excellent teaching and make the profession more attractive to bright, talented college students seeking a professional career" (paragraph 2). "The Department of Defense Dependents School has accepted the challenge for educational reform; the Master Teacher Program is one small step in an overall plan for excellence. In this endeavor, active teacher participation is vital to the success of a master teacher program" (paragraph 7).

19. **D** The answer to this question is in the following statement in paragraph 5: "First and foremost, the master teacher would have comprehensive knowledge about his or her subject."

20. **C** The answer to this question is based on the following statement in paragraph 3: "Fewer than 10 percent of all teachers aspire to be administrators."

21. **B** The answer to this question is found in the profile of a master teacher in paragraphs 5 and 6. All of the attributes are mentioned except administrative skill.

22. **A** The answer to this question is based on the following statement in paragraph 4: ". . . public health policy should ensure safety, not harass industry or needlessly terrify the public."

23. **B** The answer to this question is found in the following statement in paragraph 1: "Consider, for a moment, these chemicals: safrole, hydrazine, tannin, and ethyl carbamate. We ingest them every day when we consume pepper, mushrooms, tea, and bread."

24. **D** The answer to this question is based on the following statement in paragraph 6: "Nosophobics think they will be sick in the future because of lurking factors in their diet and general environment."

25. **C** This inference is based on the following statements in paragraphs 2 and 3 plus the overall tone of the article: "The numbers can be made to show that a substance is killing us—even when there isn't the remotest possibility" (paragraph 2). "If you listen to every restrictive environmental report that has received media attention, you know that in addition to apples, you shouldn't eat most other fruits, not to mention meats, fish, fowl, vegetables, eggs, or milk products" (paragraph 3).

26. **C** The answer to this question is based on the following statement in paragraph 7: "Yesterday's invisible hazards give rise to monster legends, claims of witchcraft, and vampire myths."

27. **B** The answer to this question can be inferred from two statements in paragraph 8 and several statements in paragraph 9. From paragraph 8 are the following statements: "The most deadly public health issues that threaten our lives have been obscured in the face of trumped-up charges against the food we eat, the water we drink, and the air we breathe. They fall under the category of hazardous lifestyles." From paragraph 9 are these statements: "Cigarette smoking claims 1,200 lives a day. . . . Another obvious example of a hazardous lifestyle habit is excessive or abusive alcohol consumption, which claims 100,000 lives annually. Add to this the use of addictive substances, such as heroin, cocaine, and crack, which claim some 50,000 lives each year."

28. **B** The answer to this question can be inferred from the following statements found in paragraph 6: "Nosophobics think they will be sick in the future because of lurking factors in their diet and general environment. They fixate on an array of allegedly health-threatening gremlins. Due to this phobia, they believe that living—and eating and drinking—in America is inherently hazardous to their health. They are sure there is a death-dealing carcinogen on every plate, a life-sapping toxin under every pillow."

29. **D** The answer to this question can be found from a statement in paragraph 9: "Cigarette smoking claims 1,200 lives a day. In just one year, over 400,000 will perish. . . ."

30. **C** The answer to this question is based on the following statements in paragraph 2: "In 1981, . . . some of the citizens of Seattle examined the hard economic questions facing their city. . . . They discovered that economic questions are not only technical and political, but ethical and religious as well. . . . When they began to discuss the economy, they felt they lacked the ability to understand and articulate the philosophical issues that lie at the heart of the social contract." In addition to these statements the tenor of the article implies this answer.

31. **A** The answer in paragraph 5 states: "Their worlds differed so much from ours. But those differences can be instructive. If we can understand why Aristotle opposed economic growth and why Adam Smith extolled it, it will prompt us to think about how decisions are actually made in modern democracies."

32. **D** The answer to this question is based on the following statement in paragraph 2: "They discovered that economic growth questions are not only technical and political, but ethical and religious as well."

33. **D** The answer to this question is based on several statements in paragraphs 3 and 4. In paragraph 3 are the statements that ". . . according to Aristotle, the pursuit of material wealth should be a means to strengthen the community, the *polis*. People who pursue material wealth for its own sake, Aristotle wrote, 'are intent upon living only and not living well.'" In paragraph 4 are these statements: "'Adam Smith . . . did not believe that the desire for wealth was in any

way unnatural or a threat to the well-being of the society. . . .'" Increasing wealth was a universal urge. . . . "'Smith had observed the process of economic growth visible in Europe in the sixteenth and seventeenth centuries. . . . (and) how a society could increase the production power over time. . . .'"

34. **B** The answer to this question is based on the following statements in paragraph 5: "'We won't find simple answers for our age in the writing of these philosophers. . . . Their worlds differed so much from ours. . . . If we can understand why Aristotle opposed economic growth and why Adam Smith extolled it, it will prompt us to think about how decisions are actually made in modern democracies.'"

35. **A** The answer to this question is based on the positive tone of the article. The article gives no criticism of the program.

36. **B** The answer to this question is supported by several statements in paragraphs 4 and 5: "Thus, according to Aristotle, the pursuit of material wealth should be a means to strengthen the community, the *polis*. People who pursue material wealth for its own sake . . . are intent upon living only and not living well" (paragraph 4). "Adam Smith . . . did not believe that the desire for wealth was in any way unnatural or a threat to the well-being of the society. . . . Smith had observed the process of economic growth . . . in Europe in the sixteenth and seventeenth centuries. He had seen how a society could increase the production power over time, expanding the supply of necessities and conveniences of life" (paragraph 5).

37. **C** The answer to this question is based on the following statement in paragraph 2: "'What is distinctive about the South,' says Robert C. Stewart, executive director of the Alabama Humanities Foundation, 'and about the Southerners' response to it, is that it remained primarily agricultural well into the twentieth century, long after the rest of the nation had become urbanized.'"

38. **B** In paragraph 7: "With Walker Percy's *The Last Gentleman* (1966) and Mary Ward Brown's *Tongues of Flame* (1986), Southern literature reaches the point at which it ceases to be distinctively Southern and becomes broadly American. . . ."

39. **D** The answer to this question is supported by the following statement from paragraph 7: "'With Walker Percy's *The Last Gentleman* (1966) and Mary Ward Brown's *Tongues of Flame* (1986), Southern literature reaches the point at which it ceases to be distinctly Southern and becomes broadly American,' says Quinlan."

40. **B** The answer to this question is based on the following statement in paragraph 5: "'The progressive South is uncomfortable with its rural heritage.'"

41. **B** The answer to this question can be inferred from statements made throughout the article. In paragraph 1 are the following statements: ". . . writers have drawn upon Southerners' almost instinctive relationship to their surroundings. Working within a land-oriented cultural ethos, Southern writers have evoked a familiar, often haunting sense of place that gives the South a distinctive regional identity." In paragraph 2 are these statements: "'What is distinctive about the South . . . and about the Southerners' response to it, is that it remained primarily agricultural . . .' and '. . . Southerners have had mixed feelings about the land rather than purely idealized reactions, with pastoral myths often giving way to hard reality.'" In paragraph 3 there is reference to the Alabama Humanities Foundation helping ". . . Alabamians examine their traditional relation to the land . . ." and a statement that the Foundation ". . . introduces participants to some of the major works of twentieth-century Southern literature and to a renewed sense of their roots in the land and its continuing vitality."

42. **C** The answer to this question is based on paragraph 6: "Participants are learning that Southern writers do not present a uniform view of 'home.' Among the works being read is William Faulkner's *The Bear* (1942), which depicts a mythic landscape. . . . Jean Toomer's *Cane* (1923) portrays the spiritual landscape and folk rhythms of black life in rural Georgia. . . . John Crowe Ransom's essay 'Reconstructed but Unregenerate' (1930) and Andrew Lytle's short story 'Jericho, Jericho, Jericho' (1984), who present the rural South. . . ."

43. **A** The answer to this question is supported by the following statement in paragraph 8: "As chronicled in the works of these and other con-temporary Southern writers, the South is moving inexorably into the urban, industrial mainstream."

44. **B** The answer to this question can be inferred from the following statements from paragraph 8: ". . . the South is moving inexorably into the urban, industrial mainstream. With fewer people living close to the land, the experiences that in many ways made Southerners 'Southern' are becoming alien. . . . 'As we move farther from the land of our parents and grandparents, we need to reflect on their special relationship with the land, whether we will have it today, and what will become of it as we move into the 1990s.'"

45. **B** The answer to this question is based on the following statements in paragraphs 2 and 4: "Diaries are the best sources of this type of inquiry, according to Brown, because they enable one 'to see a person whole, to see how print and oral communication fit together in a person's life to determine which is more important and exactly how both are used'" (paragraph 2). "Because keeping a diary was a good deal more common during the eighteenth and nineteenth centuries than at present. . ." (paragraph 4).

46. **C** Though it may be true that newspapers were better written in 1850 than in 1700, there is nothing in the article to indicate this. On the other hand, the article states that more people read the newspaper in 1850, implying that more people could read. The writer states that there was an explosion of newspapers in the 1780s and 90s, implying that more people used newspapers as a source of information. In the final paragraph, the writer mentions that the American Revolution encouraged the concept that the people should be well informed.

47. **D** The answer to this question is based on the following statements in paragraph 6: "'The radical difference between the America of 1700 and 1850 was the extraordinary abundance of information. People gradually became selectors of information according to their individual temperament, their occupation, their social class.'"

48. **B** The answer to this question is based on the following statements from paragraph 4: "In particular, Brown sought out generic types . . . rather than notables. There were, however, a few major figures—Sewall, Bentley, John Adams,

William Byrd II—whose diaries . . . could not be ignored."

49. **B** The answer to this question is based on the following statements in paragraph 3: "'People in Sewall's time did not read newspapers for news. Word of mouth was much faster. What newspapers did provide was the text of official documents, such as laws or treaties, and the speeches of high officials.'"

50. **D** The answer to this question is supported by statements in paragraph 7: "'By the nineteenth century a dramatic change had occurred,' Brown says. 'The ideology of the Revolution required that the people—that is, all sorts of people, who run the nation in a democracy—be well-informed.'"

51. **A** The answer to this question is supported by the following statement in paragraph 5: "'During much of the eighteenth century, information was a scarce commodity . . . a community's leaders controlled important communications and diffused them by word of mouth to other people.'"

52. **D** The answer to this question is based on the following statement in paragraph 2: "Initially, sulphur and sulphuric compounds were selected for study because they were known to be capable of causing damage over large areas of eastern North America and because of the prospect for substantial increases in the atmospheric sulphur load in connection with the United States' plans to increase the use of coal."

53. **D** The answer is based on inferences from the first and last paragraphs: ". . . programs that examine possible control measures and increase scientific knowledge have been developed and are being carried out cooperatively by the United States and Canada." And ". . . Canada looks forward to close cooperation with the United States. . . ."

54. **A** The answer to this question is based on the following statement in paragraph 2: "Initially, sulphur and sulphuric compounds were selected for study because they were known to be capable of causing damage over large areas of eastern North America. . . ."

55. **B** The answer to this question is based on the following statement in paragraph 4:

"Long-range transport of air pollution represents a serious environmental problem for Canada."

56. **A** The answer to this question can be inferred by the following statement in paragraph 3: "Results of these early studies enabled the two countries to recognize and clarify the time-sensitive nature and the ultimate irreversibility of the impact of acid rain."

57. **A** The answer to this question is based on the following statement in paragraph 4: "Action by Canada alone will be insufficient in view of the continental dimension of the problem and the climatic behavior that favors transport of United States' pollutants over Canada."

58. **B** The answer to this question is supported by the following statement in paragraph 4: "Such action not only should prevent further increases in emissions but also should reduce emissions from their current levels."

59. **D** The passage makes no reference at all to the Industrial Revolution nor its effect on classical learning.

60. **D** The answer to this question is based on the following statements in paragraph 9: "He imagined *The Age of Fable* not in a classroom, but in the 'parlor.' His audience was not to be schoolchildren, but 'the reader of English literature, of either sex,' others 'more advanced' who may require mythological knowledge when they visit museums or 'mingle in cultivated society,' and also readers 'in advanced life.'"

61. **B** The answer to this question is based on the following statements in paragraph 6: "Bulfinch drew his 188 'citations' from the work of forty poets. All were British except for three."

62. **C** The answer to this question is inferred because all of the other reasons listed as possible answers are stated in the reading. This answer is not stated but, in addition, the author of the reading specifically states that this book was not written for the classroom (see the answer to question 60 and paragraph 8).

63. **B** The answer can be inferred from several statements throughout the reading and by one particular statement in paragraph 8. The reading's general implication is that during Bulfinch's time an educated individual was ex-

pected to be knowledgeable about classical literature, as shown in the following statements: ". . . in the American mind, the name of Bulfinch is indelibly associated with classical mythology" (paragraph 1). "Without a doubt, *The Age of Fable* formed the image that millions of Americans had of the classical gods and heroes. . . . The mythology learned by Americans was Bulfinch's mythology. . . . Bulfinch recreated dozens of myths . . . " (paragraph 2). "*The Age of Fable* consists of prose narratives of classical myths" (paragraph 3). "Bulfinch's strong background in classical literature, especially Roman, accounts for his success in adapting Ovid for American readers" (paragraph 4). The answer is best inferred from the following statement in paragraph 8: "He [Bulfinch] was responding, in particular, to the rise of science and technology, a decline in classical learning and increasing educational opportunities. . . ."

64. **D** The answer to this question is based on statements made by the author listing all of the other reasons given as answers. While the author mentions the high number of British writers used, the author does not give this as a reason for the popularity of the book.

65. **D** The answer to this question is based on the following statements made in paragraphs 2 and 7: "Thus we hope to teach mythology,' he explains in his preface, 'not as a study, but as a relaxation from study; to give our work the charm of a story-book, yet by means of it to impart a knowledge of an important branch of education'" (paragraph 2). "In using poetry as a counterpoint in *The Age of Fable*, Bulfinch was tapping into an interest of the general educated public" (paragraph 7).

PHYSICAL SCIENCES

66. **C** Look for negative values of the standard free energy, since these imply spontaneity.

67. **A** Remember to use the fourth column and to use the factors of 2 in the equation. Note that $\Delta S°$ for an element in its standard state does not equal zero.

68. **D** Since gas-phase carbon has a molar heat capacity that is about 2.5 times as great as that of graphite, the heat needed to raise the gaseous sample by 10 K will raise the graphite sample by 25 K. (To work the problem more formally, set "$nC_p\Delta T$" for each sample equal to each other and solve for ΔT for the graphite.)

69. **B** Be careful to select only the three "saturated" hydrocarbons, i.e., those having the maximum number of hydrogens for a given number of carbon atoms: CH_4, C_2H_6 and C_3H_8.

70. **D** Item II is ruled out because the heat capacities are similar for the two compounds.

71. **C** $\Delta G°$ decreases as the number of Cl's increases: $\Delta H°$ follows an irregular trend.

72. **D** The balanced equation is $C_2H_6 + \frac{7}{2} O_2 \rightarrow 3H_2O + 2CO_2$. Be certain to use $\Delta G°$ values from column 3, paying attention to coefficients.

73. **D** I is reflected in the lower values of $\Delta G°$ for the solid. II (but not III) is reflected in the higher $S°$ for the gas.

74. **C** The standard free energy of formation is 0 for both C and H_2, while for methane the value is -50.6. Thus, the free energy of the system decreases by 50.6 kJ/mol when methane is formed, as indicated in choice C.

75. **B** Use $\ln K = -\Delta G°/RT$, where $\Delta G° = -258$ kJ/mol

76. **C** The speed is lower for a heavier molecule:

$$\frac{v_{O_2}}{v_{H_2}} = \sqrt{\frac{m_{H_2}}{m_{O_2}}} = \sqrt{\frac{2}{32}} = \frac{1}{4}$$

77. **D** Speed is proportional to $T^{1/2}$, where T is in K. So $v_2/v_1 = (T_2/T_1)^{1/2}$.

78. **D** Choose the point on the horizontal axis that corresponds to the peak of the "600K" curve.

79. **D** Estimate the fraction of the area under the curve that lies to the right of 1600 m/s.

80. **D** Since the most probable speed at 600K is about 2,300 m/s, most probable speed at 1200K will be given by $(2,300)(1200/600)^{1/2} = 3,200$ m/s

81. **B** Speed is the absolute value of velocity, so it is always zero or positive.

82. **A** The spread is greater for higher temperatures, not lower, and the most probable speed is proportional to the square root of the absolute temperature.

83. **B** 0.05 liter $\times$ 0.20 mol/liter = 0.010 mol NaOH added at endpoint.

84. **C** $V_aC_a = V_bC_b$ at endpoint, since moles of hydroxide added must equal moles of monoprotic weak acid initially present.

85. **D** The pH increases by 1 unit, from 3 to 4. Thus, $[H^+]$ decreases from 10^{-3} to 10^{-4}, a factor of 10.

86. **D** The ratio requested is the reciprocal slope of the curve.

87. **B** We will have added 50 mL of NaOH past the endpoint, so $[OH-]$ will be the original concentration of NaOH diluted by a factor of 2, or 0.10. Then pOH = 1 and pH = 13.

88. **B** Halfway through the titration, at the 25 mL mark, pH closely approximates pK_a. Look for a pK_a close to 3.7 and you find formic acid.

89. **B** This route to the halfway point in the titration involves going all the way to the endpoint of a second sample, and then going halfway back: pH = pK_a.

90. **B** All but 20 percent of the original weak acid has been converted to weak base at 40 mL, since 40 mL is 80 percent of the way to the endpoint.

91. **C** Since the curve is so steep, either indicator should signal the value of V_{OH-} at the endpoint with equal accuracy.

92. **D** Although one of the four values of ΔH is negative, indicating that heat is released and that the reaction is *likely* to be spontaneous, we cannot answer the question with certainty unless we learn the value of the *entropy* for each reaction. A reaction is spontaneous if $\Delta G < 0$, where $\Delta G = \Delta H - T\Delta S$.

93. **A** The question refers to Experiment 3, but in this case the products of the reaction as written are being converted to the reactants; thus heat will be given off. There are 20 moles of Cl atoms compared with the 2 moles in the original equation, so ΔH_{diss} must be multiplied by 10 to determine the heat released.

94. **C** In pure water, $[Ag^+] = [Cl^-] = x$
$$x^2 = K_{sp} = 1.8 \times 10^{-10}$$
$$x = 1.3 \times 10^{-5} M$$

95. **C** To answer this question we need to add the equations referring to the sublimation of Ag(s) and the ionization of Ag(g):

$Ag(s) \rightarrow Ag(g)$	286 kJ/mol
$Ag(g) \rightarrow Ag^+ + e^-$	728 kJ/mol

$Ag(s) \rightarrow Ag^+ + e^-$	1010 kJ/mol

Since only 0.10 mol of silver ion is produced, the energy required is (0.10)(1014) = 101.4 kJ/mol

96. **B** We need to add the following reactions to obtain the reaction desired:

$AgCl(s) \rightarrow Ag(s) + 1/2\,Cl_2(g)$ $\Delta H_f = 128$ kJ/mol	
$Ag(s) \rightarrow Ag(g)$ $\Delta H_{subl} = 286$ kJ/mol	
$\frac{1}{2}Cl_2(g) \rightarrow Cl(g)$ $\Delta H_{diss} = 120$ kJ/mol	

$AgCl(s) \rightarrow Ag(g) + Cl(g)$ $\Delta H = 534$ kJ/mol	

Since 0.5 mol AgCl(s) reacts, the result is (0.5)(534) = 267 kJ/mol of heat that must be added.

97. **A** Since sublimation is the process by which a solid is changed directly to a gas, without passing through the liquid phase, we look for a point on the boundary between solid and gas.

98. **C** To see why the negatively-sloping solid-liquid boundary explains the fact that water expands when it freezes (i.e., is denser as a liquid than as a solid), consider liquid water in equilibrium with its solid form at 1.00 atm and 0°K:

$$H_2O(s) = H_2O(l)$$

Suppose we increase the pressure—as when the blade of an ice skate presses on ice. Then the equilibrium will shift in a direction that will best relieve the pressure, which in this case will be the state having the smaller volume per mole or, put another way, the greater density. Thus an increase in pressure causes solid water to melt to form the liquid. This effect is illustrated by the solid-liquid boundary of Fig. 1.

99. **A** As nuclear charge increases from 13 (aluminum) to 14 (silicon), it pulls the outer electrons more closely toward the nucleus. (The extra electron added to the outer shell of the atom does not completely shield this additional nuclear charge.)

100. **D** The coordinates of temperature and percent silicon that are given place the point in the left-hand region of solid 1.

101. **D** To see that 1 is true, examine the downward-sloping line at the top of the diagram. To verify II, examine the line that begins at the lower left corner and continues up and to the right. To rule out III, examine the line that starts at the upper left, slants down and to the right, then changes its slope to become approximately flat as it moves to the right. Note that the uppermost downward sloping line is not the one specified here.

102. **D** Spontaneity is determined by $\Delta G = \Delta H - T\Delta S$. We know nothing about the enthalpy changes, and so we cannot determine the spontaneity of these reactions.

103. **C** For confirming instances, look for reactions which (*a*) have $\Delta S° > 0$ and (*b*) have more product species than reactant species in their balanced reactions.

104. **A** Reaction 1 shows solid copper changing directly to copper vapor, without passing through the liquid phase. This is analogous to the carbon dioxide sublimation described.

105. **D** Since the entropy change for the (evidently spontaneous) process is favorable, the enthalpy change is not well determined.

106. **D** From the discussion, we need to know both the entropy and enthalpy of fusion of ice at its melting point.

107. **C** Entropy measures disorder, hot stability.

108. **D** II could be an explanation for the difference since it predicts a lower $\Delta S°$ for $MgCl_2$ than NaCl. I predicts the reverse effect, and III is a statement about enthalpy, not entropy.

109. **C** The relation between the initial and final masses of an isotope with a half-life is:

$$m_{final} = (1/2^n)m_{initial}$$

where *n* is the number of half-lives. Using this calculation we get:

$$2 \text{ g}/32 \text{ g} = 1/16 = 1/2^4$$

There were four half-lives in the ten-minute period, therefore each half-life is 2.5 minutes. In this problem it is just as easy to count up the half-lives. That is, it takes one half-life to get from 32 g to 16 g, a second to get from 16 g to 8 g; a third to get from 8 g to 4 g, and finally, a fourth to get from 4 g to 2 grams.

110. **B** The second particle has a mass of 0 amu (atomic mass units) and a positive charge. This fits the description of the antielectron, or positron.

111. **A** The mass number is given by the superscript *A*. The law of conservation of mass requires that the sum of mass numbers before the decay equal the number after the decay. Therefore:

$$30 = A + 0 \text{ so that } A = 30$$

112. **B** The number of neutrons in the nucleus must be the mass number, *A*, minus the atomic number, *Z*, where $Z = 15 - 1 = 14$. This gives $30 - 14 = 16$.

113. **D** The atomic number is the number of protons in the nucleus, *Z*. Conservation of mass requires that $15 = Z + 1$, so that $Z = 14$.

114. **B** The emitted particle decreases the number of protons by 1, while keeping the number of neutrons constant. Therefore, n/p increases so that the radioactive isotope $^{30}_{15}P$ lies below the belt of stability.

115. **C** All nuclei of phosphorus have the same atomic number. A different atomic number means a different element.

116. **B** Distance traveled is the product of the average speed and the time traveled. $D = v_{average}t$. The average speed in turn is found by taking the average of the velocity at the beginning and at the end of the interval:

$$v_{aver} = (2.3 \text{ m/min} + 0 \text{ m/min})/2 = 1.15 \text{ m/min}$$
$$d = (1.15 \text{ m/min}) \text{ 2 min} = 2.3 \text{ m} \sim 2 \text{ m}$$

117. **B** Kinetic energy is directly proportional to the square of the velocity. The maximum velocity for any of the intervals listed is 4 m/min, which occurs during the interval 2 min to 3 min.

118. **A** During this interval, the velocity is constant. Therefore, the acceleration is zero, so that the net force acting on the box must be zero over this interval of time.

119. **D** Momentum is the product of mass and velocity = (4.0 kg)(4 m/min) = 16 kg m/min.

120. **B** Since the velocity is constant over this interval, the acceleration is zero, which means the force acting on the box must be zero. Since work is force times distance, the work over this interval must also be zero.

121. **B** Ohm's law states that the voltage is equal to the product of the current and the resistance. Since the axes given are for voltage and current, this rearranges to $R = V/I$. V and I are both linear, so the graph will be a straight line. They are also directly proportional so that the slope will be positive.

122. **D** The force of gravity is given by:

$$F_{grav} = G \, M_{earth} m / r^2$$

The force is inversely related to the square of the radial distance. Since the term for r is **NOT** linear, the graph will be a curve. Since the relation between F and r^2 is inversely proportional, the slope of the curve will be negative.

123. **B** For any body thrown vertically upward near the surface of the earth, due to gravity the initial velocity is working in opposition to the acceleration. This means the upward velocity will decrease as the height above the ground increases. At the maximum height, the velocity is zero and the body will then start to fall back toward the ground. Velocity and time are linearly related, so the graph will be a straight line. They are also inversely related, so that the slope will be negative.

124. **B** Be careful. The variables are mass and energy, which are linear and directly proportional, so the graph is a straight line with a positive slope. c^2 is the constant value of the slope.

125. **A** Since equilibrium requires that no net force act on the body, a body in dynamic equilibrium must be moving with a constant velocity.

126. **B** Boyle's Law $PV = k$ is shown by this graph for a particular temperature.

127. **B** Because $P = F/A$ for a given area, P and F are directly proportional.

128. **C** These quantum numbers refer to the $5d$ electrons. The value of n is not used directly to answer the question. From $+2$ through -2, m can have 5 values. Each m value can have 2 values of m_s associated with it, for a total of 10 states.

129. **C** In answer C the electronegativity between the bonded atoms decreases from HF through H_2. Note that the answers in D are atoms, not molecules, so no dipole moment is defined for them. Note also that the dipole moment is zero for each of the homonuclear diatomic molecules in A.

130. **D** II is ruled out because the solubility product, unlike the solubility, does not depend on concentration.

131. **C** CO_3^{2-} from the $BaCO_3$ reacts with H^+ to form HCO_3^- (and, if enough strong acid is available, H_2CO_3), causing the $MgCO_3$ to dissociate more than it would in neutral water.

132. **B** If doubling of a concentration leads to quadrupling of the rate, then the reaction is 2nd-order in that concentration. If changing another concentration has no effect, then the rate must be 0th order in that concentration.

133. **B** The p_z orbital has a nodal plane in the xy-plane. D is unfavorable but not impossible.

134. **B** HNO_3 is a strong acid, so $[H^+] = 0.1$ Therefore: pH $= -\log (.1) = 1$

135. **D** Use $P_i = X_i P_T$ where $X(N_2) = 3/(3 + 1)$ and $X(H_2) = 1/(3 + 1)$

136. **A** The angle between the light ray and the normal to the medium's surface decreases as the speed of the light decreases. The ray is traveling fastest in medium I (largest angle with respect to the normal) and slowest in medium IV (smallest angle to normal).

137. **A** Vertical motion is independent of horizontal motion, and for both balls the vertical acceleration is due to gravity. The balls hit the ground at the same time.

138. **C** This is the definition of the Newton, N, which is a unit of force, not work or energy.

139. **D** The speed of sound in air at 0°C is 330 meters/s, so it takes 2 seconds for sound to travel 660 meters. Light has a speed of 3.00×10^8 m/s, so in 2.0 seconds it would cover 6.0×10^8 meters.

140. **B** $P_{av} = \dfrac{\Delta w}{t}$, but the work done ($\Delta w$) is mgh, therefore:

$$P_{av} = \frac{(70 \text{ kg})(9.8 \text{ m/s}^2)(2 \text{ m})}{2 \text{ s}} = 686 \frac{\text{kg m}^2}{\text{s}^3}$$

$$P_{av} = 686 \text{ J/s} = 686 \text{ W}$$

This problem can be more readily answered by estimating the value

$$P_{av} \sim \frac{(70 \text{ kg})(10 \text{ m/s}^2)(2 \text{ m})}{2 \text{ s}} = 700 \text{ W}$$

which is closest to choice **B**.

141. **B** Conservation of energy means the sum of the kinetic and potential energies must be the same at the start of the jump and at its maximum height

$$1/2 \ mv_0^2 + mgh_0 = 1/2 \ mv^2 + mgh$$

where subscript 0 stands for the initial state. This becomes $1/2 \ mv_0^2 + 0 = 0 + mgh$.

Thus: $h = \dfrac{v_0^2}{2 \ g} = \dfrac{(9.8 \text{ m/s}^2)}{2(9.8 \text{ m/s}^2)} = 4.9 \text{ m}$

The mass of the vaulter cancels out.

142. **A** The speed is constant but the direction of the car is constantly changing, thus the velocity is constantly changing, which in turn means the car undergoes acceleration. Since only the direction, but not the magnitude of the velocity, is changing, only the radial acceleration component is nonzero. The tangential acceleration component is zero.

$$a_r = \frac{v^2}{r} = \frac{(20 \text{ m/s})^2}{200 \text{ m}} \ 2.0 \text{ m/s}^2$$

BIOLOGICAL SCIENCES

143. **C** Following the arrow in the flow chart immediately reveals that fatty acids can be converted to acetyl CoA.

144. **D** You must know that the net gain in ATP molecules by the complete metabolism of glucose during cellular respiration is 36. Because fatty acids are richer in hydrogens (it is the treatment of hydrogens during the electron transport chain that provides most of the ATP), the best estimate would be, *higher than 36*.

145. **C** Recognizing the names of some amino acids is helpful, but not essential. The flow chart shows that after deamination (when NH_3 is formed), amino acids can be converted to pyruvic acid or acetyl CoA, or they can feed into the Krebs cycle. They do not feed into the transport chain.

146. **B** Basic knowledge of metabolic processes and/or urine content is required. Ammonia is too toxic to be transported directly. Urea is the nitrogenous waste resulting from the metabolism of amino acids. Uric acid is produced during metabolism of nucleic acids, and creatinine results from the metabolism of creatine (creatine phosphate can be used as a source of energy in muscle cells).

147. **A** General understanding of the location of each stage of cellular respiration is needed. Glycolysis occurs in the cytoplasm (cytosol), the Krebs cycle takes place within the mitochondrial matrix, and the transport chain is found along the mitochondrial cristae. Since the flow chart shows glycerol entering the pathway at glycolysis, it must be in the cytoplasm.

148. **D** You should understand that catabolic intermediates can often be used as building blocks during anabolic processes (synthesis). Acetyl CoA is found on the flow chart at the juncture where protein, carbohydrate, and fat metabolism can all intersect. Since starch is a polysaccharide carbohydrate that is eventually broken down to glucose, all routes mentioned in the question can lead to each other.

149. **D** The supernatant at the top will contain the lighter viral protein coats that did not enter the host cell, while the much larger and heavier

bacterial cells (now also containing the injected viral DNA) will be in the pellet on the bottom.

150. **A** The radioactive sulfur used in Experiment 1 will be found in protein material (sulfur is not found in nucleic acids). Since the radioactive labeling involved the virus and not the bacteria, only viral proteins (which remained outside the host cell and were dislodged by agitation) will be labeled.

151. **C** Experiment 2 used radioactive phosphorus, a component of nucleic acids like DNA. As stated in the passage (and in Question 150), only the virus was labeled. Upon infection, the viral DNA is injected into the host cell. Therefore, C is the only possible answer.

152. **D** Two general points must be understood to answer this question properly: (1) Bacterial growth for many generations involves many cycles of cell division, and (2) DNA replication occurs with each cycle of division in a semiconservative manner. The infected bacterial cells have a limited amount of viral DNA inside them as they begin to be cultured. *No new strands* of DNA can be labeled since the bacterial medium contains only normal nutrients. As division continues for generations, a higher and higher percentage of cells will have their DNA synthesized only from ingredients in the fresh medium (and lower and lower percentages will contain labeled DNA that was present in the first generation of cells placed in the medium).

153. **B** The abilities to formulate hypotheses and to see which variable is being examined in an experimental design are important here. If the ability to produce a specific substance is lost, and that inability prevents growth on minimal medium, then adding that particular substance should enable the cells to grow again. Choice B is the only procedure that will identify the "lost" ability. Growing different strains together will always confound which strain needs what! Similarly, growing one strain on different media (when they are not minimal media) can be unfruitful and endless.

154. **B** The question states that different strains lack the ability to synthesize the same substance. By definition, different strains have mutations at different points in the genetic material. Therefore, since it is known that the synthesis of this "lost" substance requires many steps, it is not

unreasonable to hypothesize that each mutation may have affected a different gene coding for a different enzyme involved with a different step in the synthetic pathway! Choices A and C are irrelevant to the information addressed in the question.

155. **A** The 90 plants with light flowers are those with the double recessive genotype (*aa*). The frequency of this genotype in the population can be represented by q^2. Therefore, $90/1000 = q^2 = .09$. If $q^2 = .09$, then $q = .3$. It is known that if the frequency of the q allele is .3, so the frequency of the p allele must be .7 ($p + q = 1$).

156. **C** From the response to question 155, it was learned that the frequency of $p = .7$. Homozygous dominant individuals have a frequency of $p^2 = (.7)(.7) = .49$. This question asks for the *number of individuals* with this genotype. Thus, $.49 \times 1000$ individuals = 490.

157. **D** The proportion of heterozygous individuals will be:

$$2pq = 2(.7)(.3) = .42.$$

158. **D** All of the factors *would* have an effect on the number of each plant type (more dark flowers being preyed upon by caterpillars; more light flowers being pollinated by insects; more dark plant pollen being dispersed). Therefore, *none* of the choices will have *no effect*!

159. **C** One individual out of 2500 (.0004) has the double recessive genotype. Thus, $q^2 = .0004$, and $q = .02$. If $q = .02$, then $p = .98$. These are the allele frequencies in the population.

160. **D** It should be understood that "carriers" are heterozygotes. If $q = .02$, and $p = .98$, then $2pq = 2(.98)(.02) = .0392$. The number of individuals of this genotype will be $.0392 \times 2500 = 98$.

161. **B** New alleles *originate* by mutation. A new allele represents a change in the DNA sequence of the former allele. Any change in the DNA sequence is considered a mutation.

162. **A** Hypothesis A proposes that viruses (and their ancestors) were present *before* other heterotrophs and autotrophs. It is implied that these other forms were cellular, since the hypothesis goes on to state that viruses then adapted to a parasitic life-style (the heterotrophs and autotrophs became the hosts).

163. **B** It is known today that viruses can reproduce only after infecting a host cell. A proposal that places viruses earlier in evolutionary time than cellular forms would also have to suggest a different method of reproduction.

164. **B** Hypothesis C suggests that different viruses may have originated in different hosts. If some genes were identical to the hosts, this would be strong supportive evidence. Simply having the same type of nucleic acid is too broad a similarity (DNA? RNA?). Hypothesis B says nothing about differing origins for different viruses (". . . viruses evolved from *a* cellular form. . . .").

165. **D** Hypothesis B proposes that viruses evolved *from* a cellular form, as does Hypothesis C (nucleic acid that escaped *from* the host cell). As discussed in the explanation of question 162, Hypothesis A suggests that viruses predated cellular forms.

166. **C** Again, *genetic* similarity with the host cell is strong evidence for Hypothesis C. If other kinds of similarities were at issue (environmental, temperature, pH, etc.), the highly specialized host-parasite relationships emphasized by Hypothesis B would gain support as well.

167. **C** Hypothesis A refers to viruses preceding photosynthetic organisms (autotrophs), feeding on nutrients in the surrounding seas (absorption), and surviving this way (taking care of business on their own). What is *implied* is that they did not need a host cell for anything!

168. **C** Curve C shows that most individuals die (no longer survive) very early in life. The straight line in curve B suggests that survival, as well as the rate of death (mortality rate), is the same at all ages.

169. **B** Logical thinking will definitely help here. If most individuals die at a young age, mating at a late age will not do the trick! Similarly, long courtships would probably result in unconsummated love! However, by producing large numbers of offspring, *some* of them will survive to reproductive age (fish eggs, frog eggs, insects, etc.). Choice D seems irrelevant.

170. **B** The rate of mortality is equivalent at all ages *only* for curve B. This suggests that random events play a role in the death of individuals. If these events were not random, some ages would have greater survival (and some, higher mortality) than others.

171. **D** Severe drops in survival (increases in mortality) are clearly shown early in curve C and late in curve A.

172. **B** Species (or life-history patterns) represented by curve A show high survival (and low mortality) in early life. All choices *except* B include some variable that will contribute to low survival of young (predation of young, many offspring with limited resources, limited care, and high predation). Only choice B fits the survival data represented by curve A.

173. **C** Species represented by curve B have the same probability of dying (or living) regardless of age. Living 50% through the average maximum life span has no effect. In species represented by curve C, if an individual makes it to the halfway mark, there is little subsequent change in the chances of dying (the curve is basically a horizontal line after that point). In curve A species, however, once the halfway mark is reached, the chances of dying start to *increase*.

174. **D** Each curve ends (maximum life span) in the same place on the graph.

175. **C** After separation, both cells were able to develop into complete organisms. Thus, their fate was not yet determined. Additionally, materials outside the cells were not even considered in Experiment 1 (the gray crescent was part of the cytoplasm *inside* the cells). Clearly, the direction of the cleavage plane *did* have a powerful influence.

176. **D** As stated in the explanation of question 175, the gray crescent was an extremely important region in the cytoplasm. Choices B and C are irrelevant.

177. **D** The only piece of information relevant to this question is that the genes determining skin pattern are all located in the implanted nucleus donated by the spotted frog. All frogs will be spotted.

178. **A** Experiment 2 showed that even the nuclei from *adult* skin cells had the potential to produce complete organisms when implanted into an egg. Experiment 2 did not address the ques-

tion of cytoplasmic factors, so choice B is incorrect. As long as one adult cell nucleus produced an entire organism, totipotency is demonstrated, and choice C is eliminated as well. Choice D only addresses the cytoplasmic issue. The question asks about *any* findings from Experiment 2 (cytoplasmic influences—*no*, totipotency—*yes!*).

179. **C** Induction refers to the phenomenon of one group of cells influencing the development of other cells. This was clearly demonstrated in Experiment 3 (cytoplasmic factors inside the cell were not examined). Answers B and D imply that genetic factors have been affected by environmental conditions. However, the experiment provided no evidence that either statement is correct. The importance of environmental factors does not negate the effects of genetic factors. There clearly must be an interaction between the inducing factors and the genes in the developing cells. Similarly, a loss of totipotency would only be demonstrated if the induced cells were removed and then used unsuccessfully to grow a complete organism.

180. **D** The effects described in the passage (formation of notochord, neural plate, neural tube, etc.) mark the process of neurulation. This development of the nervous system begins after gastrulation, early in organogenesis.

181. **D** Cytoplasmic factors inside the cell (Experiment 1) and induction processes due to surrounding tissues outside the cell (Experiment 3) were shown to have significant effects on the genetic potential underlying development.

182. **C** Efficiency, in terms of modes of locomotion, is solely based on the energy costs of each mode at a particular size (body mass). At all sizes, swimming "costs" less than running and flying. The slopes of the lines suggest the rate of change in energy costs related to size.

183. **B** All that is needed to answer this question is the ability to read the graph. First, find 1 g on the *x*-axis (body mass), then look to see where the "flying line" intersects the *y*-axis (energy cost).

184. **B** On the graph, humans have a body mass just under 1000 g. At this body mass, the swimming line reflects the lowest energy cost (less than 1 J/kg/m).

185. **B** An examination of the graph reveals that for any single mode of locomotion, the energy costs decrease as body mass increases. This holds true for all three modes of locomotion.

186. **B** If each potential answer is identified on its appropriate line graph, the 1-g flyer has the greatest energy cost. This should in no way imply that the smaller animal spends more *total* energy. Efficiency refers to energy cost/body mass (J/kg/m).

187. **C** A large swimmer clearly is the most efficient "mover" among the possible choices. Again, in terms of J/kg/m, the blue whale wins it "flippers down."

188. **B** Pyrrole, pyridine, and pyrimidine contain the aromatic sextet. In pyrrole, the sigma bonds around N are formed by sp^2 hybrid orbitals. An N electron participates in each of the sigma bonds. The remaining N electrons are in an N 2p orbital which overlaps with the carbon 2p orbitals in the ring to form π bonds and the aromatic sextet. In pyridine, the nitrogen atom donates one electron to each of the two sigma bonds by use of sp^2 orbitals. The third sp^2 orbital contains two electrons, which are available for acids. One electron of N is present in a p orbital, which interacts with the carbon p orbitals to form the π structure and give rise to the aromatic sextet. The bonding of the N atoms in pyrimidine is equivalent to that in pyridine.

189. **D** See the explanation of question 188.

190. **D** See the explanation of question 188.

191. **A** Attack at position 2 gives three resonance structures.

Attack at position 3 gives only two.

192. **A** The pyridine ring behaves much like a benzene ring that is joined to strongly electron-withdrawing groups. Nucleophilic substitution occurs most readily at the 2— and 4— positions. Attack at the 4— position gives the following resonance stabilized carbanion:

The structure in which N carries the negative charge is particularly stable. A similar structure can be drawn for attack of the nucleophile at the 2 position.

193. **C** Piperidine is a secondary amine like dimethylamine. Pyridine is a stronger base than pyrrole but is much weaker than aliphatic amines.

194. **A** This bond must be broken in order to account for the labeled alcohol oxygen appearing in the ester.

195. **B** The mechanism of acidic hydrolysis must be the exact reverse of the mechanism of esterification catalyzed by acid. If a labeled oxygen of an alcohol appears in the ester. hydrolysis of the ester will form the labeled alcohol back again.

196. **C** Protonation of an ester yields:

The carbon is then rendered more susceptible to attack by a nucleophile because the oxygen will not need to carry a negative charge. The nucleophile in acidic hydrolysis is H_2O while in esterification the alcohol is the nucleophile.

197. **A** Special methods are often needed to prepare esters of tertiary alcohols or esters of acids containing bulky groups.

198. **D**

acyl group

199. **A**

200. **D** 3350 cm^{-1} —OH stretch (H—bonded)
1000 cm^{-1} C—O stretch
According to the table provided, the above two bonds are associated with alcohols.

201. **A** The ultraviolet spectrum of an unknown compound is used chiefly to identify conjugation or the presence of an aromatic group.

202. **C** Proton exchange occurs very rapidly in the presence of an acid or base. Consequently, the hydroxyl proton sees only an averaged chemical environment and thus gives rise to a singlet. If proton exchange is slowed, the hydroxyl proton signal will be split by nearby protons. The hydroxyl proton will also cause splitting in the signals of these nearby protons.

203. **B**

204. **C** IR is the best method to detect a $-\overset{|}{C}=O$ group. The strong band due to C=O stretching is generally seen at about 1700 cm^{-1} where it seldom is hidden by other absorptions.

205. **C** A fundamental understanding of the relationship between genes and cell function is required. The uncoiled DNA exposes the nucleotide sequence of the gene so that it can be transcribed and translated into the gene product: a protein (or protein subunit). Since different parts of the genome are constantly being activated (depending on the needs of the cell and the needs of the organism), the chromosomes must constantly have their active genes exposed (uncoiled).

206. **C** Basic knowledge of respiratory anatomy and the gas laws are required. When the diaphragm contracts (moves downward), the volume in the thoracic cavity (and lungs) increases, causing the pressure to decrease. As a result, the air outside the body is under higher pressure than the air in the lungs, and air rushes in (inspiration).

207. **B** A general understanding of blood pressure concepts, and the factors which influence blood pressure, is required. If peripheral resistance reflects friction between the blood and the walls of the blood vessels, both narrower blood vessels (vasoconstriction) and a thicker, more viscous blood will increase peripheral resistance.

208. **B** Basic knowledge of central nervous system (CNS) anatomy and the protective coverings of the CNS are required. The organs of the CNS (brain and spinal cord) have hollow regions (ventricles and spinal canal, respectively). The CNS also has three layers of protective covering (the meninges). The question states that cerebrospinal fluid circulates in these areas. Thus B is the correct answer. The spinal nerves and cranial nerves are not considered part of the CNS.

209. **B** The question requires a solid foundation in Mendelian genetics and a familiarity with the interpretation of pedigrees. By process of elimination, the trait must be an autosomal recessive trait. The affected female in the second generation (third from the right on the second line) could not have an autosomal dominant trait if neither parent has the allele (both parents are unaffected). Similarly, the same affected female could not result from such a cross if the trait is either sex-linked dominant or sex-linked recessive (the father would also have to be affected in either case). Only an autosomal recessive trait successfully works its way through the pedigree in the pattern presented.

210. **C** A basic knowledge of the immune system is required. Although specific defense vs. nonspecific defense is defined in the question, one still must have some understanding of the roles of the various choices. Phagocytosis by macrophages, inflammation, and interferon are all general, nonspecific responses by the immune system. Each type of antibody, on the other hand, is normally produced in response to a specific antigen (usually associated with a specific invading organism).

211. **A** This question calls for a general understanding of the function of enzymes, as well as the characteristics of chemical reactions. Enzymes catalyze reactions by lowering the activation energy required to initiate them. They speed reactions rather than slow them. Enzymes do not produce energy, nor can they make an endergonic reaction exergonic.

212. **D** Familiarity with brain structure and function is required. Although most information in the question relates to the effects of Parkinsonism, the question really asks which part of the brain is associated with "intelligence, vision, and hearing . . . unaffected by this disorder. . . ."

213. **B** A familiarity with the events of meiosis and the factors that influence sex determination are helpful, but a clear understanding about the pattern of inheritance for sex-linked traits is essential. Since normal females have two X-chromosomes, Turner's Syndrome females (XO) *do not* have the same probabilities of inheriting sex-linked disorders (they actually have the same chances as males).

214. **C** A basic understanding of the events involved with muscle contraction is required. Choices A, B, and D are all necessary for a muscle cell to return to its resting state. The troponin-tropomyosin complex must return to its original position on the actin (the position it occupied before calcium was released from the sarcoplasmic reticulum). When the complex *detaches*, muscle *contraction* occurs.

215. **C** If only $(CH_3)_3CCHO$ and a strong base are present, no reaction can occur. For an aldol condensation to occur, the aldehyde or ketone must contain an α-hydrogen. The α-hydrogen is acidic and will combine with the base to form a carbanion. The carbanion is the nucleophile in the reaction that attacks the carbonyl carbon of another aldehyde or ketone molecule. The generally accepted mechanism follows, using acetone as an example.

216. **D** The amino acid residues are joined by amide linkages:

$$-NH-\overset{\overset{\displaystyle O}{\|}}{C}-$$

217. **D** Glycerol: a fat is a triglyceride.

$$
\begin{array}{l}
H_2C-O-\overset{\overset{\displaystyle O}{\|}}{C}-R \\
\,\,\,\,| \\
HC-O-\overset{\overset{\displaystyle O}{\|}}{C}-R' \\
\,\,| \\
H_2C-O-\overset{\overset{\displaystyle O}{\|}}{C}-R''
\end{array}
$$

218. **B**

219. **D**

PRACTICE EXAM III

	<u>Time</u>
Verbal Reasoning Questions 1–65	85 minutes
Physical Sciences Questions 66–142	100 minutes
Writing Sample 2 Essays	60 minutes
Biological Sciences Questions 143–219	100 minutes

PRACTICE EXAM III

Time:

Verbal Reasoning   85 minutes
Questions 1–65

Physical Sciences   100 minutes
Questions 66–142

Writing Sample   60 minutes
2 Topics

Biological Sciences   100 minutes
Questions 143–219

ANSWER SHEET
PRACTICE EXAM III

VERBAL REASONING

1. Ⓐ Ⓑ Ⓒ Ⓓ
2. Ⓐ Ⓑ Ⓒ Ⓓ
3. Ⓐ Ⓑ Ⓒ Ⓓ
4. Ⓐ Ⓑ Ⓒ Ⓓ
5. Ⓐ Ⓑ Ⓒ Ⓓ
6. Ⓐ Ⓑ Ⓒ Ⓓ
7. Ⓐ Ⓑ Ⓒ Ⓓ
8. Ⓐ Ⓑ Ⓒ Ⓓ
9. Ⓐ Ⓑ Ⓒ Ⓓ
10. Ⓐ Ⓑ Ⓒ Ⓓ
11. Ⓐ Ⓑ Ⓒ Ⓓ
12. Ⓐ Ⓑ Ⓒ Ⓓ
13. Ⓐ Ⓑ Ⓒ Ⓓ
14. Ⓐ Ⓑ Ⓒ Ⓓ
15. Ⓐ Ⓑ Ⓒ Ⓓ
16. Ⓐ Ⓑ Ⓒ Ⓓ
17. Ⓐ Ⓑ Ⓒ Ⓓ
18. Ⓐ Ⓑ Ⓒ Ⓓ
19. Ⓐ Ⓑ Ⓒ Ⓓ
20. Ⓐ Ⓑ Ⓒ Ⓓ
21. Ⓐ Ⓑ Ⓒ Ⓓ
22. Ⓐ Ⓑ Ⓒ Ⓓ
23. Ⓐ Ⓑ Ⓒ Ⓓ
24. Ⓐ Ⓑ Ⓒ Ⓓ
25. Ⓐ Ⓑ Ⓒ Ⓓ
26. Ⓐ Ⓑ Ⓒ Ⓓ
27. Ⓐ Ⓑ Ⓒ Ⓓ
28. Ⓐ Ⓑ Ⓒ Ⓓ
29. Ⓐ Ⓑ Ⓒ Ⓓ
30. Ⓐ Ⓑ Ⓒ Ⓓ
31. Ⓐ Ⓑ Ⓒ Ⓓ
32. Ⓐ Ⓑ Ⓒ Ⓓ
33. Ⓐ Ⓑ Ⓒ Ⓓ
34. Ⓐ Ⓑ Ⓒ Ⓓ
35. Ⓐ Ⓑ Ⓒ Ⓓ
36. Ⓐ Ⓑ Ⓒ Ⓓ
37. Ⓐ Ⓑ Ⓒ Ⓓ
38. Ⓐ Ⓑ Ⓒ Ⓓ
39. Ⓐ Ⓑ Ⓒ Ⓓ
40. Ⓐ Ⓑ Ⓒ Ⓓ
41. Ⓐ Ⓑ Ⓒ Ⓓ
42. Ⓐ Ⓑ Ⓒ Ⓓ

43. Ⓐ Ⓑ Ⓒ Ⓓ
44. Ⓐ Ⓑ Ⓒ Ⓓ
45. Ⓐ Ⓑ Ⓒ Ⓓ
46. Ⓐ Ⓑ Ⓒ Ⓓ
47. Ⓐ Ⓑ Ⓒ Ⓓ
48. Ⓐ Ⓑ Ⓒ Ⓓ
49. Ⓐ Ⓑ Ⓒ Ⓓ
50. Ⓐ Ⓑ Ⓒ Ⓓ
51. Ⓐ Ⓑ Ⓒ Ⓓ
52. Ⓐ Ⓑ Ⓒ Ⓓ
53. Ⓐ Ⓑ Ⓒ Ⓓ
54. Ⓐ Ⓑ Ⓒ Ⓓ
55. Ⓐ Ⓑ Ⓒ Ⓓ
56. Ⓐ Ⓑ Ⓒ Ⓓ
57. Ⓐ Ⓑ Ⓒ Ⓓ
58. Ⓐ Ⓑ Ⓒ Ⓓ
59. Ⓐ Ⓑ Ⓒ Ⓓ
60. Ⓐ Ⓑ Ⓒ Ⓓ
61. Ⓐ Ⓑ Ⓒ Ⓓ
62. Ⓐ Ⓑ Ⓒ Ⓓ
63. Ⓐ Ⓑ Ⓒ Ⓓ
64. Ⓐ Ⓑ Ⓒ Ⓓ
65. Ⓐ Ⓑ Ⓒ Ⓓ

PHYSICAL SCIENCES

66. Ⓐ Ⓑ Ⓒ Ⓓ
67. Ⓐ Ⓑ Ⓒ Ⓓ
68. Ⓐ Ⓑ Ⓒ Ⓓ
69. Ⓐ Ⓑ Ⓒ Ⓓ
70. Ⓐ Ⓑ Ⓒ Ⓓ
71. Ⓐ Ⓑ Ⓒ Ⓓ
72. Ⓐ Ⓑ Ⓒ Ⓓ
73. Ⓐ Ⓑ Ⓒ Ⓓ
74. Ⓐ Ⓑ Ⓒ Ⓓ
75. Ⓐ Ⓑ Ⓒ Ⓓ
76. Ⓐ Ⓑ Ⓒ Ⓓ
77. Ⓐ Ⓑ Ⓒ Ⓓ
78. Ⓐ Ⓑ Ⓒ Ⓓ
79. Ⓐ Ⓑ Ⓒ Ⓓ
80. Ⓐ Ⓑ Ⓒ Ⓓ
81. Ⓐ Ⓑ Ⓒ Ⓓ
82. Ⓐ Ⓑ Ⓒ Ⓓ
83. Ⓐ Ⓑ Ⓒ Ⓓ
84. Ⓐ Ⓑ Ⓒ Ⓓ
85. Ⓐ Ⓑ Ⓒ Ⓓ
86. Ⓐ Ⓑ Ⓒ Ⓓ
87. Ⓐ Ⓑ Ⓒ Ⓓ
88. Ⓐ Ⓑ Ⓒ Ⓓ
89. Ⓐ Ⓑ Ⓒ Ⓓ
90. Ⓐ Ⓑ Ⓒ Ⓓ
91. Ⓐ Ⓑ Ⓒ Ⓓ
92. Ⓐ Ⓑ Ⓒ Ⓓ
93. Ⓐ Ⓑ Ⓒ Ⓓ
94. Ⓐ Ⓑ Ⓒ Ⓓ
95. Ⓐ Ⓑ Ⓒ Ⓓ
96. Ⓐ Ⓑ Ⓒ Ⓓ
97. Ⓐ Ⓑ Ⓒ Ⓓ
98. Ⓐ Ⓑ Ⓒ Ⓓ
99. Ⓐ Ⓑ Ⓒ Ⓓ
100. Ⓐ Ⓑ Ⓒ Ⓓ
101. Ⓐ Ⓑ Ⓒ Ⓓ
102. Ⓐ Ⓑ Ⓒ Ⓓ
103. Ⓐ Ⓑ Ⓒ Ⓓ
104. Ⓐ Ⓑ Ⓒ Ⓓ
105. Ⓐ Ⓑ Ⓒ Ⓓ
106. Ⓐ Ⓑ Ⓒ Ⓓ
107. Ⓐ Ⓑ Ⓒ Ⓓ

BIOLOGICAL SCIENCES

108. Ⓐ Ⓑ Ⓒ Ⓓ	143. Ⓐ Ⓑ Ⓒ Ⓓ	192. Ⓐ Ⓑ Ⓒ Ⓓ
109. Ⓐ Ⓑ Ⓒ Ⓓ	144. Ⓐ Ⓑ Ⓒ Ⓓ	193. Ⓐ Ⓑ Ⓒ Ⓓ
110. Ⓐ Ⓑ Ⓒ Ⓓ	145. Ⓐ Ⓑ Ⓒ Ⓓ	194. Ⓐ Ⓑ Ⓒ Ⓓ
111. Ⓐ Ⓑ Ⓒ Ⓓ	146. Ⓐ Ⓑ Ⓒ Ⓓ	195. Ⓐ Ⓑ Ⓒ Ⓓ
112. Ⓐ Ⓑ Ⓒ Ⓓ	147. Ⓐ Ⓑ Ⓒ Ⓓ	196. Ⓐ Ⓑ Ⓒ Ⓓ
113. Ⓐ Ⓑ Ⓒ Ⓓ	148. Ⓐ Ⓑ Ⓒ Ⓓ	197. Ⓐ Ⓑ Ⓒ Ⓓ
114. Ⓐ Ⓑ Ⓒ Ⓓ	149. Ⓐ Ⓑ Ⓒ Ⓓ	198. Ⓐ Ⓑ Ⓒ Ⓓ
115. Ⓐ Ⓑ Ⓒ Ⓓ	150. Ⓐ Ⓑ Ⓒ Ⓓ	199. Ⓐ Ⓑ Ⓒ Ⓓ
116. Ⓐ Ⓑ Ⓒ Ⓓ	151. Ⓐ Ⓑ Ⓒ Ⓓ	200. Ⓐ Ⓑ Ⓒ Ⓓ
117. Ⓐ Ⓑ Ⓒ Ⓓ	152. Ⓐ Ⓑ Ⓒ Ⓓ	201. Ⓐ Ⓑ Ⓒ Ⓓ
118. Ⓐ Ⓑ Ⓒ Ⓓ	153. Ⓐ Ⓑ Ⓒ Ⓓ	202. Ⓐ Ⓑ Ⓒ Ⓓ
119. Ⓐ Ⓑ Ⓒ Ⓓ	154. Ⓐ Ⓑ Ⓒ Ⓓ	203. Ⓐ Ⓑ Ⓒ Ⓓ
120. Ⓐ Ⓑ Ⓒ Ⓓ	155. Ⓐ Ⓑ Ⓒ Ⓓ	204. Ⓐ Ⓑ Ⓒ Ⓓ
121. Ⓐ Ⓑ Ⓒ Ⓓ	156. Ⓐ Ⓑ Ⓒ Ⓓ	205. Ⓐ Ⓑ Ⓒ Ⓓ
122. Ⓐ Ⓑ Ⓒ Ⓓ	157. Ⓐ Ⓑ Ⓒ Ⓓ	206. Ⓐ Ⓑ Ⓒ Ⓓ
123. Ⓐ Ⓑ Ⓒ Ⓓ	158. Ⓐ Ⓑ Ⓒ Ⓓ	207. Ⓐ Ⓑ Ⓒ Ⓓ
124. Ⓐ Ⓑ Ⓒ Ⓓ	159. Ⓐ Ⓑ Ⓒ Ⓓ	208. Ⓐ Ⓑ Ⓒ Ⓓ
125. Ⓐ Ⓑ Ⓒ Ⓓ	160. Ⓐ Ⓑ Ⓒ Ⓓ	209. Ⓐ Ⓑ Ⓒ Ⓓ
126. Ⓐ Ⓑ Ⓒ Ⓓ	161. Ⓐ Ⓑ Ⓒ Ⓓ	210. Ⓐ Ⓑ Ⓒ Ⓓ
127. Ⓐ Ⓑ Ⓒ Ⓓ	162. Ⓐ Ⓑ Ⓒ Ⓓ	211. Ⓐ Ⓑ Ⓒ Ⓓ
128. Ⓐ Ⓑ Ⓒ Ⓓ	163. Ⓐ Ⓑ Ⓒ Ⓓ	212. Ⓐ Ⓑ Ⓒ Ⓓ
129. Ⓐ Ⓑ Ⓒ Ⓓ	164. Ⓐ Ⓑ Ⓒ Ⓓ	213. Ⓐ Ⓑ Ⓒ Ⓓ
130. Ⓐ Ⓑ Ⓒ Ⓓ	165. Ⓐ Ⓑ Ⓒ Ⓓ	214. Ⓐ Ⓑ Ⓒ Ⓓ
131. Ⓐ Ⓑ Ⓒ Ⓓ	166. Ⓐ Ⓑ Ⓒ Ⓓ	215. Ⓐ Ⓑ Ⓒ Ⓓ
132. Ⓐ Ⓑ Ⓒ Ⓓ	167. Ⓐ Ⓑ Ⓒ Ⓓ	216. Ⓐ Ⓑ Ⓒ Ⓓ
133. Ⓐ Ⓑ Ⓒ Ⓓ	168. Ⓐ Ⓑ Ⓒ Ⓓ	217. Ⓐ Ⓑ Ⓒ Ⓓ
134. Ⓐ Ⓑ Ⓒ Ⓓ	169. Ⓐ Ⓑ Ⓒ Ⓓ	218. Ⓐ Ⓑ Ⓒ Ⓓ
135. Ⓐ Ⓑ Ⓒ Ⓓ	170. Ⓐ Ⓑ Ⓒ Ⓓ	219. Ⓐ Ⓑ Ⓒ Ⓓ
136. Ⓐ Ⓑ Ⓒ Ⓓ	171. Ⓐ Ⓑ Ⓒ Ⓓ	
137. Ⓐ Ⓑ Ⓒ Ⓓ	172. Ⓐ Ⓑ Ⓒ Ⓓ	
138. Ⓐ Ⓑ Ⓒ Ⓓ	173. Ⓐ Ⓑ Ⓒ Ⓓ	
139. Ⓐ Ⓑ Ⓒ Ⓓ	174. Ⓐ Ⓑ Ⓒ Ⓓ	
140. Ⓐ Ⓑ Ⓒ Ⓓ	175. Ⓐ Ⓑ Ⓒ Ⓓ	
141. Ⓐ Ⓑ Ⓒ Ⓓ	176. Ⓐ Ⓑ Ⓒ Ⓓ	
142. Ⓐ Ⓑ Ⓒ Ⓓ	177. Ⓐ Ⓑ Ⓒ Ⓓ	
	178. Ⓐ Ⓑ Ⓒ Ⓓ	
	179. Ⓐ Ⓑ Ⓒ Ⓓ	
	180. Ⓐ Ⓑ Ⓒ Ⓓ	
	181. Ⓐ Ⓑ Ⓒ Ⓓ	
	182. Ⓐ Ⓑ Ⓒ Ⓓ	
	183. Ⓐ Ⓑ Ⓒ Ⓓ	
	184. Ⓐ Ⓑ Ⓒ Ⓓ	
	185. Ⓐ Ⓑ Ⓒ Ⓓ	
	186. Ⓐ Ⓑ Ⓒ Ⓓ	
	187. Ⓐ Ⓑ Ⓒ Ⓓ	
	188. Ⓐ Ⓑ Ⓒ Ⓓ	
	189. Ⓐ Ⓑ Ⓒ Ⓓ	
	190. Ⓐ Ⓑ Ⓒ Ⓓ	
	191. Ⓐ Ⓑ Ⓒ Ⓓ	

Writing Sample 1

END OF PART 1

Writing Sample 2

_____

_____

_____

_____

_____

_____

_____

_____

_____

_____

_____

_____

_____

_____

_____

_____

_____

_____

_____

_____

_____

_____

_____

_____

END OF PART 1

VERBAL REASONING

Time: 85 Minutes
Questions 1–65

Directions: There are nine passages in this test. Each passage is followed by questions based on its content. After reading a passage, choose the one best answer to each question and indicate your selection by blackening the corresponding space on your answer sheet.

Passage I (Questions 1–7)

When some 12.5 million tomato seeds returned to earth in February 1985 after almost a year in space, several thousand American students from fifth grade through university level anxiously awaited their arrival
(5) with pots and trowels at the ready. They wanted to find out whether tomatoes grown from the tiny space travelers would be any different from their earthbound counterparts.

All 12.5 million of the seeds were carried aboard
(10) Space Shuttle Mission 41-C in April 1984 and placed in orbit inside NASA's Long Duration Exposure Facility (LDEF), a free-flying, 12-sided structure loaded with experiments designed to test results of continuous exposure to outer space. When the LDEF was recovered
(15) early in 1985, the seeds—after the first known opportunity for long-duration exposure of living tissue—were divided up in packets of fifty among hundreds of schools across America. Students in science classes were to plant them and compare their growth results with earthbound
(20) plants. Control planting of earthbound tomato seeds began in the fall of 1984. Similar plants of the "seeds from Zero G"—the space-exposed specimens—began about the fall of 1985.

There were no "cookbook" rules governing how
(25) the experiments were to be carried out or observed by the students, other than the requirement of strictly scientific methodology. At the conclusion of the experimentation, student reports describing each school's results were tabulated in a summary report by NASA
(30) headquarters and made generally available upon request. The two-year experiment, named SEEDS (Space Exposed Experiment Developed for Students), was jointly sponsored by NASA and the Park Seed Company of Greenwood, South Carolina, supplier of the
(35) seeds.

Like all great ideas, this one was born in the mind of one imaginative individual. Back in 1978, George B. Park, president of the Park Seed Company of Green-

wood, S.C., was reading an article in *Scientific Ameri-*
(40) *can* magazine about the space shuttles, called "Getaway Specials," that NASA was preparing to launch from time to time into outer space, filled with scientific experiments. His inquiries led him to the Goddard Space Flight Center's Clark Porty, administrative officer for
(45) the Getaway Specials. Porty accepted Park's idea for a two-part container as a valid experiment. One of the seed containers was to be open to vacuum exposure, the other not.

Soon after that experiment, in the summer of
(50) 1983, Park had a visit from Bill Kinard of the Langley Research Center, Science Director for the LDEF projects. Kinard wanted to know if Park's company would be willing to enter into a joint venture with the Langley Research Center to put a large number of seeds
(55) onto the LDEF as a project involving the students of America, with part of the payload to be the company's own. Says Park, "I said 'yes' immediately, without thinking."

Control experiments back on earth included not
(60) only the earthbound seeds planted by the students, but also a batch of similar seeds kept in Greenwood at the seed company, and another batch in an air-conditioned area at the Kennedy Space Center at Cape Canaveral.

Park adds that one of the many benefits of the
(65) experiment for exobiologists (scientists who study possibilities of life in outer space) is knowledge gained about whether life forms could travel by passive means from one ecosystem or planet to another without a spaceship. If the seeds exposed to both vacuum and
(70) high radiation come through with little or no damage, it opens up questions (and may provide some answers) about the origins and destinations of primitive life forms. For example, scientists could extrapolate from the results of the experiment how many years organic
(75) matter might float in space and still be viable. Says Park, "If only *one* primitive life form, say a spore, or a bacterium or a virus, can live for 100,000 years, then it could get from one system to another."

But this is only one possible avenue of thought (80) arising from the experiment. What new connections might be made by the thousands of students participating in SEEDS? Their horizons are as unlimited as outer space.

1. According to the article, an exobiologist is a scientist who studies:

   A. seeds.
   B. the effects of space radiation on living things.
   C. the possibility of life in outer space.
   D. the external structures of living things.

2. The reason for sending the seeds into outer space was to test the effects on the seeds of:

   A. continuous exposure to outer space.
   B. ultraviolet light.
   C. weightlessness.
   D. low-level radiation.

3. Upon their return to earth, the seeds were distributed to:

   A. 12.5 million students from fifth grade to college level.
   B. fifty schools across America.
   C. a laboratory jointly operated by Park Seed Company and Langley Research Center.
   D. several thousand American students.

4. Which of the following rules were students to follow when doing their experiments?

   I. They were to compare growth rates only.
   II. They were to report their results honestly.
   III. They were to follow scientific methodology.

   A. I only
   B. II only
   C. III only
   D. I and II only

5. Results of the student experiments with space-exposed seeds were:

   A. submitted to *Scientific American* magazine.
   B. used by Park Seed Company to develop new strains of tomato plants.

C. tabulated in a summary report by NASA.
D. closely guarded until the end of the two-year experimental period.

6. According to the article, which of the following are the two most important facts to be learned from sending seeds into outer space?

   A. Some seeds are more able to survive space than others, and that seeds exposed to radiation in space are dangerous to humans.
   B. Astronauts can raise their own food in space, and such food has the same nutritional value as that grown on earth.
   C. Life forms other than seeds can survive in space, and they can survive for an indefinite period of time.
   D. Seeds can survive the vacuum of space and the high levels of radiation in space with little or no damage.

7. Based on the article, it would be reasonable to assume that the author's attitude toward other similar projects would be:

   A. strongly opposed.
   B. mildly opposed.
   C. mildly supportive.
   D. strongly supportive.

Passage II (Questions 8–14)

James Madison College of Michigan State University offers students a liberal education concentrated on public affairs. The college received support from the National Endowment for the Humanities in 1984 to (5) bring more humanities study into the upper level courses in social sciences.

The proposal demonstrates that a foundation for the project exists in the successful integration of the humanities and the social sciences in some parts of the (10) Madison College curriculum. In one field of concentration, for example—justice, morality, and constitutional democracy—great books form the core of the curriculum. Students read Plato, Aristotle, Machiavelli, Hobbes, Rousseau, Hegel, and Nietzsche or Weber. By (15) pairing faculty seminars and other faculty development activities with a revision of upper level courses, the Madison faculty is working to increase the humanities content of other areas of the curriculum.

Faculty seminars have been conducted by (20) Sheldon Wolin, who assigned readings by Hannah Arendt, Martin Heidegger, and Michael Oakeshott, and by philosopher Alan Bloom, who led faculty in an examination of liberal education and the study of the texts.

Although a separate, well-defined plan was pre-
(25) sented for each activity, the proposal made clear that the project was being undertaken as an integrated effort to revitalize the college's dedication to providing a liberal arts education to its students. The proposal states, "We expect these activities to sharpen our collective
(30) understanding of the role of the humanities in the study of public affairs, contribute to faculty development, improve individual courses, and make our upper level curricula more vital and coherent. Accordingly, at the outset of the project, we emphasize those activities that
(35) deepen our common perspective and enhance our individual expertise; in the later stages, we emphasize those that are aimed at course and curricular revision." Panelists' reactions demonstrated their admiration for the strong, unified goal toward which all activities of the
(40) project were directed.

8. Which of the following is mentioned as one approach to the development of an integrated curriculum at James Madison College?

   A. Use classics in a core course.
   B. Have faculty seminars as coursework for lower level freshmen and sophomore students.
   C. Rotate faculty members who lecture in order to revitalize the classes.
   D. Increase the public affairs content of upper level courses.

9. The proposal to expand humanities study for upper division students at James Madison College of Michigan State University confirms the commitment by the college to:

   A. widen students' knowledge by focusing on specific great works of literature and philosophy.
   B. further increase the core courses in the humanities through faculty involvement in curriculum and team teaching.
   C. enhance student understanding and appreciation of the curriculum with its strong emphasis on challenging readings and sensitized faculty.
   D. upgrade its standards in offering a liberal arts education.

10. It can be inferred from the article that the author:

    A. does not like the integration of curriculum that is taking place at Madison College.
    B. is impressed by what is being done with the curriculum at Madison College.
    C. has no clear opinion about what is being done at Madison College.
    D. believes that despite some positive aspects to what has been done to the curriculum at Madison College, negative aspects outweigh the positive.

11. The foundation of the project described in the article is to integrate:

    A. public affairs with a liberal education.
    B. English with humanities.
    C. humanities and social science.
    D. humanities and public education.

12. Which of the following are recognized as goals of the project?

    I. Increased faculty development activities
    II. Increased attention to individual student needs
    III. Extensive revision of upper level curricula

    A. I only
    B. III only
    C. I and II only
    D. I and III only

13. The attitude of the panelists toward the integrated curriculum is best described by which of the following statements?

    A. The panelists were in favor of the integrated curriculum proposal.
    B. The panelists were opposed to the integrated curriculum proposal.
    C. The panelists supported the idea of an integrated curriculum but believed the current curriculum needed adjustment.
    D. The panelists preferred a curriculum that integrated science and humanities.

14. The article provides an example of a field of concentration in which students read works by each of the following **EXCEPT:**

A. Spinoza and Kant.
B. Machiavelli and Hobbes.
C. Nietzsche and Weber.
D. Plato and Aristotle.

Passage III (Questions 15–20)

The possibility of climate change presents a unique challenge for American electric utilities. If there is, indeed, a significant warming of the earth's climate due to rising concentrations of greenhouse gases, utili-
(5) ties may be affected at three distinct levels. First, they will inevitably play an important role in any broad societal response to climate change and will have an opportunity to forge a new relationship with their customers to achieve common goals. Second, utilities rec-
(10) ognize that their industry will be among those whose operations are most deeply affected by a changing climate, perhaps within the time frame of current planning for construction of new facilities. Finally, electric utilities are concerned that costly and potentially coun-
(15) terproductive regulations may be promulgated before a rational basis for policy making is achieved.

An overriding consideration in each of these three areas is the number of uncertainties that remain in the scientific understanding of the Greenhouse Effect and
(20) the likely effectiveness of various countermeasures. In particular, the apparent 0.6 degree C, 1 degree F rise in average global temperature over the last century lies within the long-term range of natural variability, although the recent rate of increase seems rapid. Current
(25) models suggest that a warming trend of this magnitude could result solely from the increases in atmospheric CO_2 and other greenhouse gases (e.g., nitrous oxide, methane, chlorofluorocarbons, and ozone). However, the observed rise in temperature over the last century
(30) has not been steady and has been marked by unexplained periods of cooling.

Research is needed to tell us not only when to act but also how to act. Although the focus of recent debates has been primarily on strategies to reduce emis-
(35) sions, it is not at all clear that the point of emissions is the best place for intervention. There is, in fact, a wide variety of options potentially available for countering the Greenhouse Effect:

(1) *Reducing greenhouse gas production:* Ex-
(40) amples are reducing energy use, fuel switching from coal to natural gas, increasing the use of nonfossil sources, and reducing the rate of deforestation.

(2) *Removing greenhouse gases from effluents*
(45) *or the atmosphere:* Examples are removing CO_2 from power plant emissions as well as starting forestation programs.

(3) *Making countervailing modifications in climate and weather:* One example is cloud seeding;
(50) another more speculative example is changing the atmosphere's reflectivity by releasing particles in the stratosphere.

(4) *Adapting to changing climate:* Examples are heating and cooling of buildings, compensa-
(55) tion of disadvantaged regions, and changing of agricultural practices.

Because of the large amounts of capital and time required to build generation and transmission facilities, electric utilities must plan for decades ahead. Recent
(60) studies indicate that if significant climate change occurs, some effects may be felt within the current planning horizon for utilities. The need for more air conditioning during longer, hotter summers, for example, would not only raise the annual demand for electric
(65) energy but increase demand peaks as well. Utility planners must therefore consider both the likelihood of having to build new power plants to meet higher peak demand and the probable need to purchase more fuel for increased generations.

(70) Planners will also need to consider potential changes in energy supply resulting from climate change. Stream flows that affect the availability of hydroelectric energy, for example, depend on both the amount and timing of precipitation, which could be altered in
(75) some regions by even small changes in the average global temperature. In addition, the reliability of electricity delivery systems could be affected by shifts in the frequency and intensity of weather extremes, such as tornadoes, hurricanes, and severe storms. Power plant
(80) operations in some coastal regions could also be hampered by even a moderate rise in the sea level resulting from thermal expansion of the oceans and possibly increased melting of glaciers and Antarctic ice.

To meet these challenges, utilities will need to adopt
(85) more sophisticated strategies of risk management. Although many of the effects of climate change remain unpredictable, the cost of adapting will be much less if some prudent contingency plans are made well in advance.

15. According to the author, which of the following **MAY** be a consequence of the Greenhouse Effect on electric utilities?

A. A reduction in the need for heat
B. Institution of many useless regulations

C. Disappearance of many of the sources for producing electricity

D. Blaming the utilities themselves for the Greenhouse Effect

16. In planning for the future, the author suggests that utility planners take into account all of the following **EXCEPT:**

A. changes in energy supplies due to climate changes.

B. building new power plants to meet higher consumer demands.

C. encouraging future generations to decrease energy usage.

D. adopting additional sophisticated approaches for risk management.

17. The author states that over the last century the earth's temperature has risen:

A. 1 degree C.

B. .6 degrees F.

C. .6 degrees K.

D. .6 degrees C.

18. Which one of the following is **NOT** considered a strategy for the reduction of gas emission into the air?

A. Heating and cooling buildings

B. Removing greenhouse gases from the atmosphere

C. Cloud seeding

D. Changing consumer consumption

19. Following the author's logic, it would be reasonable to assume that:

A. awareness of the Greenhouse Effect must take the form of consumer advocacy.

B. the future of the electrical supply is in imminent danger.

C. a concerted effort between government and utility planning must be a joint venture.

D. the utility industry must gear up for intense research.

20. According to the article, which of the following are considered greenhouse gases?

I. Oxygen and hydrogen
II. Helium, radon and carbon monoxide, hydrocarbon
III. Nitrous oxide, methane, chlorofluorocarbons, and ozone

A. I only

B. II only

C. III only

D. I and II only

Passage IV (Questions 21–26)

Like so many other areas of American life, the field of aging offers opportunities to go into business for yourself. Gerontological consulting is coming into its own with the growing demand for information about (5) older persons' spending patterns, use of leisure time, housing preferences, eating habits, and the like.

So intense is the interest in the older consumer that many of America's largest companies have launched advertising campaigns targeted at adults over (10) 50. But their perceptions of older people leave a lot to be desired, observes David Wolfe in the July 1987 issue of *American Demographics*. "Few marketers understand older Americans," he says, "and their advertising campaigns repel the very people they're trying (15) to attract." Age-grading of products and services intended for older people usually backfires, he warns. A marketing strategy that presents the product or service as an opportunity for personal growth is far more likely to succeed.

(20)   In an effort to link gerontologists with the business community—showing advertisers how to avoid age stereotypes, for example—the American Society on Aging has organized a Business Forum on Aging that includes representatives from Bank of America, Sandoz (25) Corporation, American Express, Marriott Corporation, Edison Electric Institute, and others.

"Turning the hunger for information about older people into a business opportunity for gerontologists requires ingenuity and an eye for a suitable market (30) niche," says Nancy Peppard of Peppard Associates. Taking her own advice, she organized her firm in two divisions. One advises corporations about marketing, advertising, and sensitivity training for employees; the other advises health-care facilities about setting up special (35) units for dementia patients.

Jean Coyle, founder of the International Association of Gerontological Entrepreneurs, warns of the challenge of setting up your own firm. The most com-

monly mentioned issue is the tremendous amount of
(40) time it takes to set up a small business. "There's just
not enough time to do it all," she says. Entrepreneurs
are hard pressed to manage the business end of the op-
eration as well as provide a professional service.

The consulting business is fiercely competitive,
(45) observes Jane Yurrow of Leo, Inc., a firm that specializes in senior housing. Her advice is to plan on putting
a lot of effort into marketing. Marketing skills are important, agrees Susan Hartenbaum of Aging Information Services. Personal style is at least as important as
(50) subject expertise in bringing in business, she adds. A
warm, outgoing, engaging personality helps in making
calls to prospective clients in their language, says Susan. Put yourself in their shoes, she advises. Your goal
as a consultant is to help clients see their situation in a
(55) new light and help them develop an appropriate solution. Imposing your own expertise is one of the pitfalls
to avoid.

Private case management offers excellent opportunities for gerontological entrepreneurs with clinical
(60) expertise. Case managers assist older persons and their
families for a fee, offering such help as information
and referral, brokering of services, and counseling. They
personalize their services, providing as much or as little
assistance as the client wants. Private case managers
(65) generally have at least some graduate education in a
human service discipline and substantial experience
working with the elderly. More often than not, they are
social workers, although nurses, psychologists, and gerontologists operate case management firms, too.

(70) Barbara Kane, a clinical social worker in private
practice with Aging Network Services in Bethesda,
Maryland, ticks off the professional skills important for
success in this field: counseling skills, notably the ability to develop trust and confidence; assessment skills;
(75) the ability to involve the client and facilitate decision
making; the ability to resolve conflicts and negotiate
agreements; and the ability to act as a liaison among
clients, service providers, and families. But business
skills such as bookkeeping, office management, and
(80) marketing are necessary, too, she warns.

According to a study conducted in 1987 by the
Inter-Study Center for Aging and Long-Term Care, the
popularity of private case management owes much to a
convergence of several trends: growth in the older popu-
(85) lation, fragmentation and complexity of the services
offered, and the growing respectability of private practice in the eyes of human service professionals. Prospects should continue to be very good, considering the
rapid growth projected in the number of people of ad-
(90) vanced age and the increased willingness of many
people to use social work and mental health services.

21. According to David Wolfe, a marketing strategy that works for older people is which one
of the following?

A. Using older people in advertisements
B. Advertising that a product will help in personal growth
C. Making old people look young and trendy
D. Focusing on the differences between the
needs of the young and the needs of the
old

22. The article implies that advertisers consider
the older consumer to be anyone:

A. over 70.
B. between 65 and 70.
C. between 60 and 65.
D. over 50.

23. According to Barbara Kane, which skills are
needed to run a successful case management
firm?

A. Interactive skills and networking skills
B. Counseling skills and assessment skills
C. Communication skills and collaborative
skills
D. Psychological skills and organizational
skills

24. The author states that case managers come
from several fields including:

I. Psychiatry.
II. Nursing.
III. Gerontology.

A. I only
B. I and II only
C. I and III only
D. II and III only

25. The prospects in the field of case management
should continue to be good because of growth
in which of the following?

A. Number of professionals doing the job
B. Number of college-trained older people
C. Number of people over 85
D. Willingness of older people to use
case-management services

26. The article implies that the growth and expansion of certain businesses such as consulting firms and firms that offer private case management for the elderly is related to:

    A. younger people's being less receptive to age-related products.
    B. the awareness that older consumers represent an untapped market for advertising.
    C. business's slow acknowledgment of the elderly as worthwhile consumers.
    D. a nationwide program encouraging sensitivity toward the elderly.

Passage V (Questions 27–35)

Scientific interest in caves began in seventeenth- and eighteenth-century Europe with the development of elaborate (but erroneous) theories of the hydrogenic cycle in which cave systems were essential elements.
(5) The beginnings of a correct understanding of the geology of caves date from about 1850 in Europe and 1900 in North America. In Europe, emphasis was on karst hydrology, particularly on subterranean streams. Early biological studies emphasized faunal surveys and de-
(10) scriptions of the degenerate eyes of cavernicolous animals (cavernicoles); only after 1900 were a few experimental studies made.

In the early twentieth century, Racovitza and Jeannel sparked the spectacular rise of modern
(15) biospeleology in Europe. This period was, in general, an interlude for cave science in the United States, during which the only additions to knowledge about North American caves and their life were made by Europeans on field trips in North America.
(20) Biospeleology advanced slowly in the United States from 1930 to 1950, even though this was the time of a lively debate over the origin of caves. The central point was whether caves form above or below the local water table. Davis proposed cave development
(25) deep below the water table, by random circulation of slowly percolating groundwater ("phreatic" origin). This view became textbook doctrine for many years. Other theories placed the zone of cave development at or above the local water table ("vadose" origin). This
(30) data and Davis's reputation as an authority had two stifling effects on cave studies: 1) the implied random pattern of cave development discouraged the search for specific hydrological mechanisms causative of cave system patterns, and 2) the argument over the location
(35) of the water table tended to reduce the research that was done to a sterile classification of some particular cave as having a vadose or phreatic origin.

Factors influencing reactivation of geological cave research and continued progress in biospeleology
(40) in the past decade include the amassing of a large body of descriptive data collected mainly by nonprofessional explorers and surveyors within the National Speleological Society; growing acquaintance with the large body of European literature that had been largely ignored by
(45) American theoreticians of the 1930s; near completion of a systematic description of many groups of cave organisms and their distribution, which permitted biologists to turn to ecological and physiological problems; and finally, involvement of younger researchers whose
(50) interest arose from exploration and field experience.

27. Davis said that caves developed:

    A. above the water table.
    B. at the level of the water table.
    C. well below the water table.
    D. both above and below the water table.

28. According to the article, early biological studies in caves emphasized the study of:

    I. Parasitic colonies found in caves that resembled coral found in the ocean.
    II. Fauna found in caves and the description of degenerate eyes of cavernicolous animals.
    III. Single-celled organisms found in caves.

    A. I only
    B. I and III only
    C. II only
    D. II and III only

29. Scientific interest in caves in Europe began in the:

    A. fifteenth and sixteenth centuries.
    B. sixteenth and seventeenth centuries.
    C. seventeenth and eighteenth centuries.
    D. eighteenth and nineteenth centuries.

30. Early scientific research on caves was based on an erroneous theory of the:

    A. hydrogenic cycle.
    B. development of subterranean streams.
    C. development of alluvial fans.
    D. development of cave rock formations.

31. Davis's theory of cave development origin is referred to in the article as:

A. vadose.
B. hydraulic.
C. phreatic.
D. cavernicoles.

32. According to the article, which of the following was **NOT** responsible for the resurgence of interest in geological cave research and advanced progress in biospeleology during the past decade?

A. The collection of a large body of descriptive data by nonprofessionals
B. A growing acquaintance with European literature of the 1930s
C. The contributions of European theoreticians on cave development
D. The involvement of younger researchers

33. Biospeleology is the study of:

A. rock formations.
B. underground water systems.
C. the development of caves.
D. underground water tables.

34. It would be reasonable to assume that the writer believes that the discussion as to whether caves formed above the water table or below had:

A. a negative effect on cave research in the United States.
B. a positive effect on cave research in the United States.
C. no discernible effect on cave research in the United States or worldwide.
D. both negative and positive effects on cave research.

35. Vadose origin refers to the development of caves:

A. below the water table.
B. at or above the water table.
C. by slowly percolating groundwater.
D. in metamorphic rock.

Passage VI (Questions 36–41)

Robert Lowell is known both as a major twentieth-century American poet and as an important translator of Homer, Sappho, Aeschylus, Roman poets, and French writers. Yet, as the anniversary of his
(5) death approaches, Lowell's work remains difficult and obscure, and the critical appraisal of both his poetry and translations remains mixed.

Lowell scholar Daniel Gillis, a Haverford College classics professor—not a professor of modern lit-
(10) erature, as most Lowell critics have been—is attempting to reform the critical view by highlighting the influence of classical literature on the poet.

"He isn't an American poet at all," Gillis explains, "but a bearer of an older, deeper tradition of European
(15) literary and poetic history, drawing on French, Italian, German, Russian, Greek, and Latin literature as nobody else can.

"I doubt it was a conscious process. Lowell knew both the Latin and Greek languages cold. He taught
(20) Greek for several years. It was second nature to him to think in terms of ancient structures and people. It didn't worry him much that some people wouldn't be able to understand everything in his poetry. At the same time, he knew he was losing his audience; maybe he was try-
(25) ing to raise their level. He wasn't about to abandon the Graeco-Roman legacy.

"In the poem 'My Last Afternoon with Uncle Devereux Winslow,' Lowell writes, 'Unseen and unseeing, I was Aggripina/in the Golden Halls of Nero.'
(30) This means nothing to readers—or critics—unless they know their Tacitus, know Aggripina was Nero's mother, and know this refers to Nero overthrowing her. Tacitus makes it very clear; she's walking around lost and doomed; it's a very dark reference. But if you don't
(35) know Tacitus and his history of Nero, it's just a woman walking through a house. This is the reader's problem, not Lowell's. He's saying something very clear. You have to equip yourself to deal with him."

Referring to Lowell's 1950 poem "Falling Asleep
(40) over the *Aeneid*," Gillis writes that "Anglo-American critics agree this is one of Lowell's memorable poems, but their writings tend to be limited to paraphrase. . . . Their shallow familiarity with the *Aeneid* does not serve them well." Few critics even notice that Lowell places
(45) Aeneas at a funeral the hero never actually attended.

The diminishing numbers of readers who can appreciate Lowell and scholars who can satisfactorily analyze the poet point up a disturbing trend in American education. The classical grounding in Latin and Greek
(50) language and literature that was prevalent in the nineteenth century has almost disappeared from today's schools. "We are a historyless people," Gillis quotes

Arthur Schlesinger, Jr. "We wake up every morning, and for us history is born anew each day."

(55) Also, Gillis laments, "We aren't a poetry-reading country anymore. The medium itself militates against wide readership. Around the time of Lowell's death, his new books sold about 300 copies. In general, poetry editions run about 1,000 copies."

(60) Lowell's translations (which Gillis argues is the wrong word to use) have also been misunderstood. "He used the word *imitations*," Gillis notes. "They're much freer than literal translations. The Latin word *emulatio*, meaning 'emulations' or even 'competitions,' is more (65) exactly what he did. He took a poem of Horace, for instance, as raw material for a new artistic product. The Latin poets, when they adapted Greek material, did an original recasting; they were unconcerned with conveying every word literally. In that sense, Lowell was much (70) a Roman working with Greek material. It's what Ezra Pound did, too."

Gillis's first encounter with Lowell occurred in 1979, while working on the book *Eros and Death in the Aeneid*. Gillis has found that studying Lowell's (75) poetry and translations has deepened his understanding of the ancient works. In "Falling Asleep over the *Aeneid*," for example, Lowell, the perceptive analyst, sheds light on Virgil's eroticism, which few commentators have addressed or noted; he "brings . . . strands (80) together with a remarkable clarity and economy of vision, suffused with warmth and an awesome sense of loss," says Gillis.

Gillis realizes that Robert Lowell's works provide an unusual opportunity. The course that the clas- (85) sicist is developing on Lowell and classical antiquity will be a bridge: It will address a modern poet from a fresh, rich perspective; it will serve as an entree for many students who are unfamiliar with classics and untrained in Latin and Greek; and it will give classics (90) students a taste of modern literature while taking advantage of their academic forte.

The hope is that studying Lowell and his ties to classical antiquity will generate interest both in a poet deserving recognition and in an academic discipline in (95) search of creative scholars.

36. Based on the article, it would be reasonable to believe that Daniel Gillis thought critics misunderstood Robert Lowell's poetry because they evaluated him as a:

    A. Latin poet.
    B. Greek poet.
    C. European poet.
    D. twentieth-century American poet.

37. Gillis strongly presents the view that Robert Lowell should be regarded as which of the following?

    A. An important translator of Roman and Greek classical literature
    B. A poet whose works were influenced by his knowledge of the classics of antiquity
    C. An avant garde poet familiar with French writers
    D. A modern poet who preferred to write only in classical Greek and Latin

38. Through his course on Lowell and classical antiquity, Gillis expects to accomplish which of the following?

    I. To generate increased interest in a deserving poet
    II. To address a modern poet from a fresh perspective
    III. To give classics students a taste of modern literature
    IV. To revive the requirement that a college education include a grounding in the classics

    A. I only
    B. I and II only
    C. I, II, and III only
    D. I, II, III, and IV

39. For a reader to understand Lowell's works, it would be necessary not only to be familiar with classic Latin and Greek literature, but also to have a background in:

    A. the ancient languages of Latin and Greek.
    B. reading ancient Latin and Greek.
    C. European literary and poetic history.
    D. Greek and Roman mythology.

40. Gillis contends that the word *translations* is a misnomer for describing Lowell's translated works since:

    I. they are mostly improvisational statements.

    II. they are commentaries about life in ancient Greece and Rome.

    III. they are freer renditions of classical works interpreted with perceptive clarity and depth.

    A. I and II only
    B. II only
    C. III only
    D. II and III only

41. According to Gillis, the appeal of Lowell's works to a very small number of contemporary readers and scholars is an indication of which of the following?

    A. Today's education fails to provide an adequate grounding in classical works of Latin and Greek.
    B. There is less interest in reading European literature today.
    C. Lowell's works fascinate only an eclectic group of readers.
    D. As an obscure poet and translator, Lowell is virtually unknown to the public.

Passage VII (Questions 42–49)

Of the many women who surely importuned their husbands for equal status in the new American nation, the most famous was Abigail Adams. On March 31, 1776, she wrote to her husband John, then in the Con-
(5) tinental Congress: ". . . remember the ladies and be more generous to them than your ancestors, in the new code of laws. Do not put such unlimited power into the hands of the husbands," she warned, or women would rebel.

Although the threatened rebellion did not come
(10) about until nearly seventy-five years later, the role of women in public affairs during the colonial and post-revolutionary periods was considerably greater than their unequal political status might indicate, says Irwin Gertzog, professor of political science at Allegh-
(15) eny College in Meadville, Pennsylvania, who investigated the subject.

Gertzog's research shows that few women were active in politics during the colonial era, but many of them influenced religious, economic, military, and com-
(20) munity developments. Managing taverns was an im-

portant economic function in the seventeenth and eighteenth centuries. New Jersey had more than 400 taverns, about one for every 500 residents in the state. Many women owned or managed taverns and inns. Some
(25) women were printers, crafts specialists, and merchants. During the Revolutionary War, a number of women joined the army, some in male disguise and some admitted as women. "There was a need for fighting strength," says Gertzog, "and women were prepared to
(30) provide it." Women also reported military preparations and troop movements and sabotaged British commercial and military activities.

Gertzog's work focused primarily on the political activities of women in New Jersey from 1788 to
(35) 1807, when they were the only female Americans legally eligible to participate in elections. "I wanted to discover why women were granted the vote, how many of them took advantage of it, and why it was taken away in 1807," says Gertzog.

(40) During the Revolution, when New Jersey was breaking away from England, the provincial congress met in June of 1776 to draft a new constitution. "The British forces had landed in New Jersey at Sandy Hook," says Gertzog, "and the delegates had to work quickly.
(45) The legitimate authority of the new regime had to be established before it could raise funds, muster an army, and advise the Continental Congress that it had established a government independent of Great Britain."

The new constitution gave the vote to "all inhab-
(50) itants" who were worth fifty pounds in real or personal property, thereby removing extensive real estate holdings as the sole economic test for voter eligibility. According to Gertzog, this more inclusive suffrage provision was prompted by petitions from men who were
(55) serving (or who would soon serve) in the army and supporting the war with taxes but who, without change, would not qualify to vote. Although the constitution did not explicitly grant female suffrage, neither did it say that voters had to be male. Gertzog found no evi-
(60) dence that women actively lobbied for the franchise.

The number of women who took advantage of the right to vote was difficult for Gertzog to estimate. The few available voting lists from the period, discovered in the archives of the New Jersey Historical Soci-
(65) ety, suggest that as many as 15 percent of the qualified women voted even though, through 1797, married women were ineligible. Under the laws governing domestic relations, a woman's property normally became her husband's as soon as they were wed. Consequently,
(70) eligible women voters were either single or widowed.

Why did women lose the vote in 1807? Gertzog is still seeking answers to this question, but some partial explanations seem evident: One is the substantial increase in competition between Republicans and Fed-
(75) eralists after the turn of the century. Whenever a party

was obliged to justify loss of a close election, it accused the opposition of fraud. Among the charges was that ineligible women, blacks, and aliens had been rounded up by the other party and herded to the polls.

(80)　　In an 1802 legislative contest, for example, a Hunterdon County Federalist won by a single vote, and his victory resulted in an equal number of Federalists and Republicans in Trenton. Soon afterward, newspapers and leading Republicans alleged that the partisan *(85)* deadlock that prevented a divided legislature from choosing a governor and U.S. senator was due to "the Federalist vote cast by an illiterate black woman."

　　An act disenfranchising women, free blacks, and aliens was promoted as a way of reducing election fraud *(90)* by making it easier to identify ineligible voters. The act was passed later that year.

　　But these events in New Jersey, Gertzog notes, were a product of national as well as local forces. All states were then stripping the franchise from marginal *(95)* groups—free blacks, noncitizens, native Americans, and in New Jersey, women—while at the same time removing obstacles to universal white male suffrage. Thus, New Jersey women were victims of political pressures that transcended local circumstances, and they *(100)* would not be able to vote again until passage of the Nineteenth Amendment more than one hundred years later.

42. According to the article, which of the following was given as a justification for disenfranchising women in New Jersey?

A. Women were not as intellectually capable as men.

B. Women voting threatened the stability of the family.

C. Disenfranchising women would reduce voter fraud.

D. Women voted for the Federalist party, preventing the Republicans from having a majority.

43. The article implies that the political activity of women during the years preceding the passage of the Nineteenth Amendment was:

A. minimal because most women were married.

B. negligible because the Constitution made no mention of women's being permitted to vote.

C. limited because women were classed alongside other powerless groups such as nonwhites and noncitizens.

D. considered unimportant by most women who believed an interest in politics to be unfeminine.

44. The reason the New Jersey constitution of 1776 was unique among the colonies was that it granted the right to vote:

　I. to free black men.
　II. to women who owned personal or real property.
　III. based on the property a person held.

A. I and II only
B. II and III only
C. II only
D. III only

45. Abigail Adams was:

A. one of the first women to vote.
B. one of the first prominent women to call for women's rights.
C. the owner of a New Jersey tavern during the Revolutionary War.
D. a lookout who reported British troop movements during the Revolution.

46. According to the article, what percentage of the women who were eligible to vote did vote?

A. 15 percent
B. 25 percent
C. 40 percent
D. 50 percent

47. The New Jersey constitution of 1776 granted the right to vote to:

A. all men who had 40 pounds' worth of real property.
B. all adults who had 40 pounds' worth of personal or real property.
C. all men who owned real property worth more than 50 pounds.
D. all inhabitants who had 50 pounds' worth of personal or real property.

48. After losing the vote in New Jersey, women did not regain the vote until:

    A. the passage of the Bill of Rights.
    B. the passage of the Fourteenth Amendment at the end of the Civil War.
    C. a Supreme Court ruling gave all women the right to vote.
    D. The passage of the Nineteenth Amendment a century later.

49. In which year did women in New Jersey lose the right to vote?

    A. 1788
    B. 1795
    C. 1802
    D. 1807

Passage VIII (Questions 50–57)

It was not only dark and stormy, but thirty degrees below zero in Vermont that night. I drove an hour north from my home to a small town called Wells River. When I arrived at the library, a converted storefront in
(5) the center of town, the woodstove was humming, and so was the audience. I was scheduled to give a forty-minute talk on Jean Rhys's novel, *Wide Sargasso Sea,* a fictional biography of Bertha, the "mad woman in the attic" in *Jane Eyre.* My lecture was part of a se-
(10) ries of five held over a ten-week period at the library. The audience had read the book in preparation for both the lecture and the discussion that followed, which was moderated by a discussion leader. My lecturn turned out to be a shoe salesperson's slanted stool set upon a
(15) card table.

I launched into the lecture on this difficult novel, very much predicated on Bronte's long novel and narrated by three voices. The discussion reminded me again of why I loved to serve as a scholar in these programs.
(20) Talk ranged from analysis of the text to insights gained from Rhys about personal lives.

Finally, a woman at least seventy years of age rose to take issue with the interpretation I had set forth in the lecture. "Right here on page 87," she began, in a
(25) voice tremulous with excitement, "are examples that show Rochester to be more human than you have depicted him." I could see that her copy of the novel was dog-eared and underlined in several colors of ink. If only my freshmen cared this much about their reading!
(30) At the conclusion of the discussion, I had some new ideas about Jean Rhys, and these have affected my subsequent scholarship. I learned, for example, to be more subtle in my analysis of point of view.

Reading and discussion programs of this nature
(35) began just a decade ago around a kitchen table in Rutland, Vermont, across the state from Wells River. Pat Bates, then program coordinator at the Rutland Free Library and currently project director for the Howard County Library in Maryland, was a newcomer to Ver-
(40) mont. She had experienced the frustration of reading a good book and having no one with whom to discuss it, of saying to a friend in the grocery store, "I just read Toni Morrison's *Sula,* and it's fantastic," and drawing a complete blank.
(45) Beginning with a reading group in her home, Bates experimented with various formats before hitting on the one that now has been successfully replicated in almost all fifty states and over one thousand libraries. Her goal was to establish a context in which a
(50) number of adults could all read the same book and later gather to discuss it. To enhance the discussion, Bates introduced the concept of opening each session with a lecture by a humanities scholar.

This scholarly component is the distinction be-
(55) tween reading and discussion programs and other reading projects like the Great Books program. The scholar's role is not to provide a tidy analysis of the text, not to deliver "the answers," but rather to enrich discussion with biographical information on the author, contex-
(60) tual perspectives from the literary tradition or historical era, and be a catalyst for discussion by raising provocative questions about the text.

I frequently served as a scholar for Bates. I spoke about humanities texts—works by Charlotte Bronte,
(65) Mary Wilkins Freeman, Margaret Atwood, Toni Morrison—to eager audiences in small libraries, community centers, and even churches. I "got hooked" on teaching this way because the audiences were hungry— the very best *metaphor*—for the scholar's information
(70) and even hungrier for the human interaction around a text.

These audiences were diverse: adolescents and octogenarians, people with high school degrees, people with Ph.D.s, individuals from all classes and careers.
(75) Each had experienced the human need for a story. Yet they had not had their needs satisfied by the often empty calories of television. Hence, the intensity of the woman in Wells River who reacted strongly to *Wide Sargasso Sea* and needed help digesting the novel. What more
(80) could a teacher-scholar ask than for "students" who are well prepared, eager to talk, willing to argue, and replete with a wealth of life experience?

50. One of the purposes of the scholarly lecture was to provide readers with:

    A. a means to participate in a cultural activity.
    B. a socializing process in isolated areas.
    C. an analysis of the text.
    D. an enriching discussion combining biographical information on the author with contextual perspectives.

51. Which of the following is a reasonable assumption based on the article?

    A. The author's college freshmen have a deeper understanding of literature than the people in these small towns.
    B. The people to whom the author speaks in these small towns have misinterpreted the literature being discussed.
    C. The author has found the talks in these small towns enriching to her own scholarly work.
    D. The people who participate in the library reading programs are culturally deprived.

52. According to the article, the presence of the humanities scholar was to:

    I. provide definitive answers to all literary questions.
    II. keep an intellectual emphasis in the discussions.
    III. provide a lively, stimulating literary ingredient to discussions.

    A. I only
    B. III only
    C. I and II only
    D. II and III only

53. The format of the discussion group that has been used successfully at over one thousand libraries is which of the following?

    A. A number of adults all read the same book, gather to discuss it, and are provided with a lecture by a humanities scholar.
    B. A number of adults select different topics to present for discussion.
    C. A number of adults read the same book and prepare open-ended discussion questions.
    D. A number of adults read the same book and select chapters to interpret and present for discussion.

54. The program discussed in this article began in:

    A. Howard County, Maryland.
    B. Rutland, Vermont.
    C. Wells River, Vermont.
    D. Portland, Maine.

55. People who participated in these programs were usually:

    A. scholars and academicians.
    B. young adults with a college education.
    C. older adults who were either retired or elderly.
    D. from a wide, diverse cross section of society.

56. One can infer that the author frequently lectures to reading groups because:

    A. she finds the audiences well prepared and eager to discuss the book at hand.
    B. she is well paid for her time.
    C. she finds the participants better behaved than her students.
    D. she enjoys the interacting with adults rather than students.

57. The author infers that the interest in such programs among adults was due to:

    A. lack of interest in watching television.
    B. the need of adults to share reactions to books they have read through discussions.
    C. the need of adults to socialize with people of similar age and interests.
    D. a desire to read the latest novels.

Passage IX (Questions 58–65)

Two projects brought together for the first time the alumni associations from nine Big Ten universities, and a variety of other institutions, for several programs available to the public.

(5) Under the leadership of Frank B. Jones, alumni associations from the University of Illinois, Michigan State University, University of Michigan, University of Minnesota, Northwestern University, Ohio State University, Purdue University, and the University of Wis-
(10) consin combined to cosponsor the first project. "The Northwest Ordinance: Liberty and Justice for All" featured educational programs held on Big Ten campuses for the general public, a publishing program including articles by humanities scholars, and a two-day schol-
(15) arly symposium to examine the state of current scholarship on the ordinance.

The symposium, held at the Indiana University campus, brought together a dozen scholars who were at work on the ordinance or some related aspect of
(20) American history. The Institute of Early American History and Culture in Williamsburg, Virginia, had expressed an interest in publishing the proceedings.

The alumni associations developed public education packs for distribution to libraries, historical so-
(25) cieties, and other interested organizations. The packs contain articles commissioned by the alumni associations, a map of the Old Northwest Territory, a copy of the ordinance, a poster, a bibliography of selected reading materials, and a suggested speakers bureau of North-
(30) west Ordinance scholars.

The second project sponsored by the Big Ten alumni associations is called Liberty's Legacy. This traveling exhibition will bring original historical documents on the Northwest Ordinance, related ordinances,
(35) and the Constitution to the general public; to elementary, secondary, and university students; and to alumni in six states.

Among the 56 items included in the Northwest Ordinance part of the exhibition are a rare first printing
(40) of *The Definitive Treaty between Great Britain and the United States (1783),* written and printed at the instruction of Ambassador Benjamin Franklin in Paris; Jefferson's Ordinance of 1784, which set up a temporary government for the West; and the Land Ordinance
(45) of 1785, which established the system for the surveying and eventual sale of the new lands to settlers in the Northwest Territory. Colorful maps that illustrate the new land system will also be included, along with pages of the original Northwest Ordinance.
(50) "These ordinances and documents rank among the most important in our early American history, both for what they accomplished and for what they inspired," says Frank Jones.

Those projects should help to engender public un-
(55) derstanding and appreciation of the Northwest Ordinance as one of the cornerstone documents of our founding. Like any enduring cornerstone, the Northwest Ordinance has been built upon again and again. It has served as a blueprint for the nation's westward expan-
(60) sion. Without the ordinance, the United States could not have grown so tall or stood so long.

58. Based on the article, it would be reasonable to assume that the author believes the Northwest Ordinance was:

A. an important document that helped lead to the development of a strong America.
B. a key component to the development of the American constitution.
C. a building block for local governments on the frontier.
D. a model for laws up to the present day in the United States.

59. Which of the following was **NOT** generated by the Northwest Ordinance project sponsored by the alumni associations of Big Ten universities?

A. Exhibitions featuring original treaties related to the government and development of the Northwest Territory
B. Scholarly research and seminars on the ordinance and related documents
C. Increased public awareness of the document's role in American history
D. Increased federal funding for similar historical efforts

60. According to the article, the Northwest Ordinance served as a plan that stimulated which of the following?

A. Westward expansion among settlers
B. Resolution of conflicts between Indian tribes in the area and incoming farmers
C. Setting up of definite boundary lines for future states
D. Involvement of the federal government in solving any land disputes

61. Which of the following was **NOT** one of the purposes behind the alumni associations' co-sponsoring of the Northwest Ordinance project?

A. To promote greater cooperation among alumni associations in the future

B. To emphasize the ordinance's historical role in American history

C. To demonstrate the ordinance's impact on westward expansion into new territories

D. To show the establishment of a system for surveying and selling new lands to settlers in the Northwest Territory

62. Two European countries mentioned in some capacity in relationship to the printing and publication of the Northwest Ordinance were:

A. England and France.

B. England and Belgium.

C. England and Spain.

D. England and the Netherlands.

63. The land ordinance discussed in the article did which one of the following?

A. It gave the land known as the thirteen colonies to the new government of the United States.

B. It divided the land of the Northwest Territory.

C. It created a system for surveying and ultimately selling land to settlers.

D. It became the foundation of the new U.S. Constitution.

64. Among the historical documents displayed with the Northwest Ordinance exhibition were which of the following?

  I. Pages from the original Northwest Ordinance document

  II. The rare first printing of *The Definitive Treaty between Great Britain and the United States* (1783)

  III. Jefferson's Ordinance of 1784 which established the surveying and sale of lands to settlers in the Northwest Territory

A. I only

B. I and II only

C. I and III only

D. I, II, and III

65. The role of the alumni associations in the Northwest Ordinance project included:

A. hiring the Institute of Early American History and Culture to publicize the proceedings.

B. developing public information packs for libraries, historical societies, and other interested organizations.

C. writing scholarly articles on the Northwest Ordinance for distribution to elementary and secondary schools.

D. selling posters and maps to raise money for future historical projects.

END OF TEST 1.

**IF YOU FINISH BEFORE THE TIME IS UP, YOU MAY
CHECK YOUR WORK ON THIS TEST ONLY.**

PHYSICAL SCIENCES

Time: 100 Minutes
Questions 66–142

Directions: This test contains 77 questions. Most of the questions consist of a descriptive passage followed by a group of questions related to the passage. For these questions, study the passage carefully and then choose the best answer to each question in the group. Some questions in this test stand alone. These questions are independent of any passage and independent of each other. For these questions, too, you must select the one best answer. Indicate all your answers by blackening the corresponding circles on your answer sheet.

A periodic table is provided at the beginning of this book. You may consult it whenever you wish.

Passage I (Questions 66–73)

1. Rationale. An investigator sets out to determine the absorption spectrum of the $Co(NH_3)_6^{3+}$ complex, and to study the effect on the spectrum of substituting different "ligands"—groups surrounding the cobalt—for the original ammonia ligand.

The investigator hopes to gain information about the molecular orbitals in the cobalt complexes. The first step in such a process is to measure the wavelength of maximum absorption for each complex, and to interpret this wavelength in terms of a transition energy.

Procedure. The experimental setup is shown in the next column. The experimenter uses the same cell for each sample, so that the path length will not vary, and each solution is made up to be $0.01\,M$. By measuring the light transmitted by the sample, a photodetector at the

output end of the spectrometer determines the absorbance at each wavelength and sends this information to the chart recorder. The latter displays absorbance as a function of wavelength; the investigator calculates the wavelength of maximum absorption for each compound.

Analysis of Data. Table 1 shows the relationships among solution colors, colors absorbed, wavelengths typical of these colors, and corresponding photon energies.

Table 1

Color of solution	clear	violet	blue/ bl green	green	yellow	orange	red	red-purple
Color absorbed	"ultraviolet"	yellow	orange/ red	purple	violet	blue	blue/ green	green
λ (nm) *of absorbed light*	< 400	400	500	530	580	610	680	700
Energy of absorbed light (kJ/mol)	> 299	299	239	226	207	196	176	171

Table 2

Complex	λ_{max} (nm)
$Co(NH_3)_6^{3+}$	430
$Co(NH_3)_5(H_2O)^{3+}$	500
$Co(NH_3)_5(CO)^+$	500
$cis\text{-}Co(NH_3)_4Cl_2^+$	560
$trans\text{-}Co(NH_3)_4Cl_2^+$	680

Table 3 shows several possible series of molecular energy levels that might be used to explain the transitions in Tables 1 and 2. When a photon matching the difference between two of the levels is absorbed, an electron can be promoted to a higher level.

Table 3 (energy in kJ/mol)

66. What is the color of a solution that absorbs light having an energy of 239 kJ/mol?

   A. orange/red
   B. blue/blue-green
   C. purple
   D. green

67. The region on the chart between 400 and 600 nm shows how many distinct, visible solution colors?

   A. 3
   B. 4
   C. 5
   D. 6

68. The highest energy transition in Table 2 corresponds to absorption by which of the following compounds?

   A. $Co(NH_3)_6^{3+}$
   B. $Co(NH_3)_5(H_2O)^{3+}$
   C. $Co(NH_3)_5(CO)^+$
   D. $cis\text{-}Co(NH_3)_4Cl_2^+$

69. The replacement of one ammonia in $Co(NH_3)_6^{+3}$ by a water molecule results in a shift in absorption from:

   A. indigo to blue-green.
   B. blue-green to indigo.
   C. yellow to orange-red.
   D. orange-red to yellow.

70. Using the data from Table 1, choose the expression that best describes the relationship between energy (in kJ/mol) and λ (in nm):

   A. $E = 0.75\ \lambda$
   B. $E = (1.20 \times 10^5)/\lambda$
   C. $E = (\lambda - 101)$
   D. $E = 0.50\lambda + 99$

71. Which of the diagrams in Table 3 could be used to explain the absorption of $cis\text{-}Co(NH_3)_4Cl_2^+$?

   A. I
   B. II
   C. III
   D. IV

72. Which of the diagrams in Table 3 explains the absorption of the complexes that appear to be blue solutions?

   A. I
   B. II
   C. IV
   D. V

73. Which of the diagrams in Table 3 predicts one or more possible transitions in the ultraviolet region of the spectrum?

   A. I
   B. III
   C. IV
   D. None of the above

Passage II (Questions 74–79)

An experimenter wishes to test the hypothesis that a concentration difference alone can produce a voltage in an electrochemical cell. In order to test her hypothesis, she constructs the cell shown below, where both sides of the cell contain $AgNO_3$, with concentrations shown in the diagram. She will use the voltmeter shown to determine what voltage, if any, exists across the electrodes at different times after the circuit is closed.

The table that follows shows the voltage in the cell as a function of the time that current has been allowed to flow in the circuit. It also displays the concentration of silver ion on each side of the cell.

t(s)	v (volts)	$[Ag^+]$ on left (mol/L)	$[Ag^+]$ on right (mol/L)
0	0.1180	0.1000	0.0010
10	0.0721	0.0953	0.0057
20	0.0567	0.0910	0.0100
30	0.0472	0.0872	0.0138
40	0.0404	0.0837	0.0173
50	0.0351	0.0805	0.0205
.			
.			
.			
1000	0.0000	0.0505	0.0505

74. The purpose of the salt bridge in the experiment is to:

   A. conduct Ag^+ ions from left to right.
   B. conduct Ag^+ ions from right to left.
   C. allow K^+ and NO_3^- ions to flow from one half cell to another in order to keep the solution electrically neutral.
   D. allow electrons to flow from left to right.

75. The reduction potential for Ag^+, $E°$, is 0.799 volts. For the net reaction that occurs in the overall cell, what is $E°_{cell}$ in v?

   A. 0
   B. 0.799
   C. −0.799
   D. 0.009

76. For how many time values listed in the chart does the value of V change by more than 0.010 v from the previous time?

   A. 1
   B. 2
   C. 3
   D. 4

77. If the apparatus was modified so that the solutions on each side could mix through a horizontal connecting tube, the measured voltages would:

   A. be unchanged from those given in the table.
   B. drop rapidly to zero.
   C. increase from those shown in the table.
   D. take a longer time to reach zero.

78. Which of the following best describes the relationship among the voltage and the concentrations on each side?

    A. As time passes, electrons flow through the salt bridge from left to right, causing the ions to equilibrate and the voltage to drop.
    B. As time passes, Ag^+ ions flow through the salt bridge from left to right, causing the voltage to drop.
    C. As time passes, electrons flow through the wire from left to right, causing the ions to equilibrate and the voltage to drop.
    D. As time passes, electrons flow through the wire from right to left, causing the concentration gradient to decrease and the voltage to drop.

79. Suppose that C_1 represents the concentration of silver ion on the left of the cell, while C_2 represents the concentration on the right. Which of the following best describes the relation between C_1 and C_2?

    A. $C_1 - C_2$ is constant, owing to conservation of charge.
    B. $C_1 - C_2$ is constant, owing to conservation of Ag^+ ion.
    C. $C_1 + C_2$ is constant, owing to conservation of charge.
    D. $C_1 + C_2$ is constant, owing to conservation of Ag^+ ion.

Passage III (Questions 80–87)

Applications of equilibrium constants to real life problems often confront a student with a reaction and ask what the products and their concentrations will be. These problems often seem to lie outside the examples frequently provided in texts. Our advice is to determine, however roughly, what the equilibrium constant is for a given reaction, and then either solve assuming total reaction (if $K_{eq} \gg 1$), or, if the reaction is seen not to proceed very far, to calculate equilibrium concentrations.

The following problems combine questions about solubility with those concerning strong and weak acids. (Note that H_2O, when it is formed, is not listed as a "major product".)

80. Which of the following best explains the result of reaction 1?

    A. Cl^- is a weak base.
    B. K_{sp} for AgCl $\gg 1$.
    C. K_{sp} for AgCl $\ll 1$.
    D. Most chloride salts are soluble.

81. Which of the following could have been the second component in reaction 2?

    A. 0.05 mol H^+
    B. 0.05 mol OH^-
    C. 0.1 mol H^+
    D. 0.1 mol OH^-

82. Which of the following could be the second component in reaction 4?

    A. 0.05 mol of acetic acid
    B. 0.05 mol of HCl
    C. 0.025 mol acetic acid
    D. 0.025 mol HCl

Reaction	1st Component	2nd Component	Major Products
1	0.1 mol Ag^+	0.1 mol Cl^-	0.1 mol AgCl(s)
2	0.1 mol H^+	?	0.05 mol H^+
3	0.1 mol acetic acid	0.1 mol OH^-	?
4	0.05 mol acetate	?	0.025 mol acetic acid, 0.025 mol acetate
5	1 mol CO_3^{2-}	?	1 mol H_2CO_3
6	1 mol HCl	1 mol formic acid	?

83. The pH of the resulting solution in reaction 3 is closest to which of the following?

A. 1
B. 4
C. 7
D. 9

84. Which of the following could be the second component in reaction 5?

A. 1 mol H^+
B. 1 mol OH^-
C. 2 mol H^+
D. 2 mol OH^-

85. An investigator wishes to predict the result when 1 mole of ammonium chloride is mixed with an equal amount of strong base. Which reaction from the chart most closely resembles this reaction?

A. Reaction 2
B. Reaction 3
C. Reaction 4
D. Reaction 5

86. The final product of which reaction would make a useful buffer?

A. 2
B. 3
C. 4
D. 5

87. After reaction 6, the original formic acid:

A. has not appreciably changed.
B. has changed about 50 percent to formate.
C. has largely changed to formate.
D. has been neutralized.

Passage IV (Questions 88–96)

Several students measure the voltages in three different cells, each made from two half-cells as indicated in the table below. The concentration of each of the ions in solution is $1.0\,M$. The average values of the measurements, as well as the relative polarities, are shown in the table below.

By combining the results in the table, the students derive the following chart showing reduction potential:

88. Based on the table, when the circuit is closed in cell A, in which direction do electrons flow through the voltmeter?

A. Toward the Ni electrode
B. Toward the Pb electrode
C. Neither direction since they are equally attracted to both electrodes
D. Cannot be determined

Cell	Half-Cell 1	Polarity	Half-Cell 2	Polarity	Voltage
A	Ni^{2+}/Ni	−	Pb^{2+}/Pb	+	0.131
B	Zn^{2+}/Zn	−	Fe^{3+}/Fe^{2-}	+	1.53
C	Ni^{2-}/Ni	+	Zn^{2+}/Zn	−	0.505

89. Based on the table, at which electrode does reduction occur in cell B?

    A. Positive
    B. Negative
    C. Neither
    D. Cannot be determined

90. By studying cells B and C, the students can determine that:

    A. Zn^{2+} is reduced by Fe^{2+}.
    B. Zn is oxidized by both Fe^{+3} and Ni^{2+}.
    C. Zn is oxidized by Fe^{3+} and is reduced by Ni.
    D. Zn is reduced by Fe^{3+} and is oxidized by Ni.

91. By studying cells A and C, the students can determine that which of the following statements is true?

    A. Pb is more readily oxidized than Ni. Zn is more readily oxidized than Ni.
    B. Pb is less readily oxidized than Ni. Zn is more readily oxidized than Ni.
    C. Pb is more readily oxidized than Ni. Zn is less readily oxidized than Ni.
    D. Pb is less readily oxidized than Ni. Zn is less readily oxidized than Ni.

92. By examining the result for cell A only, what can the students find the reduction potential for Pb^{2+}/Pb to be?

    A. 0.131 v
    B. −0.131 v
    C. 0.131 v greater than for Ni^{2+}/Ni
    D. 0.131 v less than for Ni^{2+}/Ni

93. By examining the results for cells A and B only, the students can find that compared to the half-cell reduction potential for Ni^{2+}, the reduction potential for Zn^{2+}/Zn:

    A. is 1.40 less.
    B. is 1.40 more.
    C. is .37 less.
    D. cannot be determined.

94. According to the chart, will Zn react spontaneously with $1\,M\,Pb^{2+}$ in solution?

    A. Yes
    B. No
    C. Only in acidic solution
    D. Cannot be determined

95. If the reduction potential for Ni^{2+}/Ni is taken arbitrarily to be 1.00 v, what is the reduction potential for Pb^{2+}/Pb?

    A. −0.87 v
    B. 0.87 v
    C. −1.131 v
    D. 1.131 v

96. If "cell D" were to be made up as cell A was, but with Pb^{2+}/Pb and Zn^{2+}/Zn as the half-cells, what would be the voltage and polarity?

    A. 0.37 v, with Zn positive
    B. 37 v, with Pb positive
    C. 0.636 v, with Zn positive
    D. 0.636 v, with Pb positive

Passage V (Questions 97–101)

A chemist is asked to identify two solutions whose labels have peeled off. One is known to contain 1.0 formula weight of NaCl for each kg of water in which it is dissolved. The other has an identical concentration of Na_2CO_3.

97. Which chemical test might best furnish an identification?

    A. Flame test for sodium
    B. Test for chloride by adding $AgNO_3$
    C. Test for pH
    D. Titration with NaOH

98. The chemist decides instead to measure the freezing point of each solution. This method will distinguish between the two compounds because:

    A. CO_3^{2-} is more effective at lowering the freezing point of a solution.
    B. Cl^- is more effective at lowering the freezing point of a solution.
    C. the freezing point is lowered more by doubly charged ions.
    D. the freezing point is lowered in proportion to the total number of ions in the solution.

99. The freezing point depression is directly proportional to the:

  A. molarity of the solution.
  B. molality of the solution.
  C. molecular weight of the solute.
  D. volume of the solution.

100. In order to distinguish between the solutions using the freezing point depression, the chemist must assume that:

  A. NaCl is much more soluble than Na_2CO_3.
  B. Na_2CO_3 is much more soluble than NaCl.
  C. each salt dissolves completely.
  D. each salt has a negligible K_{sp}.

101. The chemist measures the freezing point depression and finds which of the following?

  A. One solution, which she should identify as NaCl, has a freezing point depression that is 50 percent greater than the other's.
  B. One solution, which she should identify as Na_2CO_3, has a freezing point depression that is 50% greater than the other's.
  C. One solution, which she should identify as NaCl, has a freezing point depression that is 33 percent greater than the other's.
  D. The freezing point depressions are equal, since each solution is completely ionized.

Passage VI (Questions 102–106)

An apparatus is devised for evaluating the properties of thin lenses. It consists of a sliding mount that holds the lens and allows it to be moved forward and backward along a track. A reference object, such as an arrow, is fixed at one end of the track. The lens position is then adjusted along the track until the object is in focus.

In one test, an arrow 0.050 meters high is fixed at point A on the track. When the center of the sample lens is 0.60 meters from the arrow, a sharp image of the arrow is formed on the opposite side of the lens at point B, which is 0.30 meters away from the center of the lens. The position of the object arrow is more than two focal lengths away from the lens.

102. What is the focal length of the test lens?

  A. 0.60 m
  B. 0.30 m
  C. 0.20 m
  D. 0.15 m

103. What is the height of the image of the arrow at position B?

  A. 0.10 m
  B. 0.30 m
  C. 0.45 m
  D. 0.60 m

104. Which statement describes the image of the arrow formed at point A?

  A. The image is real and erect.
  B. The image is virtual and erect.
  C. The image is real and inverted.
  D. The image is virtual and inverted.

105. The image is formed because light from the object is:

  A. polarized.
  B. reflected.
  C. refracted.
  D. diffracted.

106. Which statement describes what happens to the image as the object is moved towards the lens?

  A. The image will increase in size and move closer toward the lens.
  B. The image will increase in size and move farther away from the lens.
  C. The image will decrease in size and move closer toward the lens.
  D. The image will decrease in size and move farther away from the lens.

Passage VII (Questions 107–111)

A racetrack is constructed so that its opposite ends are semicircles attached to each other by long straight stretches of road. The radius of curvature of one end is 50.0 meters. The radius of curvature of the opposite end is twice that. The track is perfectly flat. A racecar with a mass of 2000 kilograms drives in a clockwise direction around the outer edge of the track at a constant speed of 20 meters per second.

107. In comparing the centripetal acceleration acting on the car as it goes around the larger curve to the centripetal acceleration as the car goes around the smaller curve at the opposite end of the track, one finds that the centripetal acceleration around the large curve will be:

    A. one-quarter the a_c associated with the small curve.
    B. half the a_c associated with the small curve.
    C. twice the a_c associated with the small curve.
    D. quadruple the a_c associated with the small curve.

108. What is the net force acting on the car as it goes around the smaller curve?

    A. 0 N
    B. 8.0×10^3 N
    C. 1.2×10^4 N
    D. 1.6×10^4 N

109. One of the two straightaways between the two curves lies between the points labeled X and Y in the diagram of the track. What is the net force acting on the car as it goes along this straightaway?

    A. 0 N
    B. 8.0×10^3 N
    C. 1.2×10^4 N
    D. 1.6×10^4 N

110. If the car travels from point X to point Y in 20 seconds, what must be the length of this section of the straightaway?

    A. 100 m
    B. 200 m
    C. 300 m
    D. 400 m

111. The kinetic energy of the car as it goes around the larger curve is:

    A. less than it is along the straightaway.
    B. greater than it is along the straightaway.
    C. exactly equal to the value along the straightaway.
    D. exactly four times greater than it is along the straightaway.

Passage IX (Questions 112–117)

Poiseuille's law is often used to describe blood flow rate through the circulating system. It is given by the equation

$$Q \frac{\pi}{8\eta l}(P_1 - P_2)R^4$$

where Q = flow rate of fluid

    η = coefficient of viscosity

    l = length of tube through which fluid flows

    R = radius of tube

P_1 and P_2 = pressures at point 1 and point 2 of tube

Poiseuille's law describes only laminar or streamline flow where layers of the fluid flow in parallel directions. If the speed of these layers increases, the flow may become turbulent where the fluid swirls and forms eddies. More pressure will then be required to maintain the flow rate because of greater frictional losses. The Reynolds number ($\Re$) is often used to determine the velocity at which laminar flow becomes turbulent.

$$\Re = \frac{2\bar{v}Rd}{\eta}$$

where $\bar{v}$ = average speed of the fluid

    d = density of the fluid

Empirical studies have shown that laminar flow occurs when $\Re$ is less than 2,000. At $\Re$ values greater than 3,000, turbulent flow occurs. Between these two values, the flow can be either laminar or turbulent.

112. A patient is given an antibiotic intravenously. According to Poiseuille's formula, which of the following will be most effective in increasing the flow rate of the antibiotic into the patient?

    A. Raise the bag of intravenous antibiotic
    B. Increase the radius of the needle
    C. Dissolve the antibiotic in another solvent
    D. Decrease the length of tubing

113. The radius of a person's artery decreases by 50 percent from arthereosclerosis. In order to maintain the same blood flow rate the person's heart must:

    A. increase the net pressure by a factor of 32.
    B. double the net pressure.
    C. triple the net pressure.
    D. increase the net pressure by a factor of 16.

114. The flow rate of blood at rest is about 5 L/min. If $\eta = 4.0 \times 10^{-3}$ N s/m^2 and $d = 1.030 \times 10^3$ kg/m^3, what is the Reynolds number for an artery with diameter 2.0 cm?

    A. 1,365
    B. 2,000
    C. 6,800
    D. 68

115. What is the average linear blood flow rate above which turbulence must occur for the 2.0-cm artery?

    A. 2.9 m/s
    B. 0.58 m/s
    C. 25 L/min
    D. 10 L/min

116. Poiseuille's law indicates that most of the pressure exerted by the heart is dissipated in the:

    A. arteries.
    B. veins.
    C. capillaries and arterioles that feed the capillaries.
    D. heart valves.

117. For a liquid flowing through a pipe of radius R, length l, and pressure drop $(P_1 - P_2)$, a decrease in temperature most likely will:

    A. decrease the flow rate.
    B. decrease the average speed of liquid layers.
    C. increase the coefficient of viscosity.
    D. All of the above

Passage X (Questions 118–123)

The experimental setup shown is used to determine osmotic pressure (π) of various aqueous solutions of glucose. The membrane is permeable to water.

118. The above diagram indicates which of the following?

    A. $\pi_A > \pi_B$;
       Concentration$_A$ > Concentration$_B$

    B. $\pi_A < \pi_B$;
       Concentration$_B$ > Concentration$_A$

    C. $\pi_A > \pi_B$;
       Concentration$_B$ > Concentration$_A$

    D. $\pi_A > \pi_B$;
       Concentration$_A$ > Concentration$_B$

119. The pressure exerted on the piston that would prevent any net flow of water from solution A to solution B is equal to:

    A. the osmotic pressure of solution B.
    B. the osmotic pressure of solution A.
    C. the difference in the osmotic pressures of the two solutions.
    D. twice the osmotic pressure of solution B.

120. If solution A were replaced by water, what would happen to the pressure required to prevent net flow of water?

    A. It would increase.
    B. It would decrease.
    C. It would remain the same.
    D. The effect cannot be predicted.

121. The osmotic pressure of a red blood cell is about 7.7 atm. A red blood cell immersed in water will most likely:

    A. shrink in size.
    B. dissolve.
    C. release water.
    D. burst.

122. The osmotic pressure of a $0.10\,M$ glucose solution is:

    A. the same as a $0.10\,M$ NaCl solution.
    B. less than a $0.10\,M$ NaCl solution.
    C. greater than a $0.10\,M$ NaCl solution.
    D. zero.

123. Which of the following phenomena best explains osmosis?

    A. Brownian motion
    B. Friction
    C. Capillary action
    D. Diffusion

Questions 124 through 142 are independent of any passage and independent of each other.

124. What is the current in a 60-W light bulb operating at 120-V household voltage?

    A. 2.0 A
    B. 1.5 A
    C. 1.0 A
    D. 0.5 A

125. A siren sounds with a frequency of 700 Hz. What frequency is heard by a driver in a car moving away from the siren with a uniform velocity of 35 m/s? (The speed of sound in air is about 350 m/s for the ambiant temperature.)

    A. 720 Hz
    B. 630 Hz
    C. 540 Hz
    D. 790 Hz

126. Fluid moves with constant speed and no turbulence through a tube of uniform diameter as illustrated below. At which point is the pressure lowest?

    A. A
    B. B
    C. C
    D. D

127. The threshold of hearing has an intensity of 10^{-12} W/m² (watts per square meter), which corresponds to a sound level β, of 0 dβ (decibels). What is the intensity of a 40 dβ sound?

    A. 40×10^{-12} W/m²
    B. 10^{-3} W/m²
    C. 10^{-8} W/m²
    D. 40×10^{-3} W/m²

128. Which of the following procedures would allow an experimenter to determine the activation energy E_a for a given reaction?

    A. Measure k at 298K.
    B. Measure k at 398K.
    C. Measure k at 298K and 398K.
    D. Measure the rate for a variety of concentrations.

129. Which of the following will **NOT** change the total pressure in a closed vessel containing N_2 gas? (Assume ideal gas behavior.)

    I. Increasing the temperature.
    II. Replacing half the N_2 molecules with gaseous helium atoms.
    III. Adding an equal amount of gaseous hydrogen.

    A. I only
    B. II only
    C. III only
    D. I and II only

130. A student wishes to find the solubility of $Ba(IO_3)_2$, for which $K_{sp} = 1.6 \times 10^{-9}$. If x represents the solubility, which equation should she solve?

    A. $1.6 \times 10^{-9} = (x)(x)$
    B. $1.6 \times 10^{-9} = (x)(2x)$
    C. $1.6 \times 10^{-9} = (x)(x)^2$
    D. $1.6 \times 10^{-9} = (x)(2x)^2$

131. For which of the gas-phase reactions below would ΔS be expected to be negative?

    I. $2H_2O \rightarrow 2H_2 + O_2$
    II. $2H \rightarrow H_2$
    III. $N_2 + 3H_2 \rightarrow 2NH_3$

    A. I only
    B. II only
    C. I and II only
    D. II and III only

132. For the reaction $2NO_2(g) \rightleftharpoons N_2O_4(g)$, which of the following is true?

    I. Removing NO_2 shifts the equilibrium to the left.
    II. Increasing the volume of the container shifts the equilibrium to the right.
    III. Adding helium gas to the container shifts the equilibrium to the right.

    A. I only
    B. II only
    C. III only
    D. I and II only

133. The pH of a solution of $0.001\ M$ NaOH is closest to which of the following?

    A. 0.001
    B. 3
    C. 7
    D. 11

134. A student wishes to prepare a buffer whose pH is 6.3, using an acid HA with a pK_a of 6.0. Which expression below will correctly express the ratio R of HA to NaA that must be mixed in order to achieve the desired pH?

    A. $6.3 = 6.0 + \log R$
    B. $6.0 = 6.3 + \log R$
    C. $10^{-6.3} = 10^{-6.0} + \log R$
    D. $6.3 = \log 6.0 + R$

135. The period of a simple pendulum can be increased by:

    A. increasing the length of the pendulum.
    B. decreasing the length of the pendulum.
    C. increasing the mass of the box.
    D. decreasing the mass of the box.

136. The depth of water in the ocean is determined by using sonar signals. Assuming that the speed of sound in water is about 1.5 km/s and it takes a total of 6 s for a sonar signal to return to the ship after being emitted, what is the estimated depth of the ocean at that point?

    A. 3.0 km
    B. 9.0 km
    C. 0.25 km
    D. 4.5 km

137. What is the work done in holding a 20-N weight at a height of 2 m above the floor for a total of 5 s?

A. 0 J
B. 8 J
C. 2 J
D. 200 J

138. Three capacitors are connected as shown to a 24-V potential voltage source:

$C_2 = C_3 = 8\mu\mathfrak{F}$ $C_2 = 3\mu\mathfrak{F}$

What is the total capacitance of this circuit?

A. $4\,\mu\mathfrak{F}$
B. $7\,\mu\mathfrak{F}$
C. $12\,\mu\mathfrak{F}$
D. $18\,\mu\mathfrak{F}$

139. Pascal's principle holds that when an external pressure is applied to an enclosed fluid, the pressure:

A. is uniformly distributed undiminished to all points in the fluid.
B. is distributed undiminished, but as a function of fluid depth.
C. is greatest at the point of application and decreases as the distance from the application point increases.
D. affects only the rate of flow in the fluid layers closest to the tube's walls.

140. Two point charges attract each other with a force of 3.6×10^{-6} N when they are 3 m apart. What is the force if the distance is increased to 6 m?

A. It is tripled.
B. It is reduced to one-ninth.
C. It is quadrupled.
D. It is quartered.

141. Two tuning forks vibrate so that the note produced by the first fork is exactly one octave above the note produced by the second fork. Compared to the speed of the wave produced by the first fork, the speed of the wave produced by the second fork is:

A. half as fast.
B. twice as fast.
C. eight times as fast.
D. the same speed.

142. Four resistors are connected as shown.

What is the current through the 40 Ω resistor?

A. 1.2 A
B. 2.0 A
C. 3.0 A
D. 4.0 A

END OF TEST 2.

**IF YOU FINISH BEFORE THE TIME IS UP, YOU MAY
CHECK YOUR WORK ON THIS TEST ONLY.**

WRITING SAMPLE

Time: 60 Minutes
2 Essays

Directions: This test consists of two parts. You will have 30 minutes to complete each part. During the first 30 minutes you may work on Part 1 only. During the second 30 minutes, you may work on Part 2 only. You will have three pages for each essay answer, but you do not have to fill all three pages. Be sure to write legibly; illegible essays will not be scored.

Part 1

Consider this statement:

Necessity is the mother of invention.

Write a unified essay in which you perform the following tasks. Explain what you think the above statement means. Describe a specific situation in which necessity does *not* lead to invention. Discuss what you think determines when necessity is the mother of invention and when it is not.

DO NOT START THE NEXT TOPIC UNTIL THE TIME IS UP.

Part 2

Consider this statement:

The key to failure is to try to please everyone.

Write a unified essay in which you perform the following tasks. Explain what you think the above statement means. Describe a specific situation in which the key to failure is in **NOT** trying to please everyone. Discuss what you think determines whether failure is accomplished when no one is pleased.

END OF SECTION 3.

DO NOT RETURN TO PART 1.

BIOLOGICAL SCIENCES

Time: 100 Minutes
Questions 143–219

Directions: This test contains 77 questions. Most of the questions consist of a descriptive passage followed by a group of questions related to the passage. For these questions, study the passage carefully and then choose the best answer to each question in the group. Some questions in this test stand alone. These questions are independent of any passage and independent of each other. For these questions, too, you must select the one best answer. Indicate all your answers by blackening the corresponding circles on your answer sheet.

A periodic table is provided at the beginning of the book. You may consult it whenever you wish.

Passage I (Questions 143–149)

Hemoglobin is a vital protein that transports oxygen in the red blood cells. It consists of four polypeptide chains, and at least seven different genes code for the subunits or chains of the molecule. Not all these genes are equally active throughout life.

All types of hemoglobin contain two alpha chains, but the remaining two chains of the molecule vary depending on age. At different times in the life of the individual, the proportion of hemoglobin molecules containing a particular type of chain (pair) may vary (see *y*-axis). The molecule found in RBCs at a particular time is designated by the types of chains present and how many of each (example: alpha$_2$beta$_2$). The figure below reflects the timing of production of the different chains during human development.

Embryonic and fetal development

143. According to the figure, most fetal hemoglobin contains:

   A. alpha and beta chains.
   B. alpha and gamma chains.
   C. alpha and epsilon chains.
   D. gamma and beta chains.

144. By extrapolating from the figure, what is the composition of most adult hemoglobin molecules?

   A. Alpha and beta chains
   B. Alpha and gamma chains
   C. Beta and delta chains
   D. Alpha and delta chains

145. The hemoglobin gene that appears to stop functioning earliest encodes the:

   A. delta chain.
   B. gamma chain.
   C. epsilon chain.
   D. beta chain.

146. At approximately what point does the beta chain start to appear in a higher proportion of hemoglobin molecules than the gamma chain?

   A. Three to six months before birth
   B. Just before birth
   C. Between birth and three months of age
   D. After six months of age

147. After determining from the figure when each type of hemoglobin is present, which types would you predict have an extremely high affinity for oxygen?

   A. $alpha_2gamma_2$ and $alpha_2delta_2$
   B. $alpha_2gamma_2$ and $gamma_2epsilon_2$
   C. $alpha_2epsilon_2$ and $gamma_2beta_2$
   D. $alpha_2gamma_2$ and $alpha_2epsilon_2$

148. Not all adult hemoglobin is of the same type. Based on information in the graph, a small proportion of adult hemoglobin is probably:

   A. $alpha_2beta_2$.
   B. $alpha_2gamma_2$.
   C. $alpha_2delta_2$.
   D. $alpha_2epsilon_2$.

149. Based on information in the figure, what is the maximum percentage of hemoglobin molecules present at any one time that can be $epsilon_2delta_2$?

   A. 0 percent
   B. 55 percent–58 percent
   C. 0 percent–5 percent
   D. Cannot be determined

Passage II (Questions 150–156)

A set of experiments designed to investigate possible mechanisms of hormone action was carried out. One experiment examined the action of epinephrine, a hormone that is an amino acid derivative. The second experiment utilized the steroid hormones, estrogen, and progesterone.

Experiment 1

It is known that epinephrine stimulates the cytoplasmic enzyme glycogen phosphorylase to hydrolyze glycogen into sugar in cells of the liver and skeletal muscles. However, when epinephrine was added to a test-tube mixture containing the enzyme and glycogen, no hydrolysis occurred. Similarly, injecting epinephrine directly into the cells did not result in the hydrolysis of glycogen either. The effects of epinephrine were observable only if the hormone was added to the extracellular solution surrounding intact cells.

Experiment 2

It is known that estrogen and progesterone are necessary for the normal development and proper functioning of the reproductive system in mammals. In an ex-

periment using rats and monkeys as subjects, target tissues along the reproductive tract and inside the brain were examined to detect the presence of these hormones. Results showed that the hormones were not only inside target cells, but inside the nucleus of these cells. In addition, they were found in association with special protein receptor molecules. When cells that are not normally affected by these hormones (spleen cells) were examined in a similar way, no trace of the hormones was found.

150. Based on the experimental observations, which hormone is least likely to have a *direct* effect on the genes?

   A. Estrogen
   B. Progesterone
   C. Epinephrine
   D. Both A and B

151. What is the probable reason that the steroid hormones could be found inside their target cells?

   A. They are lipid soluble and can normally pass through cell membranes.
   B. They are water soluble and can normally pass through cell membranes.
   C. They are lipid soluble and carrier molecules transport them across cell membranes.
   D. They are water soluble and carrier molecules transport them across cell membranes.

152. If steroids can enter cells, what is a reasonable hypothesis as to why there was no trace of the hormones in nontarget cells such as the spleen?

   A. They passed in and passed out again.
   B. No special protein receptor molecule was present.
   C. Both A and B
   D. Neither A nor B

153. Which statement is compatible with the observations in Experiment 1?

   A. Epinephrine stimulates glycogen phosphorylase by contact inside cells.
   B. Epinephrine stimulates glycogen phosphorylase by contact outside cells.
   C. Epinephrine stimulates glycogen phosphorylase when the hormone is outside and the enzyme is inside a cell.
   D. All of the above

154. Which conclusion is implied by the observations made in Experiment 1?

    A. Epinephrine interacts with the membrane of its target cells.

    B. Epinephrine does not interact with the membrane of nontarget cells.

    C. Epinephrine interacts with the membrane of liver cells and skeletal muscle cells.

    D. All of the above

155. It is now known that most peptide hormones and hormones that are derivatives of amino acids bind to specific protein receptors in the membrane, which then activate a "second messenger" responsible for affecting activities inside the cell. What might be a major difference between a target cell and nontarget cell with respect to a particular hormone of this type?

    A. Nontarget cells do not have the appropriate membrane receptors.

    B. Nontarget cells have the membrane receptors but do not have the "second messenger."

    C. Nontarget cells have the same "second messenger" as target cells, but may have membrane receptors for a different hormone.

    D. Both A and C

156. It has been stated that the surface of a target cell has approximately 10,000 protein receptor molecules. Yet this accounts for only 1/10,000 of the total number of proteins that help make up the cell's membrane structure. Based on this estimate, approximately how many proteins are on a typical cell membrane?

    A. 10^7

    B. 10^8

    C. 10^9

    D. 10^{10}

Passage III (Questions 157–163)

    There are three major "fluid compartments" of the human body. The regions of fluid are found inside the cells (intracellular fluid), outside or in between the cells (interstitial fluid), and in the blood (plasma). The two latter regions make up the extracellular fluid. Although the three compartments may contain many of the same materials in solution, each contains a different combination of concentrations. These differences in solute con-

centration contribute to the functioning of living systems, and must be maintained in order to ensure that normal cellular activities proceed. The figure below compares some of the dissolved constituents of the three fluid regions.

157. An important difference between extracellular fluids and intracellular fluid is that outside the cells there is:

    A. more sodium.

    B. more chloride.

    C. less potassium.

    D. All of the above

158. The charge difference that exists between the inside and outside of cellular membranes (especially obvious in the resting potential of nerve and muscle cells) is due, in part, to the concentration differences noted in question 157. A major factor shown in the figure that contributes to the final charge difference is:

    A. the higher magnesium concentrations inside the cells.

    B. the higher bicarbonate concentrations outside the cells.

    C. the higher biphosphate and protein concentrations inside the cells.

    D. the similarities in carbonic acid concentrations.

159. Magnesium is an important intracellular electrolyte that is essential for the proper functioning of the sodium-potassium pump. Based on this information, which symptom would most likely result from a magnesium deficiency?

    A. Endocrine gland malfunctions
    B. Neuromuscular irritability
    C. Lowered body temperature
    D. Low blood sugar

160. Movement of fluid between the plasma and interstitial compartment takes place across the capillaries. Since blood hydrostatic pressure is higher than blood colloid osmotic pressure at the arteriole end of the capillaries, fluid (water and small proteins) leaks out. Most, but not all, returns at the venule end. Fluid not reabsorbed into the capillaries is eventually returned by the:

    A. urinary system.
    B. liver.
    C. spleen.
    D. lymphatic system.

161. Homeostatic regulation of electrolytes such as sodium, potassium, calcium, and phosphate is monitored and controlled by the:

    A. liver.
    B. endocrine system.
    C. brain.
    D. none of the above

162. If an individual drinks sea water, the blood plasma becomes hypertonic. What will be the primary effect of this change on the intracellular fluid?

    A. Water will move from cells to blood.
    B. Water will move from blood to cells.
    C. Solutes will move from blood to cells.
    D. Solutes will move from cells to blood.

163. The bicarbonate ion is an important component of the blood buffer system. Buffers, the respiratory system, and the urinary system work together to help maintain homeostatic levels of:

    A. glucose.
    B. water.
    C. gases.
    D. pH.

Passage IV (Questions 164–169)

Meiosis is the basis by which chromosome number is reduced by half and gametes are formed. Because sexual reproduction involves the union of two such haploid gametes, genetic variability is maintained.

An immense source of variability during meiosis is the process whereby linked genes (genes at different loci on the same chromosome) undergo crossing over. Homologous chromosomes break and exchange equivalent segments, forming chromosomes with brand-new combinations of genes to be passed on in the gametes (recombinant gametes) to prospective offspring. The appearance of recombinant offspring provides evidence that a chromosome break and crossing over has taken place between linked loci, and the frequency of such recombinant offspring suggests how often the chromosome breaks occurred. By monitoring new combinations of traits that result from crossover events, one can ultimately estimate the distance between the gene loci controlling those traits (the further apart two loci are on a chromosome, the more frequently breaks can occur between them).

In the fruit fly, *Drosophila melanogaster,* gray body and normal wings are two linked dominant traits. The recessive alleles for these genes are black body and vestigial wings, respectively. Flies homozygous for gray body and normal wings were crossed with flies having black bodies and vestigial wings. The F_1 offspring were then crossed with individuals having both recessive phenotypes with the following results in the F_2:

gray body, normal wings:	335
black body, vestigial wings:	305
gray body, vestigial wings:	75
black body, normal wings:	85

164. Between which loci did crossing over occur?

    A. Gray body and black body
    B. Normal wings and vestigial wings
    C. Body color and wing type
    D. Both A and B

165. How many map units apart are the two gene loci?

    A. Less than 10
    B. Between 10 and 11
    C. 20
    D. 25

166. In fruit flies, the genes for normal bristles and normal eye color have been mapped to be about 20 units apart on the same chromosome. In a cross between heterozygotes for both traits and recessive individuals, how many offspring (out of 600) would be expected to have recombinant phenotypes?

    A. 100
    B. 120
    C. 30
    D. 150

167. The crossover frequency between linked genes A and B is 40 percent, between B and C is 65 percent, and between A and C is 25 percent. What is the sequence of genes on the chromosome?

    A. A-B-C
    B. C-A-B
    C. A-C-B
    D. C-B-A

168. If all the chromosomes are to be mapped, how many linkage groups should there be in an organism with 64 chromosomes per somatic cell?

    A. 64
    B. 32
    C. 16
    D. 48

169. In a cross between a heterozygote for the linked genes A, B, and D and a partner with the recessive phenotype for all three traits, what would be the phenotypes of the *double-crossover* recombinant offspring, if the map order of the loci is A-D-B?

    A. A-D-B and a-d-b
    B. A-D-b and a-d-B
    C. A-d-B and a-D-b
    D. A-d-b and a-D-B

Passage V (Questions 170–175)

Clotting or coagulation is part of a larger process called hemostasis (stoppage of bleeding) and occurs to close wounds that would otherwise cause blood loss. The clot itself, a network of insoluble fibers (fibrin), is the end result of a multistep sequence of events involving numerous coagulation factors, most of which are present in the plasma (plasma proteins and other factors desig-

nated by roman numerals) or are released by blood platelets (Pf_{1-4}).

Two parallel clotting systems are present. Both the *extrinsic system* and *intrinsic system* share a number of the same coagulation factors, even though each pathway is initiated by a different mechanism. The extrinsic system is triggered when a blood vessel is ruptured. The surrounding damaged tissues release tissue thromboplastin, and a series of reactions involving plasma coagulation factors eventually leads to the production of extrinsic thromboplastin (Stage 1). The intrinsic system (all components are present in the blood itself) is triggered when the rough surface of a ruptured vessel contacts platelets, causing them to release various platelet factors that eventually lead to the formation of intrinsic thromboplastin (Stage 1).

Steps involved in both systems are outlined in the following figure.

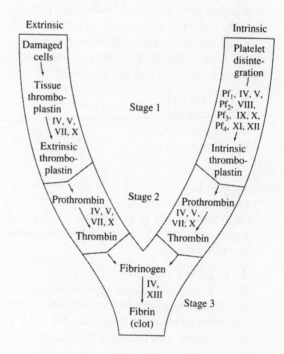

170. Based on information presented in the figure, which statement is correct about the two clotting systems?

    A. Differences are seen only in Stage 1.
    B. Both types of thromboplastin lead to the conversion of prothrombin to thrombin.
    C. Plasma factor IV (calcium) is used in all steps of each system.
    D. All of the above

171. Most plasma coagulation factors in the figure are made in the:

    A. blood vessel walls.
    B. liver.
    C. spleen.
    D. bone marrow.

172. Heparin is a substance produced by basophils (a type of white blood cell) and mast cells (a connective tissue cell). It interferes with the formation of thromboplastin and fibrin. The correct term for such a compound is:

    A. agglutinin.
    B. agglutinogen.
    C. antigenic.
    D. anticoagulant.

173. Hemophilia is a sex-linked group of heredity disorders in which affected individuals lack one of the coagulation factors. If a normal woman whose father was a hemophiliac marries a normal man, what is the probability of producing a hemophiliac child (regardless of sex)?

    A. 100 percent
    B. 75 percent
    C. 50 percent
    D. 25 percent

174. Vitamin K is required for the synthesis of numerous coagulation factors. The pharmaceutical *dicumarol* acts as an antagonist to Vitamin K. For which condition might this compound be recommended?

    A. A patient with slow clotting time
    B. A patient with excess heparin production
    C. A patient prone to forming thromboses (clots in unbroken blood vessels)
    D. A patient with internal hemorrhaging

175. A secondary effect of thrombin (besides converting fibrinogen to fibrin) is to cause platelets to adhere to each other and disintegrate. This added effect:

    A. feeds back and reinforces the intrinsic system.
    B. feeds back and reinforces the extrinsic system.
    C. Both A and B
    D. Neither A nor B

Passage VI (Questions 176–181)

An experiment designed concurrently to examine many variables was carried out. The goal of the experiment was to determine the appropriate environment for the proper functioning of two protein-digesting enzymes, pepsin (an enzyme that converts proteins to peptides in the stomach), and chymotrypsin (a pancreatic enzyme that converts proteins to peptides in the small intestine).

The Experiment

Each enzyme was placed separately in nine beakers containing identical mixtures of food proteins. To each beaker, a solution of buffering agents was added so that the activity of the enzymes could be compared at three different pH levels (pH: 2–4, 4–6, 6–8). *Three replicates* of the three pH environments were established for each enzyme.

One replicate beaker of each pH environment was then maintained in a water bath at each of three different temperature settings (temperatures: 22°C, 37°C, 62°C). At regular time intervals, samples identical in size were removed from each beaker to monitor the amounts of intact protein and peptides present.

Results are shown in Tables 1 and 2 on page 197.

176. The most appropriate environment for chymotrypsin activity is:

    A. 37°C, pH: 4–6
    B. 22°C, pH: 6–8
    C. 37°C, pH: 6–8
    D. 22°C, pH: 4–6

Table 1. Protein and Peptide Levels of "Pepsin" Samples Maintained in Different Environments.

Temperature	pH		
	2–4	4–6	6–8
22°C	moderate protein moderate peptide	high protein no peptide	high protein no peptide
37°C	low protein high peptide	high protein no peptide	high protein no peptide
62°C	high protein no peptide	high protein no peptide	high protein no peptide

Table 2. Protein and Peptide Levels of "Chymotrypsin" Samples Maintained in Different Environments.

Temperature	pH		
	2–4	4–6	6–8
22°C	high protein no peptide	high protein no peptide	moderate protein moderate peptide
37°C	high protein no peptide	moderate protein moderate peptide	low protein high peptide
62°C	high protein no peptide	high protein no peptide	high protein no peptide

177. Which statement most correctly reflects the data in Tables 1 and 2?

   A. Both enzymes have some pH flexibility, but no temperature flexibility.

   B. Both enzymes have some temperature flexibility, but no pH flexibility.

   C. Both enzymes have some pH flexibility, but only pepsin has temperature flexibility.

   D. Both enzymes have some temperature flexibility, but only chymotrypsin has pH flexibility.

178. Which environment appears to be incompatible with both enzymes?

   A. pH: 4–6

   B. pH: 2–4

   C. 22°

   D. 62°

179. Pepsin digests proteins in the specific environment of the stomach. What is the most reasonable explanation for why pepsin does not digest the proteins that make up part of the stomach's own walls?

    A. The environment of the entire stomach is highly acidic.
    B. The wall of the stomach is maintained at approximately 62°C.
    C. Food proteins are surrounded by an acidic environment, while mucous secretions keep the walls alkaline.
    D. Food proteins are surrounded by an alkaline environment, while mucous secretions keep the walls acidic.

180. The soupy material (chyme) released from the stomach into the small intestine is highly acidic. What occurs to ensure that digestion of proteins by pancreatic enzymes continues in the intestinal environment?

    A. The pancreas releases different enzymes with different pH ranges for digesting proteins.
    B. The pancreas delays its release of enzymes until alkaline food arrives in the intestine.
    C. The pancreas sends sodium bicarbonate to adjust intestinal pH.
    D. The small intestine passes the acidic chyme to the large intestine while retaining undigested food molecules.

181. After both pepsin and chymotrypsin successfully digest proteins to peptides, what takes place in the small intestine that allows body tissues to benefit from these nutrients?

    A. The peptides are absorbed into the blood.
    B. The peptides are combined to form polypeptides for more efficient protein synthesis by cells.
    C. The peptides are digested further to amino acids.
    D. All of the above

Passage VII (Questions 182–187)

The kidneys help remove metabolic waste products from the blood. They further contribute to the maintenance of homeostasis by regulating the volume, composition, and pH of the blood. The nephrons of the kidney carry out these various roles through the processes of filtration, reabsorption, and secretion. Filtration takes place from glomerular capillaries into Bowman's capsule. Materials forced out of the blood this way make up the resulting fluid, the filtrate. Substances in the filtrate include waste products, water, nutrients, and electrolytes. Vital substances needed by the body are reabsorbed from filtrate to peritubular capillaries, while wastes and materials not needed continue in the filtrate and are excreted in the urine. Additional changes can be made by transporting materials from peritubular capillaries to filtrate (secretion).

The following table shows some of the chemical constituents of the plasma, as well as how much of each chemical is filtered and reabsorbed in the nephron in one day (all values, except for water, are expressed in grams).

Chemical Constituents in Plasma; Filtered and Reabsorbed in 24 Hrs.

CHEMICAL	PLASMA	FILTRATE IMMEDIATELY AFTER GLOMERULAR CAPSULE	REABSORBED FROM FILTRATE
Water	180,000 mL	180,000 mL	178,000–179,000 mL
Proteins	7,000–9,000	10–20	10–20
Chloride (Cl−)	630	630	625
Sodium (Na+)	540	540	537
Bicarbonate (HCO3−)	300	300	299.7
Glucose	180	180	180
Urea	53	53	28
Potassium (K−)	28	28	24
Uric acid	8.5	8.5	7.7
Creatinine	1.5	1.5	0

182. In a single day, approximately what percentage of water filtered from the plasma leaves the body as urine?

   A. 0.05 percent–0.1 percent
   B. 0.5 percent–1 percent
   C. 1.5 percent–2 percent
   D. 5 percent–10 percent

183. According to information in the table, all plasma constituents are filtered completely **EXCEPT:**

   A. chloride ions.
   B. sodium ions.
   C. urea.
   D. proteins.

184. The afferent arteriole leading into the glomerulus has a wider diameter than the efferent arteriole, which carries blood away to the peritubular capillaries. This arrangement:

   A. increases the efficiency of reabsorption.
   B. represents a countercurrent mechanism.
   C. increases pressure in the glomerulus.
   D. allows red blood cells to pass into the filtrate.

185. Normally, glucose from the plasma is filtered into Bowman's capsule and then completely reabsorbed by active transport in the proximal convoluted tubules. Which of the following is a probable reason that diabetics have high glucose levels in the urine?

   A. The level of glucose that is filtered is higher than normal.
   B. The number of glucose carrier molecules is limited.
   C. Both A and B
   D. Neither A nor B

186. The kidney helps maintain pH balance with a variety of urinary adjustments. If an individual's blood pH is too high, which of the following would be an appropriate urinary system response?

   A. Secrete bicarbonate ions.
   B. Reabsorb additional bicarbonate ions in the distal convoluted tubules.
   C. Filter additional acidic proteins.
   D. Allow the larger alkaline proteins through the glomerulus.

187. The kidney can increase red blood cell production by releasing the hormone erythropoietin. It can also cause additional reabsorption of sodium ions through the renin-angiotensin system's stimulatory effects on aldosterone production. Why do both of these actions help raise blood pressure?

   A. Both lead to a decrease in plasma water content.
   B. Both lead to vasodilation of blood vessels.
   C. Both lead to an increase in blood volume.
   D. Both lead to an increase in secretion at the collecting tubules.

Passage VIII (Questions 188–192)

An organic chemistry student heats benzil with a strong base to form the benzilate anion:

When methoxide ion in methanol is used instead of base, the methyl ester of benzilic acid is formed. Two mechanisms are considered:

Mechanism A.

$$C_6H_5-C=O \quad \underset{\underset{\text{fast}}{(1)}}{\overset{OH^-}{\underset{\longleftarrow}{\longrightarrow}}} \quad C_6H_5-\overset{\overset{O^\ominus}{|}}{\underset{|}{C}}-OH$$

Mechanism diagram A showing subsequent steps (2) slow and (3) fast.

Mechanism B.

Mechanism diagram B showing steps (1) fast, (2) slow, and (3) fast, yielding $+ H_2O$.

---

188. Both mechanisms involve a(n):

   A. reversible step.
   B. molecular rearrangement.
   C. nucleophilic substitution.
   D. electrophilic substitution.

189. If the methoxide ion in methanol is substituted for OH^-/H_2O, step (1) of Mechanism A will most likely yield which of the following?

   A.
   $$C_6H_5-\overset{\overset{OCH_3}{|}}{C}=O$$
   $$C_6H_5-C=O$$
   $$\underset{OCH_3}{|}$$

   B.
   $$C_6H_5-CH-OCH_3$$
   $$C_6H_5-CH-OCH_3$$

   C.
   $$C_6H_5-\overset{\overset{O^-}{|}}{\underset{|}{C}}-OCH_3$$
   $$C_6H_5-C=O$$

   D.
   $$C_6H_5-\overset{\overset{OCH_3}{|}}{C}=O$$
   $$C_6H_5-C=O$$

190. Which of the following studies can be used to help determine the correct mechanism?

   A. Carry out the same reaction using O^{18}-labeled water.
   B. Measure the rate of formation of benzilate anion for different initial concentrations of benzil.

C. Measure the rate of formation of benzilate anion for different pH values.

D. Carry out the same reaction using a deuterated phenyl group.

191. Aliphatic diketones like $CH_3-\overset{\overset{O}{\|}}{C}-\overset{\overset{O}{\|}}{C}-CH_3$ do not undergo similar reactions in alkaline solution because:

A. they never undergo nucleophilic addition reactions.

B. they do not react with bases.

C. they undergo condensation reactions due to the presence of α-hydrogen atoms.

D. the central carbon-carbon bond undergoes cleavage in alkaline solution.

192. Which of the following reactions is unlikely?

A. benzilic acid + $CH_3NH_2 \rightarrow$ amide formation

B. benzilic acid + $CH_3OH \rightarrow$ esterification

C. benzilic acid + $CH_3COOH \rightarrow$ acylation of alcohol group

D. benzilic acid + HCN $\rightarrow$ substitution of OH– by CN–

Passage IX (Questions 193–197)

The reactivity of carbon-carbon double bonds toward nucleophilic addition is increased by the presence of an electron-withdrawing substituent. Thus α, β-unsaturated ketones, acids, esters, and nitriles undergo nucleophilic addition reactions that simple alkenes do not undergo. On the other hand, electron-withdrawing substituents deactivate the carbon-carbon double bond toward electrophilic addition as well as determine the orientation of the addition. (See Reaction 1 below.) The following reactions are known to occur:

Reaction 1.

$$CH_2{=}CH{-}CHO + HCl(g) \rightarrow \underset{\underset{Cl \quad\; H}{|\quad\; |}}{CH_2{-}CH{-}CHO}$$

Reaction 2.

193. From the above reactions, it appears that a basic molecule or ion adds to α, β-unsaturated carbonyl compounds in the:

A. α position.

B. β- position.

C. carbonyl oxygen.

D. carbonyl carbon.

194. An H^+ ion will most likely attack the α, β-unsaturated carbonyl compound at the:

A. α carbon.

B. β carbon.

C. carbonyl oxygen.

D. carbonyl carbon.

195. What product(s) will be formed from the following reaction?

A.

B.

C.

D.

196. A plausible explanation for the fact that electron-withdrawing groups activate nucleophilic addition is that:

  A. they stabilize an anionic intermediate by dispersing the negative charge.
  B. they increase the negative charge on the carbon atoms of the double bond, increasing their susceptibility to attack by nucleophiles.
  C. they destabilize the transition state.
  D. they stabilize an anionic intermediàte by dispersing the negative charge through inductive effects only.

197. Given compounds A, B, and C below, rank them in order of increasing reactivity toward :CN-

$$\begin{array}{ccc} H\ H & H\ H\ O & O\ H\ H\ O \\ |\ \ | & |\ \ |\ \ \| & \|\ \ |\ \ |\ \ \| \\ H-C=C-CH_3 & H-C=C-C-H & H-C-C=C-C-H \\ \\ A & B & C \end{array}$$

  A. A < C < B
  B. B < C < A
  C. A < B < C
  D. C < B < A

Passage X (Questions 198–202)

An organic chemist is interested in studying free radical addition to conjugated dienes. The following reactions are performed:

Experiment 1.

Step (1) Peroxide decomposes to form a free radical

peroxide → R•

Step (2) The free radical abstracts bromine from $BrCCl_3$

$$R• + BrCCl_3 → R—Br + •CCl_3$$

Step (3) The •CCl_3 adds to the conjugated system

$$•CCl_3 + CH_2=CH—CH=CH_2 → \text{allylic free radical}$$

Step (4) allylic free radical

$$\text{allylic free radical} \xrightarrow{BrCCl_3} Cl_3C—CH_2—CH—CH=CH_2 + $$
$$\qquad\qquad\qquad\qquad\qquad\qquad | $$
$$\qquad\qquad\qquad\qquad\qquad\qquad Br $$
$$Cl_3C—CH_2—CH=CH—CH_2—Br$$

Experiment 2.

$BrCCl_3$ is also reacted with a 50:50 mixture of 1,3-butadiene and 1-octene. $BrCCl_3$ reacts mostly with 1,3-butadiene.

198. Based on the above reactions, which of the following statements is false?

  A. Conjugated dienes undergo addition by free radicals.
  B. Alkenes undergo addition by free radicals.
  C. Simple alkenes undergo free radical addition reactions faster than conjugated dienes.
  D. Conjugated dienes undergo free radical addition reactions faster than simple alkenes.

199. Which radicals are formed by the addition of •CCl_3 to 1,3-butadiene?

  A. $Cl_3C—CH_2—\overset{\bullet}{C}H—CH=CH_2$

  $Cl_3C—CH_2—CH=CH—\overset{\bullet}{C}H_2$

  B. $Cl_3C—\overset{\bullet}{C}H—CH_2—CH=CH_2$

  $Cl_3C—CH_2—\overset{\bullet}{C}H—CH=CH_2$

  C. $Cl_3C—CH_2—CH=CH—\overset{\bullet}{C}H_2$

  $Cl_3C—\overset{\bullet}{C}H—CH_2—CH=CH_2$

  D. $Cl_3C—CH_2—\overset{\bullet}{C}H—CH=CH_2$

  $Cl_3C—\overset{\bullet}{C}H—CH=CH—CH_3$

200. Which statement is supported by Experiment 2?

A. The transition state of the diene is more stable than the transition state of the simple alkene.

B. The diene is more stable than the simple alkene.

C. The activation energy for the diene is lower than the activation energy for the simple alkene.

D. The activation energy for the diene is higher than the activation energy for the simple alkene.

201. Both alkenes and dienes undergo free radical polymerization. Polymers formed from dienes, however, differ from polymers of alkenes in that polymers formed from dienes:

A. contain double bonds.

B. are saturated.

C. require an initiator to begin the polymerization.

D. are all substituted.

202. Dienes like simple alkenes undergo electrophilic addition. Butadiene when treated with bromine forms which of the following?

A. 3,4-dibromo-1-butene only

B. 1,4-dibromo-2-butene only

C. 3,4-dibromo-1-butene and 1,4-dibromo-2-butene

D. 1-bromo-2-butene only

Questions 203 through 219 are independent of any passage and independent of each other.

203. The α and β forms of D-glucose are:

A. enantiomers.

B. epimers.

C. meso structures.

D. anomers.

204. Chromatography can be used to:

A. separate nonvolatile liquids.

B. separate volatile liquids.

C. separate a nonvolatile liquid from a volatile liquid.

D. All of the above

205. Human blood types are most often examined in reference to the ABO gene locus. The I^A and I^B alleles are both dominant to the I^O allele. If blood from a type AB individual were donated to three individuals who were, respectively, types A, B, and O, which of the recipients' blood would agglutinate?

A. The recipients with blood types A and B

B. The recipient with blood type O

C. None of the recipients

D. All of the recipients

206. The conversion of threonine to isoleucine is a five-step enzymatic pathway. The end product, isoleucine, fits into the allosteric site of the enzyme at step 1, preventing its normal function. This is an example of:

A. enzyme specificity.

B. competitive inhibition.

C. enzyme enhancement.

D. feedback inhibition.

207. The cerebellum is the part of the brain that helps coordinate skeletal muscles and helps maintain posture and balance. To perform this complex function, the cerebellum must receive input from:

A. the cerebrum and proprioceptors.

B. the cerebrum and the inner ear.

C. proprioceptors and the inner ear.

D. the cerebrum, proprioceptors, and the inner ear.

208. The following figure shows relative hormone concentrations during the menstrual cycle. As estrogen levels go up, Follicle Stimulating Hormone (FSH) is inhibited. Luteinizing hormone (LH), after stimulating ovulation, also stimulates the corpus luteum to produce high levels of progesterone. Progesterone helps maintain the preparedness of the uterus in case fertilization takes place. As LH levels decrease, corpus luteum activity slows down and progesterone levels rapidly drop. This causes a disintegration of uterine tissues, resulting in the menstrual flow. If fertilization occurs, Human Chorionic Gonadotropin (HCG) is produced by embryonic cells. This hormone maintains the corpus luteum and the pregnancy proceeds. HCG seems to mimic the actions of:

A. estrogen.
B. FSH.
C. LH.
D. progesterone.

209. Chromosome puffs can be observed along giant polytene chromosomes in the salivary gland cells of insect larvae. They appear to be regions of DNA that uncoil or decondense. The locations of puffs change at different times during larval development in response to hormonal signals. This phenomenon is an example of:

A. gene regulation at the transcriptional level.
B. a polygenic trait.

C. posttranscriptional RNA processing.
D. gene expression at the translational level.

210. Curare is a chemical used in arrow poisons as well as in pharmaceutical compounds. It competes with acetylcholine for receptor sites along the motor end plate. The immediate physiological effects of high doses of curare can include:

A. decreased ability to relax muscles.
B. inability to contract muscles and paralysis.
C. inability to repolarize muscles.
D. abnormal heat production in the affected muscle cells.

211. Arrector pili muscles are smooth muscles associated with hair follicles in the skin. When contracted, the muscles pull the hairs erect and "goosebumps" appear as the skin around the hair shafts slightly elevates. What stimulates the arrector pili muscles to contract?

A. Somatic motor neurons
B. Autonomic motor neurons
C. Exocrine secretions
D. Endocrine secretions

212. A variety of organs with similar functions among the vertebrates are thin, moist, highly vascular, and cover a relatively large surface area. These are necessary characteristics for an efficient:

A. heart.
B. blood-brain barrier.
C. neuromuscular interface.
D. respiratory membrane.

213. If a muscle cell is stimulated a second time before it has time to relax completely, a stronger contraction results. What is this phenomenon called?

A. Tetany
B. Partial (incomplete) tetany
C. Summation
D. Threshold stimulation

214. The inflammatory response results from the release of histamine by mast cells or basophils. The redness, heat, pain, and swelling associated with inflammation are due to which physiological effects of histamine?

A. Dilation of local blood vessels/Less fluid leakage from capillaries
B. Dilation of local blood vessels/More fluid leakage from capillaries
C. Constriction of local blood vessels/Less fluid leakage from capillaries
D. Constriction of local blood vessels/More fluid leakage from capillaries

215. Toluene will show peaks in its:

A. IR spectrum only.
B. UV and IR spectrum only.
C. IR, UV, and NMR spectrum.
D. UV spectrum only.

216. Acetone and acetaldehyde in the presence of a strong base will yield which of the following?

A. Two different β-hydroxyaldehydes
B. Four different β-hydroxycarbonyl compounds
C. Two different β-hydroxyketones
D. Three different β-hydroxycarbonyl compounds

217. Which of the following compounds will not react with acetyl chloride?

A. NH_3
B. CH_3NH_2
C. $(CH_3)_2NH$
D. $(CH_3)_4N^+Cl^-$

218. Aldehydes react with alcohols in acidic solution to form:

A. hemiacetals and acetals.
B. hemiacetals only.
C. ketals only.
D. hemiketals only.

219. Basic hydrolysis of the dipeptide

Ala-Gly :
$$H_2N-\underset{\underset{CH_3}{|}}{CH}-\underset{\overset{\|}{O}}{C}-\underset{\underset{H}{|}}{N}-\underset{\underset{H}{|}}{CH}-COOH \text{ gives:}$$

A. $H_3\overset{+}{N}-\underset{\underset{CH_3}{|}}{CH}-\underset{\overset{\|}{O}}{C}-O^- + H_3\overset{+}{N}-CH_2-COO^-$

B. $H_2N-\underset{\underset{CH_3}{|}}{CH}-COOH + H_3\overset{+}{N}-CH_2-COO^-$

C. $H_2N-\underset{\underset{CH_3}{|}}{CH}-COO^- + H_2N-CH_2-COO^-$

D. $H_2N-\underset{\underset{CH_3}{|}}{CH}-COOH + H_2N-CH_2-COOH$

END OF TEST.

IF YOU FINISH BEFORE THE TIME IS UP, YOU MAY
CHECK YOUR WORK ON THIS TEST ONLY.

PRACTICE EXAM III ANSWER KEY

VERBAL REASONING		PHYSICAL SCIENCES		BIOLOGICAL SCIENCES	
1. C	45. B	66. B	110. D	143. B	187. C
2. A	46. A	67. C	111. C	144. A	188. B
3. D	47. D	68. A	112. B	145. C	189. C
4. C	48. D	69. C	113. D	146. C	190. A
5. C	49. D	70. C	114. A	147. D	191. C
6. D	50. D	71. C	115. B	148. C	192. D
7. D	51. C	72. A	116. C	149. A	193. B
8. A	52. B	73. D	117. D	150. C	194. C
9. D	53. A	74. C	118. B	151. A	195. D
10. B	54. B	75. A	119. C	152. C	196. A
11. C	55. D	76. B	120. A	153. C	197. C
12. D	56. A	77. B	121. D	154. D	198. C
13. A	57. B	78. D	122. B	155. D	199. A
14. A	58. A	79. D	123. D	156. B	200. C
15. B	59. D	80. C	124. D	157. D	201. A
16. C	60. A	81. B	125. B	158. C	202. C
17. D	61. A	82. D	126. D	159. B	203. D
18. D	62. A	83. D	127. C	160. D	204. D
19. D	63. C	84. C	128. C	161. B	205. D
20. C	64. B	85. B	129. B	162. A	206. D
21. B	65. B	86. C	130. D	163. D	207. D
22. D		87. A	131. D	164. C	208. C
23. B		88. B	132. A	165. C	209. A
24. D		89. A	133. D	166. B	210. B
25. D		90. B	134. B	167. B	211. B
26. B		91. B	135. A	168. B	212. D
27. C		92. C	136. D	169. C	213. C
28. C		93. D	137. A	170. D	214. B
29. C		94. A	138. B	171. B	215. C
30. A		95. D	139. A	172. D	216. B
31. C		96. C	140. D	173. D	217. D
32. C		97. C	141. D	174. C	218. A
33. C		98. D	142. B	175. A	219. C
34. A		99. B		176. C	
35. B		100. C		177. D	
36. D		101. B		178. D	
37. B		102. C		179. C	
38. C		103. A		180. C	
39. A		104. C		181. C	
40. C		105. C		182. B	
41. A		106. B		183. D	
42. C		107. B		184. C	
43. C		108. D		185. C	
44. C		109. A		186. A	

PRACTICE EXAM III EXPLANATORY ANSWERS

VERBAL REASONING

1. **C** The answer to this question is based on the following statement in paragraph 7: "Park adds that one of the many benefits of the experiment for exobiologists (scientists who study possibilities of life in outer space) is knowledge gained about whether life forms could travel. . ."

2. **A** The answer to this question is based on the following statement made in paragraph 2: "All 12.5 million of the seeds were carried aboard Space Shuttle Mission 41-C . . . and placed in orbit inside . . . (LDEF), a free-flying, 12-sided structure loaded with experiments designed to test results of continuous exposure to outer space."

3. **D** The answer to this question is based on the following statement in paragraph 1: "When some 12.5 million tomato seeds returned to earth in February 1985 after almost a year in space, several thousand American students . . . anxiously awaited their arrival . . ." And on this statement from paragraph 2: "the seeds . . . were divided up . . . among hundreds of schools."

4. **C** The answer to this question is based on the following statement made in paragraph 3: "There are no 'cookbook' rules governing how the experiments are to be conducted other than the requirement of strictly scientific methodology."

5. **C** The answer to this question is based on the following statement in paragraph 3: "At the conclusion of the experimentation, student reports . . . are to be tabulated in a summary report by NASA headquarters and made generally available upon request."

6. **D** The answer to this question is based on paragraph 7: ". . . one of the many benefits of the experiment . . . is knowledge gained about whether life forms could travel by passive means from one ecosystem or planet to another without a spaceship. If the seeds exposed to both vacuum and high radiation come through with little or no damage, it opens up questions . . . about the origins and destinations of primitive life forms."

7. **D** The answer to this question can be inferred from the following statements found in paragraphs 4 and 8 and the generally positive tone of the article: "Like all great ideas this one was born in the mind of an imaginative individual" (paragraph 4). "What new connections might be made by the thousands of students participating in SEEDS? Their horizons are as unlimited as outer space" (paragraph 8).

8. **A** The answer to this question is based on the following statement in paragraph 2: "In one field of concentration, for example—justice, morality, and constitutional democracy—great books form the core of the curriculum. Students read Plato, Aristotle, Machiavelli, Hobbes, Rousseau, Hegel, and Nietzsche or Weber."

9. **D** The answer is based on the statement in paragraph 4: ". . . the proposal made clear that the project was being undertaken as an integrated effort to revitalize the college's dedication to providing a liberal arts education to its students."

10. **B** The answer to this question can be inferred from the fact that the author does not include any criticism of the program in the article, but does quote a number of positive statements such as this one from paragraph 4: "Panelists' reactions demonstrated their admiration for the strong, unified goal toward which all activities of the project were directed."

11. **C** The answer to this question is based on a statement in paragraph 2: "The proposal demonstrates that a foundation for the project exists in the successful integration of the humanities and the social sciences in some parts of the Madison College curriculum."

12. **D** The answer to this question is based on the following statement in paragraph 4: "We expect these activities to . . . contribute to faculty development, improve individual courses, and make our upper level curricula more vital. . . ." There is no mention of individual student needs.

13. **A** The answer to this question is supported by the following statement in paragraph 4: "Panelists' reactions demonstrated their admiration for

the strong, unified goal toward which all activities of the project were directed."

14. **A** The answer to this question is based on a statement from paragraph 2: "Students read Plato, Aristotle, Machiavelli, Hobbes, Rousseau, Hegel, and Nietzsche or Weber."

15. **B** The answer to this question is found in the following statement from Paragraph 1: "Finally, electric utilities are concerned that costly and potentially counterproductive regulations may be promulgated before a rational basis for policy making is achieved."

16. **C** The answer to this question can be chosen by ruling out choices A, B, and D, all of which are referred to in the article. That leaves choice C as the only possible answer. Choice A is referred to in paragraph 5: "Planners will need to consider potential changes in energy supply resulting from climate change." Choice B is referred to in paragraph 4: "Utility planners must therefore consider both the likelihood of having to build new power plants to meet higher peak demand and the probable need to purchase more fuel for increased generation." Choice D is referred to in a statement in paragraph 6: "To meet these challenges, utilities will need to adopt more sophisticated strategies of risk management."

17. **D** The answer to this question is based on the following statement in paragraph 2: "In particular, the apparent 0.6 degree C, 1 degree F rise in average global temperature over the last century lies within the long-term range of natural variability, although the recent rate of increase seems rapid."

18. **D** The answer to this question can be chosen on the basis of ruling out A, B and C leaving D as the answer. Choice A is referred to in paragraph 4 (point 4): "Adapting to changing climate: Examples are heating and cooling of buildings, compensation of disadvantaged regions, and changing of agricultural practices." Choice B is referred to in paragraph 4 (point 2): "Removing greenhouse gases from effluents or the atmosphere: Examples are removing CO_2 from power plant emissions as well as starting forestation programs." Choice C is referred to in paragraph 4 (point 3): "Making countervailing modifications in climate and weather: One example is cloud seeding; another

more speculative example is changing the atmosphere's reflectivity by releasing particles in the stratosphere."

19. **D** The answer to this question is based on the following statement in paragraph 3 and by the constant references in the article for the need for better understanding of the Greenhouse Effect: "Research is needed to tell us not only when to act but also how to act."

20. **C** The answer to this question is supported by this statement in paragraph 2: "Current models suggest that a warming trend of this magnitude could result solely from the increases in atmospheric CO_2 and other greenhouse gases (e.g., nitrous oxide, methane, chlorofluorocarbons, and ozone)."

21. **B** The answer to this question is based on the following statement in paragraph 2: "A marketing strategy that presents the product or service as an opportunity for personal growth is far more likely to succeed."

22. **D** The answer to this question is based on the following statement in paragraph 2: "So intense is the interest in the older consumer that many of America's largest companies have launched advertising campaigns targeted at adults over 50."

23. **B** The answer to this question is based on the following statement in paragraph 8: "Barbara Kane . . . ticks off the professional skills important for success in this field: counseling skills . . . (and) assessment skills."

24. **D** The answer to this question is based on the following statement in paragraph 7: "More often than not, they are social workers, although nurses, psychologists, and gerontologists operate case management firms, too."

25. **D** The answer to this question can be inferred from the following statement in paragraph 9: "Prospects should continue to be very good, considering the rapid growth in the number of people of advanced age and the increased willingness of many people to use social work and mental-health services."

26. **B** The second paragraph discusses the emergence of an increasing elderly market and the need for advertising targeting that market. It also

notes the poor perception of advertisers of just how to appeal to the elderly and the need for marketing consultants to advise them.

27. **C** The answer to this question can be found in the following statement in paragraph 3: "Davis proposed cave development deep below the water table . . ."

28. **C** The answer to this question is supported by the following statement in paragraph 1: "Early biological studies emphasized faunal surveys and descriptions of the degenerate eyes of cavernicolous animals (cavernicoles) . . ."

29. **C** The answer to this question is based on the following statement in paragraph 1: "Scientific interest in caves began in seventeenth- and eighteenth-century Europe . . ."

30. **A** The answer to this question is contained in the following statement from paragraph 1: ". . . with the development of elaborate (but erroneous) theories of the hydrogenic cycle in which cave systems were essential elements."

31. **C** The answer to this question is supported by the following statement from paragraph 3: "Davis proposed cave development deep below the water table, by random circulation of slowly percolating groundwater ('phreatic' origin)."

32. **C** The answer to this question is based on ruling out A, B, and D, which are supported by statements in the article, leaving C, which is not supported by any statement. In paragraph 4 are the following statements that support A, B, and D: "Factors influencing reactivation of geological cave research and continued progress in biospeleology in the past decade include amassment of a large body of descriptive data collected mainly by nonprofessional explorers and surveyors (A) . . . growing acquaintance with the large body of European literature that had been largely ignored by American theoreticians of the 1930s (B) . . . and finally, involvement of younger researchers whose interest arose from exploration and field experience (D)."

33. **C** The answer to this question is based on the following statement in paragraph 3: "Biospeleology advanced slowly in the United States from 1930 to 1950, even though this was the time of a lively debate over the origin of caves."

34. **A** The answer is clear from the statement: "The argument over location of the water table tended to reduce the research that was done to a sterile classification of some particular cave as having vadose or phreatic origin."

35. **B** The answer to this question is supported by the following statement from paragraph 4: "Other theories place the zone of cave development at or above the local water table ('vadose' origin)."

36. **D** The answer to this question can be inferred from several statements in paragraph 1 and a statement in paragraph 3: "Robert Lowell is known both as a major twentieth century American poet and as an important translator" and "Lowell's work remains difficult and obscure" are from paragraph 1. Another statement that implies the answer is in paragraph 3: "'He isn't an American poet at all,' Gillis explains, 'but a bearer of an older, deeper tradition of European literary and poetic history . . .'"

37. **B** The answer to this statement can be inferred from several statements in paragraph 2: "Lowell scholar Daniel Gillis . . . is attempting to reform the critical view (of Lowell) by highlighting the influence of classical literature on the poet" and paragraph 3 points out that Lowell is a "bearer of an older, deeper tradition of European literary and poetic history . . . and Latin literature. . . ."

38. **C** The answer to this question is based on the following statements from paragraphs 11 and 12: "The course . . . will address a modern poet from a fresh, rich perspective; . . . it will give the classics students a taste of modern literature while taking advantage of their academic forte" (paragraph 11). "The hope is that studying Lowell and his ties to classical antiquity will generate interest both in a poet deserving recognition and in an academic discipline in search of creative scholars" (paragraph 12). While the author laments the lack of a classical grounding in today's education, he does not expect his course to change this fact.

39. **A** The answer to this question can be inferred from the following statement found in paragraph 7: "The diminishing numbers of readers who can appreciate Lowell and scholars who can satisfactorily analyze the poet point up a disturbing trend in American education. The classical grounding in Latin and Greek language and

literature that was prevalent in the nineteenth century has almost disappeared from today's schools."

40. **C** The answer to this question is based on the following statement made in paragraph 9: "Lowell's translations (which Gillis argues is the wrong word to use) have also been misunderstood. 'He used the word imitation,' Gillis notes. 'They're much freer than literal translations.'"

41. **A** The answer to this question is based on the statement from paragraph 7, which was cited as the answer to question 39.

42. **C** The answer to this question is based on the following statement from paragraph 10: "An act disenfranchising women, free blacks, and aliens was promoted as a way of reducing election fraud by making it easier to identify ineligible voters."

43. **C** The answer is in the last paragraph. "All states were then stripping the franchise from marginal groups—free blacks, noncitizens, native Americans, and in New Jersey, women—while at the same time removing obstacles to universal white male suffrage."

44. **C** The answer to this question is based on the following statement in paragraph 6: "The new constitution gave the vote to 'all inhabitants' who were worth fifty pounds in real or personal property, thereby removing extensive real estate holdings as the sole economic test for voter eligibility."

45. **B** The answer to this question is based on several statements in paragraph 1: "Of the many women who surely importuned their husbands for equal status in the new American nation, the most famous was Abigail Adams . . . (who) wrote to her husband John to ' . . . remember the ladies and be more generous to them than your ancestors, in the new code of laws. Do not put such unlimited power into the hands of the husbands. . . .'"

46. **A** The answer to this question is supported by the following statement in paragraph 7: "The few available voting lists from the period . . . suggest that as many as 15 percent of the qualified women voted . . ."

47. **D** The answer to this question is based on the following statement in paragraph 6: "The new constitution gave the vote to 'all inhabitants' who were worth fifty pounds in real or personal property. . . ."

48. **D** The answer to this question is based on the following statement in paragraph 11: "Thus, New Jersey women were victims of political pressures that transcended local circumstances, and they would not be able to vote again until the passage of the Nineteenth Amendment more than one hundred years later."

49. **D** The answer to this question is supported by the following statement in paragraph 8: "Why did women lose the vote in 1807?"

50. **D** The answer to this question is based on the following statement in paragraph 6: "The scholar's role is not to provide a tidy analysis of the text, not to deliver 'the answers,' but rather to enrich discussion with biographical information on the author, with contextual perspectives from the literary tradition or historical era . . ."

51. **C** The answer to this question is based on several statements from paragraphs 2 and 3. In paragraph 2 are the following statements: "The discussion reminded me again of why I loved to serve as a scholar in these programs. Talk ranged from analysis of the text to insights gained from Rhys about personal lives." In paragraph 3, are these statements: "If only my freshmen cared this much about their reading! At the conclusion of the discussion, I had some new ideas about Jean Rhys, and these have affected my subsequent scholarship. I learned, for example, to be more subtle in my analysis of point of view."

52. **B** The answer to this question can be inferred from several statements. In paragraph 5 is this statement: "To enhance the discussion, Bates introduced the concept of opening each session with a lecture by a humanities scholar." In paragraph 6, is the statement: "The scholar's role is . . . to enrich discussion with biographical information on the author . . . and to be a catalyst for discussion by raising provocative questions about the text."

53. **A** The answer to this question is supported by the following statements in paragraph 5: "Her

goal was to establish a context in which a number of adults could all read the same book and later gather to discuss it. To enhance the discussion, Bates introduced the concept of opening each session with a lecture by a humanities scholar."

54. **B** This answer to this question is based on the following statement in paragraph 4: "Reading and discussion programs of this nature began just a decade ago around a kitchen table in Rutland, Vermont, across the state from Wells River."

55. **D** The answer to this question is based on the following statement in paragraph 8: "These audiences were diverse: adolescents and octogenarians, people with high school degrees, people with Ph.D.s, individuals from all classes and careers."

56. **A** The answer to this question can be inferred from statements in paragraphs 7 and 8. In paragraph 7, is the statement: "I spoke about humanities texts . . . to eager audiences. . . (who) were hungry . . . for the scholar's information and even hungrier for the human interaction around a text." In paragraph 8 is the statement: "What more could a teacher-scholar ask than for 'students' who are well prepared, eager to talk, willing to argue, and replete with a wealth of life experience?"

57. **B** The answer to this question is supported by a number of statements. In paragraph 4, we learn that the program grew out of the "frustration of reading a good book and having no one with whom to discuss it." In paragraph 7, the author states, "I spoke about humanities texts . . . to eager audiences in small libraries, community centers, and even churches . . . because the audiences were hungry . . . for the scholar's information and even hungrier for the human interaction around a text."

58. **A** The answer to this question is supported by the following statements in paragraph 8: "These projects should help to engender public understanding . . . of the Northwest Ordinance as one of the cornerstone documents of our founding. Like any enduring cornerstone, the Northwest Ordinance has been built upon again and again. It has served as a blueprint for the nation's westward expansion."

59. **D** The answer to this question is based on ruling out A, B, and C as they are supported by statements in the article, leaving D as the remaining answer. A is supported by the following statement in paragraph 6: "Among the items included . . . are a rare first printing of *The Definitive Treaty between Great Britain and the United States (1783)* . . . Jefferson's Ordinance of 1784, which set up a temporary government for the West; and the Land Ordinance of 1785, which established the system for surveying and eventual sale of the new lands." B is supported by the following statement in paragraph 2: "The Northwest Ordinance: Liberty and Justice for All (project) featured . . . a two-day scholarly symposium to examine the state of current scholarship on the ordinance." It is also supported by the following statement in paragraph 3: "The symposium . . . brought together a dozen scholars who were at work on the ordinance or some related aspect of American history." C is inferred by the following statements found in paragraphs 1, 2, and 4. From paragraph 1, is the statement: "Two projects brought together for the first time by the alumni associations from nine Big Ten universities, and a variety of other institutions, for several programs available to the public." From paragraph 2 comes the following statement: "[the first project entitled] Northwest Ordinance . . . featured education programs . . . for the general public." The statement: "The alumni associations developed public educational packs for distribution . . ." is from paragraph 4.

60. **A** The answer to this question is supported by the following statement in paragraph 8: "[The Northwest Ordinance] has served as a blueprint for the nation's westward expansion . . ."

61. **A** The answer is based on ruling out B, C, and D. They are supported by statements in the article, leaving A the remaining answer as it is not supported by any statements. From paragraph 7, is the following statement that supports B: "These ordinances and documents rank among the most important in our early American history, both for what they accomplish and for what they inspired. . . ." C is supported by the following statements from paragraph 8: "Like any enduring cornerstone, the Northwest Ordinance has been built upon again and again. It has served as a blueprint for the nation's westward expansion." From paragraph 6, is the following sentence that supports D: "Among the

56 items included in the Northwest Ordinance part of the exhibition [is] . . . the Land Ordinance of 1785, which established the system for surveying and eventual sale of the new lands to settlers in the Northwest Territory."

62. **A** The answer to this question can be inferred from paragraph 6: "Among the 56 items included in the Northwest Ordinance part of the exhibition are a rare first printing of *The Definitive Treaty between Great Britain and the United States (1783),* written and printed at the instruction of Ambassador Benjamin Franklin in Paris . . ."

63. **C** The answer to this question is based on the following statement in paragraph 6: ". . . the Land Ordinance of 1785, which established the system for the surveying and eventual sale of the new lands to settlers in the Northwest Territory."

64. **B** The answer to this question is based on the following statements in paragraph 6: "[Included are] a rare first printing of *The Definitive Treaty between Great Britain and the United States (1783)*" and ". . . along with pages of the original Northwest Ordinance."

65. **B** The answer to this question is based on the following statement in paragraph 4: "The alumni associations developed public education packs for distribution to libraries, historical societies, and other interested organizations."

PHYSICAL SCIENCES

66. **B** Note that one scale measures color observed in solution, while the other measures color absorbed—the complement of the first.

67. **C** Violet, blue, blue green, green, yellow.

68. **A** The hexamminecobalt (III) complex ion has the shortest wavelength of maximum absorption, hence the greatest transition energy.

69. **C** The absorbed wavelength shifts from 430 nm to 500 nm. The *absorption* colors shift from yellow to orange-red.

70. **C** Only choice C describes an inverse relationship between energy and wavelength.

71. **C** The absorption at 560 nm corresponds to an energy gap slightly *higher* than the gap associated with the 580-nm absorption, given in the table as 207 kJ/mol. When we search for such a gap, we find one of 211kJ/mol between the bottom and top levels of III.

72. **A** A blue solution absorbs light in the orange-red region, around 239 kJ/mol. The gap between the middle and bottom levels shown in (I) could produce this absorption.

73. **D** None of the pairs of levels shown could lead to an energy gap greater than kJ/mol, which is needed for the onset of ultraviolet light.

74. **C** Sodium and nitrate ions flow through the bridge, not silver ions or electrons.

75. **A**
$$E°_{cell} = E°_{RED} + E°_{OXID}$$
$$= 0.799 \text{ v} + (- 0.799 \text{ v})$$
$$= 0$$

76. **B** The second and third time values recorded show a voltage drop of more than 0.010 v.

77. **B** As shown, a potential develops owing to the difference in concentration between the two sides; current flows so as to diminish this difference by oxidation on one side and reduction on the other. Physical mixing allows the concentration difference to be eliminated without the need for a flow of electrons between the cells.

78. **D** The salt bridge does not allow electrons to pass; the wire does. The electrons go from right to left, since in that way oxidation occurs at the dilute solution, increasing the silver ion concentration. Simultaneously, reduction occurs at the concentrated side, lowering the silver ion concentration.

79. **D** Any silver ion that appears on the right due to oxidation is balanced by a like amount that disappears on the left due to reduction.

80. **C** Since K_{sp} is small, and since K_{eq} for the reaction describing the combination of the two ions is $1/K_{sp}$, the reaction goes essentially to completion.

81. **B** The second reactant must have been a strong

base, since some of the H⁺ is used up and there is no other major product.

82. **D** You start with a weak base, and need to convert half of its original amount to its conjugate acid. You'll need 0.025 moles of a strong acid to do this.

83. **D** The solution is mostly sodium acetate, which is slightly basic owing to hydrolysis of the acetate ion.

84. **C** Each mole of carbonate requires 2 moles of H⁺ to convert it to carbonic acid.

85. **B** Ammonium chloride dissociates to form ammonium ion, which is a weak acid. (Don't confuse ammonium ion with its conjugate base, ammonia.)

86. **C** This reaction results in an equal mixture of a weak acid with its conjugate base; such a solution is a buffer.

87. **A** Its slight dissociation before the HCl was added will be decreased owing to the excess of hydrogen ion.

88. **B** Electrons flow through the circuit toward the *positively* charged electrode.

89. **A** Electrons flow spontaneously toward the positive electrode, combining with and reducing Fe^{3+} ions at the electrode surface.

90. **B** Zn is the negative electrode, thus electrons flow from it and it is the anode in cells B and C.

91. **B** Nickel is the negative electrode, hence more readily oxidized in cell A; similarly, it is more readily reduced in cell C.

92. **C** The data give no indication of *absolute* potential, so A and B cannot be correct. Since the Pb electrode is positive, it must be reduced, with a potential that is 0.131 v greater than that for the reduction of Ni^{2+}.

93. **D** Cell A has no half-reaction in common with cell B, so no comparison can be made.

94. **A** The chart shows that the half-reaction for Pb^{2+}/Pb has the greater reduction potential, so Pb^{2+} will be reduced while Zn will be oxidized.

95. **D** $1.00 \text{ v} + 0.131 \text{ v} = 1.13 \text{ v}$.

96. **D** According to the chart, Pb^{2+} is more readily reduced than Zn^{2+} by $0.505 + 0.131 = 0.636$ v.

97. **C** Since CO_3^{2-} is a weak base, the solution of sodium carbonate should have a pH above 7, while that of NaCl should be 7. The chloride test using silver ion would be inconclusive, since Ag_2CO_3 would also precipitate. Titration with a strong base would give no reaction with either negative ion.

98. **D** Although each solution has the same number of formula weights of salt per weight of solvent, each Na_2CO_3 entity furnishes 3 ions when it dissolves, while each NaCl furnishes only 2.

99. **B** Freezing point depression and boiling point elevation represent one of the few uses of molality general encountered in introductory chemistry.

100. **C** Use of the freezing point depression to distinguish the solutions will assume that each salt dissociates completely, as sodium salts generally do.

101. **B** Since f.p.d. is proportional to total molality of ions, the depression for the sodium carbonate will be 1.5 times larger than that for sodium chloride.

102. **C** The reciprocal of the focal length is equal to the sum of the reciprocals of the object and image distances:

$$1/F = 1/d_{object} + 1/d_{image}$$

$$= 1/0.60 \text{ m} + 1/0.30 \text{ m} = 3/0.60 \text{ m}$$

$$F = 0.20 \text{ meters}$$

103. **A** The ratio of the object to image size is equal to the ratio of the object to image distance:

$$S_{object}/S_{image} = d_{object}/d_{image}$$

$$S_{image} = (0.60 \text{ m})(0.050 \text{ m})/(0.30 \text{ m}) = 0.10 \text{ m}$$

104. **C** Since the surface on both sides of the lens is convex, the lens is a converging lens. For any converging lens, an object that is more than two focal lengths away from the lens will produce an image that is real, inverted and smaller than the object.

105. **C** Light is bent or refracted when it passes from

one medium (air) into another (the material of the lens).

106. **B** For a converging lens: 1) If the object is more than two focal lengths away, the image will be smaller than the object and appear on the opposite side of the lens at a distance between one and two focal lengths from the lens; 2) If the object is two focal lengths away, the image on the opposite side of the lens will be the same size as the object and appear at a distance of two focal lengths from the lens. The net effect of moving the object toward the lens is to increase the size of the image on the opposite side of the lens and to increase its distance from the lens.

107. **B** Centripetal acceleration is inversely proportional to the radius of the curve: $a_c = v^2/r$. Since the radius of the larger curve is twice that of the smaller curve, the centripetal acceleration at the larger curve will be half as great as that at the smaller curve.

108. **D** The force is given by Newton's second law, where:

$$F = ma_c = mv^2/r$$
$$= (2000 \text{ kg})(20 \text{ m/s})^2/50.0 \text{ m}$$
$$= 1.6 \times 10^4 \text{ N}$$

109. **A** Along the straightaway, the car travels at a constant speed, so there is no acceleration and therefore no force acting on the car. In the turns, although the speed is still constant, the direction of the car is changing so that the presence of a force is required.

110. **D** The distance is the product of the velocity and the time required to cover the distance: $d = vt = (20 \text{ m/s})(20 \text{ s}) = 400 \text{ m}$.

111. **C** Kinetic energy is $1/2\ mv^2$. Since the mass of the car is constant and its velocity is constant, its kinetic energy must be the same along the straightaway as it is going around the curves.

112. **B** Poiseuille's formula shows an R^4 dependence of the flow rate. Thus increasing the bore of the needle (R) will have the most marked effect on the flow rate.

113. **D** $Q \sim \dfrac{P}{R^4}$ If the radius is halved then $(1/2)4 = 1/16$. To maintain Q, $(1/2)4\ P$ must increase by a factor of 16.

114. **A** 5L/min = 5000 cm^3/min
$$= 8.333 \text{ M} \quad 10^{-5} \text{ m}^3/\text{s};$$

$$Q = \bar{v}A \text{ and } \bar{v} = Q/A$$
$$= 8.333 \times 10^{-5}/3.14 \quad (1.0 \times 10^{-2})^2$$
$$= 0.265 \text{ m/s};$$
$$\mathfrak{R} = 2\bar{v}Rd/\eta$$
$$= \frac{2 \quad 0.265 \quad 0.010 \quad 1030}{0.0040}$$
$$= 1,365$$

115. **B** $\bar{v} = \eta\mathfrak{R}/2d$
$$= (0.0040)(3000)/2(0.010)(1030)$$
$$= 0.58 \text{ m/s}$$

116. **C** Because the flow rate must necessarily be the same in the arteries, veins, and capillaries, Poiseuille's formula shows the pressure drop will increase with decreasing R.

117. **D** A decrease in temperature usually increases friction between fluid layers, thus increasing the viscosity coefficient. As $\eta \uparrow$, $\bar{v} \downarrow$ and $Q \downarrow$.

118. **B** Because a pressure of 2.0 atm must be exerted on the piston to prevent water from entering solution B, $\pi_B > \pi_A$ and the concentration of solution B is more concentrated than solution A: π = molarity $\times RT$ (T = temperature; R = universal gas constant).

119. **C** See question 118.

120. **A** Osmotic pressure difference would increase requiring more pressure on the piston to prevent water from entering solution B.

121. **D** Water will enter the RBC causing hemolysis (bursting).

122. **B** Osmotic pressure is a colligative property, meaning it depends on the moles of particles. A 1.0 M solution of NaCl contains more particles in solution than 1.0 M glucose solution.

$$NaCl(s) \rightarrow Na^+(aq) + Cl-(aq)$$

123. **D** Osmosis results from the diffusion that occurs across a membrane. Diffusion is the spreading of molecules from high concentration to low concentration due to random collisions. More water molecules per unit volume are in the dilute solution than in the more concentrated solution. Thus, more water molecules of the dilute solution will collide with the membrane per unit time, causing a net flow of water molecules from the dilute to the concentrated solution.

124. **D** 60 W represents the power usage of the bulb. Power is the product of current and voltage. Thus,

$$I = P/V = \frac{60 \text{ W}}{120 \text{ V}} = 0.5 \text{ A}$$

125. **B** The Doppler effect is given by

$$v = v_1 \frac{(v - v_0)}{(v)}$$

where v_i is the actual frequency and v is the frequency perceived; v is the velocity of sound in air, and v_0 is the velocity of the observer

$$= 700 \text{ Hz} \frac{(350 - 35)}{(350)} = 700 \text{ Hz } (0.90) = 630 \text{ Hz}$$

Choices A and D can be eliminated immediately because as the source and observer move apart, the frequency drops.

126. **D** Bernoulli's equation states that the sum of the pressure (P), the kinetic energy component per unit volume ($ev^2/2$), and the potential energy component per unit volume (egh, where e is the fluid density) is constant.

$$P + \frac{ev^2}{2} + egh = \text{constant}$$

Since the diameter of the tube is uniform, the flow rate (volume per second, m^3/s) must be constant. The volume unit can be resolved into area times distance so flow rate becomes:

$$\frac{\text{Volume}}{\text{time}} = \frac{\text{Area} \quad \text{distance}}{\text{time}} \text{ and } \frac{d}{t} \text{ is velocity.}$$

Thus, the velocity is constant. This makes the kinetic energy component constant ($ev^2/2$). The pressure at any given point depends on its height. The greater the height, the greater the value of egh and the smaller the value of P. The pressure is greatest at point B and lowest at point D.

127. **C** Using the relation $d\beta = 10 \log_{10}(I/I_0)$ where

$$I_0 = 10-^{12}W/m^2$$

Therefore,

$$40 \text{ d}\dagger = 10 \log_{10}(I/10^{-12} \text{ W/m}^2)$$
$$4 = \log_{10}(I/10^{-12})$$

Taking the antilog (exponential) of both sides gives:

$$10^4 = I/10^{-12}$$
$$I = 10^4 \times 10^{-12} \text{ W/m}^2 = 10^{-8} \text{ W/m}^2$$

128. **C** To use $k = A \exp(- E_a/RT)$, where neither k nor A is known, requires two equations, obtained by measuring different values of k at two different temperatures.

129. **B** The pressure exerted by a gas depends on the total number of molecules, not on its molecular weight or the number of atoms per molecule. Changes in T, however, *will* affect the pressure.

130. **D** If "x" equals the solubility of Ba(IO$_3$)$_2$, then

$[Ba^{2+}] = x$ and $[IO_3^-] = 2x$.

131. **D** In each of II and III, the number of moles of gaseous products is less than that of gaseous reactants; thus "disorder" decreases.

132. **A** The reaction shifts to the left in response to the loss of NO$_2$. Increasing the volume has the reverse effect from that stated in II—there's more room for the more numerous NO$_2$'s. Adding an inert gas raises the *total* pressure, but only partial pressures of reactants and products figure into the equilibrium expression, so the equilibrium will not shift in III.

133. **D** pH = 14 − pOH = 14 − 3 = 11; alternatively, find [H$^+$] using [H$^+$] = K_w/[OH$^-$] = 1 × 10^{-14}/ (0.001) = 1 × 10^{-11}; pH = 11

134. **B** Rearrange this expression to get the familiar Henderson-Hasselbalch equation; the trick is that the H—H equation uses the ratio of conjugate base to conjugate acid, the reciprocal of R as defined here. So,

$6.3 = 6.0 + \log (1/R)$

$6.0 = 6.3 - \log (1/R)$
$6.0 = 6.3 + \log R$

If you do not notice this, you'll probably choose A.

135. **A** The period, T, is equal to:

$$T = 2\pi \sqrt{L/g}$$

Thus, the period is directly proportional to the square root of the length. Any increase in L will produce an increase in T. The mass of the box does not influence the period.

136. **D** Six seconds represents the round trip time of the sonar signal. Therefore, it takes 3 s for a signal traveling at 1.5 km/s to reach the ocean floor. Since distance equals speed times time,

$$(1.5\frac{\text{km}}{\text{s}})(3 \text{ s}) = 4.5 \text{ km}$$

137. **A** Work is force times distance moved. A body held at a given height is not in motion, so work is no longer being performed on it.

138. **B** Capacitors C_2 and C_3 are connected in series and can be replaced by a single equivalent capacitor of

$$\frac{1}{C_{eq}} = \frac{1}{C_2} + \frac{1}{C_3} = \frac{1}{4}$$

So $C_{eq} = 4\ \mu\text{F}$. The equivalent capacitor and C_1 are connected in parallel and can be replaced by a single equivalent capacitor given by:

$C_{EQ} = C_{eq} + C_1 = 4\ \mu\text{F} + 3\ \mu\text{F} = 7\ \mu\text{F}$.

139. **A** This is the definition of Pascal's Principle.

140. **D** The force is inversely proportional to the square of the distance between the point charges. Since the distance is doubled, the force must be quartered.

141. **D** The speed of sound in air is constant at any given temperature regardless of the frequency of the sound.

142. **B** This is a parallel circuit diagram. The voltage drop is the same across both branches, but the current is divided between them. The resistors on each branch are connected in series. The equivalent resistance in the 40 Ω branch is 60 Ω. The current through that loop and through each R in that loop is:

$$I = V/R = \frac{120 \text{ V}}{60\ \Omega} = 2.0 \text{ amperes}$$

BIOLOGICAL SCIENCES

143. **B** The fetal stage begins in the third month of pregnancy. The graph shows that starting at that time and through birth, 90 percent–100 percent of all hemoglobin molecules contain the alpha and gamma chains.

144. **A** If extended beyond the graph, only the alpha, beta, and delta chains could possibly continue to adulthood. Clearly, the alpha and beta chains would predominate.

145. **C** The epsilon chain is produced in the first trimester only. It no longer is made after the fetus reaches three months (after conception).

146. **C** The graphic lines representing the beta and gamma chains cross each other between birth and three months of age. Hereafter, the gamma chain decreases in percentage while the beta chain increases in the percentage of hemoglobin molecules in which it is found.

147. **D** Although the alpha and beta chains are present in the adult (and adults need efficient oxygen transport), the gamma and epsilon chains are those present prior to birth when the embryo and fetus must have hemoglobin with an extremely high oxygen affinity in order to be able to draw oxygen from the mother's blood supply.

148. **C** Again, as described in question 144, the delta chain can be extrapolated to extend (although at a very low percentage) beyond birth towards adulthood.

149. **A** Since the epsilon chain is no longer produced after the first three months of pregnancy, and the delta chain is not produced *until* at least four to five months later, no hemoglobin molecule can contain both types of chain at the same time.

150. **C** None of the three hormones actually has a *direct* effect on the genes. However, since the two steroid hormones can freely enter cells and eventually reach the nucleus, while the water-soluble epinephrine cannot even cross the cell membrane, the latter is the LEAST likely to affect the genes *directly*.

151. **A** Steroids are lipids that can freely cross the cell membrane without the need for carrier molecules to help them.

152. **C** Since steroid hormones can freely cross cell membranes, they should be able to enter all cells (as well as leave all cells). The description of Experiment 2 states that in target cells, these hormones were bound to receptor proteins inside. Why aren't such hormones found in non-target cells of the spleen? They entered, there was no receptor to bind with them, and they passed out freely!

153. **C** Injecting epinephrine into the cells has no effect. Epinephrine and glycogen phosphorylase in contact in a beaker has no effect. Only C is a reasonable answer.

154. **D** The description of Experiment I indicates that epinephrine has an effect only when in solution *surrounding intact* cells (see explanation for question 153). This suggests a form of membrane interaction. Thus, all three conclusions make logical sense.

155. **D** Receptors on the cell membrane can make target cells "noticed" by insoluble hormones passing by in the blood, whereas nontarget cells would lack such a recognition site (therefore, A is a correct answer). However, the question states in a very general way that after a hormone binds to a cell's membrane, the "second messenger" is responsible for "affecting activities inside a cell." This suggests a more general mechanism of action (other hormones bind to special membrane receptors, leading to the same "second messenger" carrying out the next steps). Thus, C is a reasonable answer as well. Choice B makes no sense (Why bind with the hormone if you don't have the next ingredient in the chain?).

156. **B** This question simply requires a familiarity with scientific notation (exponents). $10,000 = 10^4$. If $10^4 = 1/10^4$ of the total number of proteins, then $10^4 = X/10^4$, and $X = 10^8$.

157. **D** "Outside" the cell includes both the plasma and the interstitial fluids. Simply examining the bar graphs reveals that all three statements are true.

158. **C** One has to know that the *resting potential* of nerve and muscle cells reflects concentration differences between the inside and outside of the cell. These concentration differences result in a more *negatively charged* environment *inside* the cells compared to outside. An anion is a negatively charged substance attracted to the positively charged anode. Thus, C is the reasonable choice since it involves higher levels of two groups of negatively charged substances inside.

159. **B** Knowledge about the role of the sodium-potassium pump is crucial to answering this question correctly. It should be understood that this pump helps repolarize nerve and muscle cells. Without it, such tissues would not be able to restore their resting states, and as a result, would depolarize inappropriately (a form of irritability).

160. **D** Basic knowledge about the function of the lymphatic system is required.

161. **B** Various hormones of the endocrine system regulate the substances mentioned in the question (sodium and potassium: aldosterone; calcium and phosphate: calcitonin and parathyroid hormone). If one chose D as the answer with the urinary system in mind, it should be understood that kidney activities with respect to most of these ions are in response to hormonal signals.

162. **A** An understanding of osmotic principles as well as of the selective permeability of the cell membrane is required. Only the water will move freely from one fluid compartment to the other. Since the blood is hypertonic (more solute), it has less water. Thus, water moves from where there is more of it, to where there is less of it (cell to blood)!

163. **D** Basic knowledge about the role of buffers in acid-base balance is required.

164. **C** Crossing over can only take place between two separate loci on the same chromosome (different loci for different traits). Gray and black body (as well as normal and vestigial wings) are *two alleles for the same trait at the same locus!*

165. **C** The distance between loci can be reflected by how often random breaks in the chromosome occur between them. Evidence that a break occurred is the appearance of a phenotype that could only have come about if a crossover event took place. The F_1 parent that is heterozygous has one chromosome with gray body together with normal wings, and the other chromosome with black body and vestigial wings together. The double recessive parent can only contribute a chromosome with black body and vestigial wings. The only way an offspring can have gray body with vestigial wings, or black body with normal wings, is if a crossover event took place in the heterozygous parent during gamete formation. 160 offspring are "recombinants" (75 + 85) out of a total of 800 (suggesting that 160 crossover events took place). 160/800 = 20 percent = 20 map units.

166. **B** 20 map units represents 20 percent recombinants out of 600. 20% × 600 = 120.

167. **B** If A and B are 40 units apart, and A and C are 25 units apart, C could be between A and B or on the outer side of A. The key information is that the distance between B and C is 65 units. C must be on the outer side of A (If C were between A and B, it would have to be 15 units from B).

168. **B** A linkage group is a group of genes with loci on the same chromosome. The number of linkage groups is the same as the haploid number of the species (since crossing over occurs between *homologous pairs* during meiosis). If there are 64 chromosomes in a somatic cell, then 64 is the diploid number and 32 is the haploid number.

169. **C** A double-crossover involves breaks at two different loci at the same time. If the map order of the loci is A-D-B, the heterozygous parent will have one A-D-B chromosome and one a-d-b chromosome. One break will be between the

A-D loci, and the other break will be between the B-D loci:

With two breaks involved, A will join with d, and d with B. Similarly, a will join with D, and D with b.

170. **D** Examination of the flow chart figure reveals that all statements are correct.

171. **B** Basic knowledge about the various functions of the liver is required. Specifically, the synthesis of prothrombin, fibrinogen, and numerous other blood proteins and clotting factors.

172. **D** Knowledge of blood topic terminology is needed. Since heparin interferes with the formation of two vital clotting factors (coagulation factors), it is referred to as an anticoagulant. An agglutinogen is another term for antigen, while agglutinin is synonymous with blood antibody.

173. **D** Knowledge of Mendelian genetics and the uniqueness of sex-linked traits is essential. If the normal woman's father was a hemophiliac, she must be a carrier for the trait ($X^H X^h$). The normal man has the normal allele on his only X-chromosome ($X^H Y$). Their offspring have an equal chance of being either of the following genotypes:

$X^H X^H$	$X^H X^h$	$X^H Y$	$X^h Y$
normal female	normal female	normal male	hemophiliac male

174. **C** If vitamin K is needed to make clotting factors, dicumarol indirectly acts as an "anticoagulant." This "anticoagulant" characteristic is helpful in preventing unwanted clots like thromboses.

175. **A** A look at the flow chart reveals that platelet disintegration leads to the release of platelet clotting factors, which is a repetition of the first step of the intrinsic system.

176. **C** Enzyme activity is reflected by proteins being digested to peptides (low protein, high pep-

tide). Table 2 reveals that chymotrypsin is most active at 37°C (body temperature) and pH: 6–8 (which is the approximate pH of the small intestine—where the enzyme is at work).

177. **D** Both enzymes show activity at two temperatures (37°C and 22°C), but only chymotrypsin shows activity at two pH ranges (pH: 6–8 and 4–6). Pepsin shows activity only at pH: 2–4 (the pH of the stomach).

178. **D** Neither enzyme shows any activity at 62°C. The other two categories of temperature and all three pH ranges show at least moderate activity by at least one of the enzymes.

179. **C** Basic knowledge of the characteristics of the stomach is helpful but not necessary. The mucous secretions of the stomach are highly alkaline. This inactivates pepsin (which is only active in a highly acidic environment) when it comes in contact with the inner walls. Table 1 shows the acidic pH required for pepsin activity. Thus, choices A and D make no sense (pepsin *would* digest the stomach if these choices were correct). Additionally, since 62°C is far too high above the body's homeostatic temperature range, choice B is ruled out.

180. **C** Basic knowledge of pancreatic and intestinal function is helpful. The small intestine releases the hormone secretin, which signals the pancreas to secrete sodium bicarbonate. This helps neutralize the acidic chyme and allows all pancreatic and intestinal enzymes to work properly. Choice A cannot be correct because any enzyme released by the pancreas through the pancreatic duct would have to work at the pH range maintained in the small intestine. Choice B cannot be correct because food arriving is always a part of the acidic soup from the stomach. Choice D seems to stretch the imagination a bit too far!

181. **C** An understanding of digestive and absorptive processes is necessary. Protein material must be digested to amino acids before absorption can occur. Cells cannot synthesize proteins unless they first receive amino acids (the polypeptides in B will be of no use since they have no way of getting to the cells).

182. **B** Data from the table indicate that out of 180 liters of water that are filtered from the plasma, 178–179 are reabsorbed. Thus, 1–2 liters leave

in the urine. $1/180 = .006$; $2/180 = .011$. These figures are read as slightly more than one-half of one percent and slightly more than one percent, respectively.

183. **D** An examination of the first two columns shows all constituents EXCEPT proteins have every gram (or mL) that is present in the plasma filtered into the filtrate.

184. **C** Any situation in which a wide vessel (or pipe) feeds fluids into an area that is drained by a narrower vessel will have fluid accumulate and pressure build up between them. Red blood cells in the filtrate is not a usual situation since they are too large normally to pass through the glomerulus. The countercurrent mechanism of the kidney refers to the directional flow of solutes and water around the Loop of Henle.

185. **C** Without proper insulin function, plasma glucose levels are high in diabetics. Therefore, higher than normal quantities will be filtered into the nephrons. However, there are only the "normal" numbers of carrier molecules to reabsorb glucose into the peritubular capillaries, and the excess glucose continues through the kidney and leaves in the urine.

186. **A** If an individual's blood pH is too high (too alkaline), the urinary system can adjust by either retaining additional sources of H^+ or by allowing additional alkaline substances out in the urine. HCO_3- is such a basic ion. Reabsorption of HCO_3- or filtering acidic substances will only increase pH further. "Larger alkaline proteins" do not normally get filtered through the glomerulus.

187. **C** Knowledge of the variables that influence blood pressure, and the role of the adrenal cortex hormone aldosterone (increasing reabsorption of Na^+), are essential. An understanding of osmotic relationships is also required, i.e., increased levels of cells and solutes in the blood will osmotically attract additional water. This will raise blood volume, which in turn raises blood pressure (vasodilation lowers blood pressure).

188. **B** Step 2 of both mechanisms involves transfer of an aryl group with its bonding electrons to the adjacent carbon atom (carbanion rearrangement).

189. **C** $^{\ominus}OCH_3$ will add to one carbonyl group form-

$$
\begin{array}{c}
O^- \\
| \\
C_6H_5-C-OCH_3 \\
| \\
C_6H_5-C=O
\end{array}
$$

ing according to Mechanism A.

190. **A** Oxygen exchange with O^{18}-labeled water will indicate that step 1 is reversible (and faster than step 2).

191. **C** The aliphatic analogs undergo aldol condensations in alkaline solution.

192. **D** Reactions include acylation of the alcohol group and reaction of the carboxyl group (amide formation, esterification).

193. **B** In Reaction 1, Cl⁻ adds, while in Reaction 2, the neutral base :NH₂OH attacks the β carbon. Attack at the β position produces the intermediate

$$
\left[
\begin{array}{c}
\text{H H} \\
| \quad | \\
-C-C=C-\overline{O}| \; ^{\ominus} \\
| \\
\text{Nu}
\end{array}
\leftrightarrow
\begin{array}{c}
\text{H H} \\
| \quad | \\
-C-C-C=O \\
| \quad \quad \;\; \ddots \\
\text{Nu} \; ^{\ominus}
\end{array}
\right]
$$

which is resonance-stabilized. By adding to an end of the conjugated system, the electro-negative oxygen can carry the negative charge.

194. **C** Addition to oxygen yields the carbocation

$$
\left[
\begin{array}{c}
| \quad | \quad | \\
-C\text{---}C\text{---}C-OH
\end{array}
\right]^+
$$

in which the positive charge is shared among three carbon atoms. Addition to carbon would give the intermediate

$$
\begin{array}{c}
| \quad | \quad | \\
-C-C\text{---}C\text{---}O \\
| \\
\text{H} \quad \quad +
\end{array}
$$

which is less stable.

195. **D** This is a nucleophilic addition of a carbanion to an α, β-unsaturated carbonyl compound. Again, attack occurs at the end of the conjugated system.

196. **A**

197. **C** The carbonyl group activates the carbon-carbon double bond toward electron-rich reactants.

198. **C** Experiment 2 shows that 1,3-butadiene reacts more rapidly than 1-octene.

199. **A** These two structures account for the 1,2- and 1,4- addition products shown in step (4).

200. **C** The magnitude of the activation energy determines the rate of the reaction. Activation energy is the *difference* in energy between the reactant(s) and the transition state.

201. **A** Free Radical• $CH_2=CH-CH=CH_2$
$CH_2=CH-CH=CH_2 \nearrow$
$[-CH_2-CH=CH-CH_2-]_n$
polybutadiene

202. **C** As with free radical addition, the 1,2- and 1,4- addition products are formed.

203. **D** The glucose anomers are diastereomers that differ in configuration about C—1.

204. **D**

205. **D** This question requires an understanding of Mendelian genetics and antigen-antibody relationships. The A and B antigens on the RBCs donated from the Type AB donor will be agglutinated by anti-B in the plasma of the Type A recipient, anti-A (in the Type B recipient), and both anti-A and anti-B (in the Type O recipient).

206. **D** A basic understanding of enzyme function is needed. When the product of an enzymatic pathway inhibits any of the previous steps in the pathway, this is referred to as feedback inhibition. Enzyme specificity refers to the conditions appropriate for an enzyme to work (substrate, pH, temperature, etc.). Competitive inhibition occurs when a substance occupies the active site that normally binds to the substrate involved in the reaction. The question states that isoleucine fits into the allosteric site.

207. **D** Knowledge of the basic functions of brain structures is necessary, as well as an understanding of the various sources of sensory and CNS information needed to coordinate movement, posture, and balance. The movement of skeletal muscles is initiated in the cerebrum. Pos-

ture and balance are influenced, in part, from sensory signals originating in the joints, tendons, and muscles themselves (proprioception), as well as from the utricle, saccule, and semicircular canals in the inner ear.

208. **C** The ability to interpret the figure showing hormonal changes during the menstrual cycle is helpful, but not essential. The paragraph contains the information needed to answer this question. HCG maintains the corpus luteum. Earlier in the paragraph, it is stated that "As LH levels decrease, corpus luteum activity slows down. . . ." Thus, HCG mimics LH.

209. **A** A basic understanding of the processes of transcription and translation is needed. If chromosome puffs represent uncoiled or decondensed regions of DNA, this suggests that the DNA sequence has to be "read," either for DNA replication (mitosis) or protein synthesis. Since the insect larva is undergoing different developmental changes in response to hormones, the synthesis of various proteins needed during each subsequent stage seems most probable. The hormone appears to be "activating" genes along the DNA so that transcription of these DNA sequences can occur.

210. **B** General knowledge of neuromuscular relationships is needed. If curare competes with acetylcholine along the motor end plate (at the neuromuscular junction), ACh cannot perform its function. ACh normally causes skeletal muscles to depolarize and contract. If this is blocked, B is clearly the correct choice. Choices A and C refer to events *after* depolarization has already taken place. Heat production results from contraction (muscle activity), which requires ACh in the first place.

211. **B** Broad knowledge of the functions of the nervous and endocrine system is helpful. The main point is that the arrector pili muscles are described as "smooth muscles." These are involuntary muscles that are under the direct control of the autonomic nervous system.

212. **D** Basic knowledge about vertebrate biology is helpful. The characteristics described are shared by structures including gills, lungs, and even the skin of frogs (which can serve as an extra respiratory organ underwater).

213. **C** Knowledge of basic concepts in muscle physiology is helpful. Since the described phenomenon involves only a second contraction, summation is the appropriate answer. If the situation involved multiple stimuli (20–30) in rapid succession, partial tetany would be correct. Tetany occurs when multiple stimuli occur so rapidly that there is no time to relax at all. Threshold refers to the level of stimulation required to initiate any response by the muscle cell.

214. **B** An understanding of the effects of histamine and the inflammatory response are helpful, but not essential. Logical thinking will come through here as well. The symptoms described, e.g., redness and heat, would result from *more* red, warm blood in the area (dilation of blood vessels). Similarly, swelling and pain would result from *additional fluids* in the area stimulating pain receptors (more fluid leakage from capillaries).

215. **C** Aromatic systems show strong absorptions in the UV region of the system. C—C and C—H bonds will absorb in the IR region. The NMR will show the inequivalent hydrogens.

216. **B** Because both reactants contain acidic α-H's, two different carbanions will form and attack the carbonyl groups in condensation reactions.

217. **D** Quaternary nitrogen atoms cannot react to form an amide because it already has four bonds.

218. **A**

$$R'—C{=}O + ROH \rightleftharpoons \underset{\underset{\text{hemiacetal}}{OH}}{R'—\overset{\overset{H}{|}}{C}—OR} \overset{H^+/ROH}{\rightleftharpoons} \underset{\underset{\text{acetal}}{OR}}{R'—\overset{\overset{H}{|}}{C}—OR}$$

219. **C** Hydrolysis breaks the amide linkage to form the amino acid residues alanine and glycine. Because the acids are in basic solution, their dibasic form predominates.

PRACTICE EXAM IV

	Time
Verbal Reasoning Questions 1–65	**85** minutes
Physical Sciences Questions 66–142	**100** minutes
Writing Sample 2 Essays	**60** minutes
Biological Sciences Questions 143–219	**100** minutes

ANSWER SHEET
PRACTICE EXAM IV

VERBAL REASONING

1. Ⓐ Ⓑ Ⓒ Ⓓ
2. Ⓐ Ⓑ Ⓒ Ⓓ
3. Ⓐ Ⓑ Ⓒ Ⓓ
4. Ⓐ Ⓑ Ⓒ Ⓓ
5. Ⓐ Ⓑ Ⓒ Ⓓ
6. Ⓐ Ⓑ Ⓒ Ⓓ
7. Ⓐ Ⓑ Ⓒ Ⓓ
8. Ⓐ Ⓑ Ⓒ Ⓓ
9. Ⓐ Ⓑ Ⓒ Ⓓ
10. Ⓐ Ⓑ Ⓒ Ⓓ
11. Ⓐ Ⓑ Ⓒ Ⓓ
12. Ⓐ Ⓑ Ⓒ Ⓓ
13. Ⓐ Ⓑ Ⓒ Ⓓ
14. Ⓐ Ⓑ Ⓒ Ⓓ
15. Ⓐ Ⓑ Ⓒ Ⓓ
16. Ⓐ Ⓑ Ⓒ Ⓓ
17. Ⓐ Ⓑ Ⓒ Ⓓ
18. Ⓐ Ⓑ Ⓒ Ⓓ
19. Ⓐ Ⓑ Ⓒ Ⓓ
20. Ⓐ Ⓑ Ⓒ Ⓓ
21. Ⓐ Ⓑ Ⓒ Ⓓ
22. Ⓐ Ⓑ Ⓒ Ⓓ
23. Ⓐ Ⓑ Ⓒ Ⓓ
24. Ⓐ Ⓑ Ⓒ Ⓓ
25. Ⓐ Ⓑ Ⓒ Ⓓ
26. Ⓐ Ⓑ Ⓒ Ⓓ
27. Ⓐ Ⓑ Ⓒ Ⓓ
28. Ⓐ Ⓑ Ⓒ Ⓓ
29. Ⓐ Ⓑ Ⓒ Ⓓ
30. Ⓐ Ⓑ Ⓒ Ⓓ
31. Ⓐ Ⓑ Ⓒ Ⓓ
32. Ⓐ Ⓑ Ⓒ Ⓓ
33. Ⓐ Ⓑ Ⓒ Ⓓ
34. Ⓐ Ⓑ Ⓒ Ⓓ
35. Ⓐ Ⓑ Ⓒ Ⓓ
36. Ⓐ Ⓑ Ⓒ Ⓓ
37. Ⓐ Ⓑ Ⓒ Ⓓ
38. Ⓐ Ⓑ Ⓒ Ⓓ
39. Ⓐ Ⓑ Ⓒ Ⓓ
40. Ⓐ Ⓑ Ⓒ Ⓓ
41. Ⓐ Ⓑ Ⓒ Ⓓ
42. Ⓐ Ⓑ Ⓒ Ⓓ

43. Ⓐ Ⓑ Ⓒ Ⓓ
44. Ⓐ Ⓑ Ⓒ Ⓓ
45. Ⓐ Ⓑ Ⓒ Ⓓ
46. Ⓐ Ⓑ Ⓒ Ⓓ
47. Ⓐ Ⓑ Ⓒ Ⓓ
48. Ⓐ Ⓑ Ⓒ Ⓓ
49. Ⓐ Ⓑ Ⓒ Ⓓ
50. Ⓐ Ⓑ Ⓒ Ⓓ
51. Ⓐ Ⓑ Ⓒ Ⓓ
52. Ⓐ Ⓑ Ⓒ Ⓓ
53. Ⓐ Ⓑ Ⓒ Ⓓ
54. Ⓐ Ⓑ Ⓒ Ⓓ
55. Ⓐ Ⓑ Ⓒ Ⓓ
56. Ⓐ Ⓑ Ⓒ Ⓓ
57. Ⓐ Ⓑ Ⓒ Ⓓ
58. Ⓐ Ⓑ Ⓒ Ⓓ
59. Ⓐ Ⓑ Ⓒ Ⓓ
60. Ⓐ Ⓑ Ⓒ Ⓓ
61. Ⓐ Ⓑ Ⓒ Ⓓ
62. Ⓐ Ⓑ Ⓒ Ⓓ
63. Ⓐ Ⓑ Ⓒ Ⓓ
64. Ⓐ Ⓑ Ⓒ Ⓓ
65. Ⓐ Ⓑ Ⓒ Ⓓ

PHYSICAL SCIENCES

66. Ⓐ Ⓑ Ⓒ Ⓓ
67. Ⓐ Ⓑ Ⓒ Ⓓ
68. Ⓐ Ⓑ Ⓒ Ⓓ
69. Ⓐ Ⓑ Ⓒ Ⓓ
70. Ⓐ Ⓑ Ⓒ Ⓓ
71. Ⓐ Ⓑ Ⓒ Ⓓ
72. Ⓐ Ⓑ Ⓒ Ⓓ
73. Ⓐ Ⓑ Ⓒ Ⓓ
74. Ⓐ Ⓑ Ⓒ Ⓓ
75. Ⓐ Ⓑ Ⓒ Ⓓ
76. Ⓐ Ⓑ Ⓒ Ⓓ
77. Ⓐ Ⓑ Ⓒ Ⓓ
78. Ⓐ Ⓑ Ⓒ Ⓓ
79. Ⓐ Ⓑ Ⓒ Ⓓ
80. Ⓐ Ⓑ Ⓒ Ⓓ
81. Ⓐ Ⓑ Ⓒ Ⓓ
82. Ⓐ Ⓑ Ⓒ Ⓓ
83. Ⓐ Ⓑ Ⓒ Ⓓ
84. Ⓐ Ⓑ Ⓒ Ⓓ
85. Ⓐ Ⓑ Ⓒ Ⓓ
86. Ⓐ Ⓑ Ⓒ Ⓓ
87. Ⓐ Ⓑ Ⓒ Ⓓ
88. Ⓐ Ⓑ Ⓒ Ⓓ
89. Ⓐ Ⓑ Ⓒ Ⓓ
90. Ⓐ Ⓑ Ⓒ Ⓓ
91. Ⓐ Ⓑ Ⓒ Ⓓ
92. Ⓐ Ⓑ Ⓒ Ⓓ
93. Ⓐ Ⓑ Ⓒ Ⓓ
94. Ⓐ Ⓑ Ⓒ Ⓓ
95. Ⓐ Ⓑ Ⓒ Ⓓ
96. Ⓐ Ⓑ Ⓒ Ⓓ
97. Ⓐ Ⓑ Ⓒ Ⓓ
98. Ⓐ Ⓑ Ⓒ Ⓓ
99. Ⓐ Ⓑ Ⓒ Ⓓ
100. Ⓐ Ⓑ Ⓒ Ⓓ
101. Ⓐ Ⓑ Ⓒ Ⓓ
102. Ⓐ Ⓑ Ⓒ Ⓓ
103. Ⓐ Ⓑ Ⓒ Ⓓ
104. Ⓐ Ⓑ Ⓒ Ⓓ
105. Ⓐ Ⓑ Ⓒ Ⓓ
106. Ⓐ Ⓑ Ⓒ Ⓓ
107. Ⓐ Ⓑ Ⓒ Ⓓ

BIOLOGICAL SCIENCES

108. (A) (B) (C) (D)	143. (A) (B) (C) (D)	192. (A) (B) (C) (D)
109. (A) (B) (C) (D)	144. (A) (B) (C) (D)	193. (A) (B) (C) (D)
110. (A) (B) (C) (D)	145. (A) (B) (C) (D)	194. (A) (B) (C) (D)
111. (A) (B) (C) (D)	146. (A) (B) (C) (D)	195. (A) (B) (C) (D)
112. (A) (B) (C) (D)	147. (A) (B) (C) (D)	196. (A) (B) (C) (D)
113. (A) (B) (C) (D)	148. (A) (B) (C) (D)	197. (A) (B) (C) (D)
114. (A) (B) (C) (D)	149. (A) (B) (C) (D)	198. (A) (B) (C) (D)
115. (A) (B) (C) (D)	150. (A) (B) (C) (D)	199. (A) (B) (C) (D)
116. (A) (B) (C) (D)	151. (A) (B) (C) (D)	200. (A) (B) (C) (D)
117. (A) (B) (C) (D)	152. (A) (B) (C) (D)	201. (A) (B) (C) (D)
118. (A) (B) (C) (D)	153. (A) (B) (C) (D)	202. (A) (B) (C) (D)
119. (A) (B) (C) (D)	154. (A) (B) (C) (D)	203. (A) (B) (C) (D)
120. (A) (B) (C) (D)	155. (A) (B) (C) (D)	204. (A) (B) (C) (D)
121. (A) (B) (C) (D)	156. (A) (B) (C) (D)	205. (A) (B) (C) (D)
122. (A) (B) (C) (D)	157. (A) (B) (C) (D)	206. (A) (B) (C) (D)
123. (A) (B) (C) (D)	158. (A) (B) (C) (D)	207. (A) (B) (C) (D)
124. (A) (B) (C) (D)	159. (A) (B) (C) (D)	208. (A) (B) (C) (D)
125. (A) (B) (C) (D)	160. (A) (B) (C) (D)	209. (A) (B) (C) (D)
126. (A) (B) (C) (D)	161. (A) (B) (C) (D)	210. (A) (B) (C) (D)
127. (A) (B) (C) (D)	162. (A) (B) (C) (D)	211. (A) (B) (C) (D)
128. (A) (B) (C) (D)	163. (A) (B) (C) (D)	212. (A) (B) (C) (D)
129. (A) (B) (C) (D)	164. (A) (B) (C) (D)	213. (A) (B) (C) (D)
130. (A) (B) (C) (D)	165. (A) (B) (C) (D)	214. (A) (B) (C) (D)
131. (A) (B) (C) (D)	166. (A) (B) (C) (D)	215. (A) (B) (C) (D)
132. (A) (B) (C) (D)	167. (A) (B) (C) (D)	216. (A) (B) (C) (D)
133. (A) (B) (C) (D)	168. (A) (B) (C) (D)	217. (A) (B) (C) (D)
134. (A) (B) (C) (D)	169. (A) (B) (C) (D)	218. (A) (B) (C) (D)
135. (A) (B) (C) (D)	170. (A) (B) (C) (D)	219. (A) (B) (C) (D)
136. (A) (B) (C) (D)	171. (A) (B) (C) (D)	
137. (A) (B) (C) (D)	172. (A) (B) (C) (D)	
138. (A) (B) (C) (D)	173. (A) (B) (C) (D)	
139. (A) (B) (C) (D)	174. (A) (B) (C) (D)	
140. (A) (B) (C) (D)	175. (A) (B) (C) (D)	
141. (A) (B) (C) (D)	176. (A) (B) (C) (D)	
142. (A) (B) (C) (D)	177. (A) (B) (C) (D)	
	178. (A) (B) (C) (D)	
	179. (A) (B) (C) (D)	
	180. (A) (B) (C) (D)	
	181. (A) (B) (C) (D)	
	182. (A) (B) (C) (D)	
	183. (A) (B) (C) (D)	
	184. (A) (B) (C) (D)	
	185. (A) (B) (C) (D)	
	186. (A) (B) (C) (D)	
	187. (A) (B) (C) (D)	
	188. (A) (B) (C) (D)	
	189. (A) (B) (C) (D)	
	190. (A) (B) (C) (D)	
	191. (A) (B) (C) (D)	

Writing Sample 1

END OF PART 1

Writing Sample 2

END OF PART 1

VERBAL REASONING

Time: 85 Minutes
Questions 1–65

Directions: There are nine passages in this test. Each passage is followed by questions based on its content. After reading a passage, choose the one best answer to each question and indicate your selection by blackening the corresponding space on your answer sheet.

Passage I (Questions 1–7)

Being the highest-ranking general in the U.S. army was an unlikely circumstance for someone who as a youngster showed no military inclination. Born in 1822 in Point Pleasant, Ohio, Hiram Ulysses Grant reluctantly went off at his father's insistence to the United States Military Academy at West Point, New
(5) York, in 1839. People called him "Ulysses," and the congressman who appointed him to the academy, assuming this to be the boy's first name and his mother's maiden name—Simpson—to be his middle one, affixed the misnomer "Ulysses S. Grant" to the appoint-
(10) ment. It stuck. Eventually, the initials "U.S." came to combine the man and his cause until some quarter of a century later, when there he was—general in chief of all Union forces—offering surrender terms to his Confederate nemesis Robert E. Lee in the McLean
(15) house parlor at Appomattox Court House, Virginia. This ended the most appalling war that Americans had ever known. The victory at Appomattox made Grant a hero in the North, and he went on to become the nation's eighteenth President, serving two terms from
(20) 1869 to 1877—the youngest man ever elected to the presidency at that point in American history. Yet despite such fame, his personality remains a riddle.

"There's always been a mystery about Grant," says John Y. Simon, editor of *The Papers of Ulysses*
(25) *S. Grant* and director of the Ulysses S. Grant Association at Southern Illinois University, Carbondale. "Both the military career and the presidency have been controversial. In battle, he's been called a butcher, a man of great luck, someone who really didn't win the
(30) Civil War but was simply on the scene when the Confederates finally were forced to abandon it. In terms of the presidency, he's been looked upon as a man who did too much and a man who did too little. On Reconstruction, for example, he was viewed as a man who
(35) pushed too hard for black civil rights and when he should have known better, and as a man who didn't do nearly enough." Moreover, says Simon, although Grant has been faulted as being the dupe of conniv-

ing politicians, much of the corruption associated with
(40) his presidency had flourished during the Civil War, had continued under Andrew Johnson's administration, and was finally uncovered during Grant's presidency.

The volumes of the Grant papers have become the essential resource in modern studies of Grant. They also
(45) shed light on Grant's commitment to the well-being of the South's freedmen, his view of Johnson's Reconstruction Policy, and his political ambitions. While Grant's urging of leniency toward former officers of the Confederacy, including Lee, is well-known, his determination to
(50) protect the South's freedmen has been disputed. In fact, says Simon, Grant never wavered in his desire to protect the former slaves. After a tour of several southern states in late 1865, Grant wrote in a letter on December 18, 1865, to president Johnson: "In some form the Freeman's
(55) Bureau is an absolute necessity until civil law is established and enforced securing to the freedmen their rights and full protection."

One of the pleasures for Simon in his work with the Grant papers is the precision and grace of Grant's
(60) prose. Simon observes a direct correlation between Grant's literary ability and his capacity for leadership. An example is Grant's three-sentence letter on February 16, 1862, demanding Confederate commander Simon Buckner's surrender of the 15,000-man garri-
(65) son of Fort Donelson in Tennessee:

Sir;

Yours of this date proposing Armistice, and appointment of commissioners, to settle terms of capitulation is just received. No terms except an un-
(70) conditional and immediate surrender can be accepted.
I propose to move immediately upon your works.
I am sir; very respectfully
Your obt. Servt.
(75) U.S. Grant
Brig. Gen.

"The letter expressed exactly what Grant wanted with the greatest economy," says Simon. "It shows a

man who is direct, clearheaded, and perhaps there's a
(80) glint of genius in his expressing things that others didn't see. No one has ever figured out the origin of his phrase 'unconditional and immediate.'" What is clear, however, is that the coincidence of the initial letters of "unconditional surrender" with Grant's own
(85) first initials was not lost on his troops. The nickname of "Unconditional Surrender" Grant, which stayed with him through the remainder of the war, imbued the man with an even more inspiriting aura of steadfastness than that implied by the patriotic sobriquet "Uncle Sam"
(90) Grant, which he had acquired at West Point. As both soldier and president, Grant helped shape the United States as a modern nation. Grant's role as the engineer of Northern victory places him indisputably among the great founders of the modern United States, says
(95) Simon. As president, Grant also helped forge the new nation. In 1870, with the passage of the Fifteenth Amendment, blacks were voting more fairly and freely throughout the South than they did until Lyndon Johnson became president. While many scholars stress
(100) the failure of Grant's government to grant to blacks what was promised to them in legislation, Grant kept up the pressure for reform. Even as Grant tried to pre-serve the ideals of the republic for which the Civil War was fought, the nation was moving in vertiginous new
(105) directions. Ironically, in 1876, at nearly the same time that General Custer and his men were being massacred in the last of the great Indian battles out West, Presi-dent Grant was attending the U.S. centennial exposi-tion in Philadelphia, which trumpeted America's might
(110) and contributions to the industrial wonders of the world. A failed bid for a third term, a plunge into fi-nancial ruin that left him penniless, the onset of the throat cancer that slowly and painfully killed him—all the outward facts of Grant's life are well docu-
(115) mented. Yet, Grant's personality remains intriguing.

1. According to the article, the "mystery" about Ulysses S. Grant refers to:

    A. the web of stories that sprang up explain-ing what the initials of his first names meant.
    B. speculation on his effortless ability to make the transition from military general to political president.
    C. the lack of reliable information document-ing his service as a general in the Civil War.
    D. the acknowledgment that little is known. about who Grant is as an individual.

2. The accepted view of Grant historically has been:

    A. as a man torn between duty to his coun-try and conflicts with his convictions.
    B. an incompetent military general and an indifferent president.
    C. a blood-thirsty general and a president who was manipulated.
    D. a revered war hero and honored states-man.

3. One scholar's reference to the Grant papers as a reflection of Grant's dual abilities to write well and demonstrate strong leadership quali-ties can be inferred as:

    A. an assumption that Grant was only viewed as a war general.
    B. the erroneous belief that Grant was seen as an intellectual rather than as a military leader.
    C. strong praise for Grant.
    D. condemnation of Grant's misuse of his abilities.

4. Which of the following did not occur during Grant's presidency as mentioned in the ar-ticle?

    A. The passage of the Fifteenth Amendment
    B. The 1876 Centennial Exposition in Phila-delphia
    C. The massacre of General Custer and his men
    D. The building of the Panama Canal

5. The author states that General Grant:

    A. was not a strong supporter of civil rights for the newly freed slaves.
    B. was a corrupt president.
    C. was key to the development of a modern nation.
    D. helped bring an end to the Indian wars.

6. In the sentence "Even as Grant tried to pre-serve the ideals of the republic for which the Civil War was fought, the nation was mov-ing in vertiginous new directions" (lines 102–105), the author is suggesting that:

    A. Grant's actions were futile since the U.S. was experiencing unstable, rapid changes.
    B. Grant's actions were heroic as the U.S.

continued to uphold the values of its founding fathers.

C. Grant's actions were reflective of his military leadership as the U.S. struggled with Reconstruction in the South.

D. Grant's actions did little to enhance recognition of U.S. leadership in the international sphere.

7. The article infers that a better understanding of Grant's presidency by modern historians is due largely to:

A. a revisionist perspective favoring Grant in a sympathetic light.

B. a recent examination of Grant's papers.

C. a current historian's biography of Grant.

D. a resurgence of contemporary interest in Grant's administration.

Passage II (Questions 8–14)

The Neanderthals *(Homo sapiens neanderthalensis)* occupied Europe before the appearance of the anatomically modern Upper Paleolithic people known collectively as the Cro-Magnon. They
(5) were powerful creatures—stocky, barrel chested, with massive bones and muscles. They were unique among all other members of the genus *homo*, extant or extinct, for their rounded skulls, forward jutting face and jaws, and heavy brow ridges. Much maligned as stooped-
(10) over, inarticulate hulks, they actually stood straight and seem to have been thoughtful as well as rugged. Their brains were larger than those of modern humans and, as far as can be told from the fossil record, no less impressive. Though they are presumed to have migrated
(15) from Africa, by the time Cro-Magnon man began to migrate from Africa to Europe Neanderthals were veteran Europeans, having inhabited the region for some 200,000 years. Yet they vanished without a trace about 32,000 years ago, replaced by the Cro-Magnon man,
(20) who were taller, more slender, and physically the weakest of all hominids.

The reasons for the success of Cro-Magnon are not fully agreed upon. The story of Cro-Magnon man started in southern Africa, the birthplace of humanity's
(25) immediate ancestors, who, judging by anatomical evidence, appeared about 100,000 years ago. Molecular evidence indicates that they may have appeared a good deal earlier, as descendants of a prehistoric Eve who may have lived 250,000 years ago. That suggestion
(30) rests on analyses of samples of maternally inherited DNA from more than 2,000 individuals from all continents. The greatest DNA diversity, an index of more

remote origins, occurs among the Africans, a conclusion supported by other genetic studies.
(35)   In any event, pioneers among human ancestors began exploring frontier lands to the north. Eventually, they wandered out of Africa and into Europe around 80,000 to 100,000 years ago, where they encountered unfamiliar natives, the Neanderthals who were previ-
(40) ous immigrants from Africa. While it has always been assumed that only one species of humans could exist in any one historic period, if the Neanderthals were, in fact, a separate species (which there is disagreement on) there was a fairly long period of time in Europe
(45) and possibly other parts of the world where more than one species of *Homo* coexisted. This coexistence was not always peaceful, but not always violent either. There is at least some evidence of trade and possibly intermarriage between the two groups. Local clashes
(50) undoubtedly occurred, but without extermination. Gradually displaced from the most abundant sites, the Neanderthals broke into small groups, and eventually became extinct by attrition over a period of 10,000 years between 30,000 and 40,000 years ago with the
(55) last groups of survivors possibly living in the mountains of Spain.

Even though they were strong, and intelligent, and knew their land intimately, the Neanderthals ultimately could not compete with the newcomers though
(60) for many thousands of years they did co-exist. It is possible that an inability to adapt lead to the ultimate extinction of the Neanderthals. Set in their ways, they may have continued to live as they had always done making the same tools century after century, hunting
(65) with the same jabbing weapons in close encounters with big game, even after the newcomers had developed weapons that could be used from greater distances. In a sense, they may have been too well adapted, inflexible and committed to traditional living
(70) patterns. It is also possible that as Cro-Magnon's weaponry improved they became more aggressive in their encounters with the Neanderthals, winning more battles and pushing the Neanderthals to the least desirable locations in Europe. This may have lead to ul-
(75) timate starvation for the group.

This is the consensus scenario, the sequence of events envisioned by most specialists, among them Christopher Stringer of the British Museum of Natural History and Erik Trinkaus of the University of New
(80) Mexico. A vocal minority, the most articulate of whom is Milford Wolpoff of the University of Michigan, offers another theory: There were no newcomers, no displacements; there was no attrition; Neanderthals were never out competed; they evolved into Cro-Magnon in
(85) Europe and their equivalents into other modern people elsewhere. A third school of thought says that Neanderthals disappeared because they interbred with Cro-

Magnon and in doing so became indistinguishable. All parties agree a hundred percent on one thing, how-
(90) ever—the need for further research is always a wise position for scientists to take.

8. Based on the passage, it would be reasonable to assume that the author:

   A. had little respect for the adaptive abilities of Neanderthals.
   B. saw Cro-Magnon man as enormously more advanced than Neanderthals.
   C. felt Neanderthals were more apelike than modern man.
   D. had a high respect for the Neanderthals' ability and intelligence.

9. The author says that the greater the DNA diversity of a species:

   A. the earlier the origin of the species.
   B. the more the species has had to make adaptations to a changing environment.
   C. the more subspeciation will take place.
   D. all of the above

10. The passage suggests that it would be reasonable to assume that two human species can coexist:

   A. as long as they have trading needs.
   B. as long as the populations are fairly geographically separated from each other.
   C. as long as resources are plentiful.
   D. as long as neither species has a clear technological advantage over the other .

11. Cro-Magnon replaced Neanderthals because of all of the following reasons but one:

   A. Cro-Magnon and Neanderthals intermarried.
   B. Cro-Magnon's technology advanced more rapidly than the Neanderthals.
   C. Cro-Magnon were more aggressive and pushed Neanderthals out of the best land leading to starvation.
   D. Neanderthals' bulky bodies and stooped posture made them no competition for Cro-Magnon.

12. The author agrees with which scientific theory in explaining the extinction of the Neanderthals?

   A. The Neanderthals were unable to repulse the aggressive Cro-Magnon in battles and were eventually wiped out.
   B. The Cro-Magnon were superior in their development of tools and weaponry and out-survived the Neanderthals.
   C. The Neanderthals' adherence to traditional customs eventually led to their demise.
   D. There is no one single theory that irrefutably explains the disappearance of the Neanderthals.

13. What distinction is implied in the passage as key to the survival between Neanderthals and Cro-Magnon, respectively?

   A. A stocky physique and a taller, slender build
   B. Peaceful nature and an aggressive nature
   C. Traditional ways and adaptability
   D. Short range weapons and long range weapons

14. Which one of the following most strongly *challenges* one of the assertions made in the passage?

   A. The Neanderthals and the Cro-Magnon lived side by side for man years.
   B. Scientists accept the theory that the Neanderthals were eventually wiped out by the Cro-Magnon.
   C. It is generally agreed that both the Neanderthals and the Cro-Magnon originated in Africa.
   D. One factor in the survival of Cro-Magnon was their development of superior hunting weapons.

Passage III (Questions 15–21)

The critical importance of understanding the Islamic world is no more evident than in daily news accounts of events in the Middle East—from the Persian Gulf to Lebanon to the West Bank of the
(5) Jordan River. Islamic scholars have long had access to the *Encyclopedia of Islam,* which is widely recognized as the major research tool for the field. It includes articles on topics that relate to history, geography, aspects of public and private life, people,
(10) dynasties and sects, art, archaeology, music, folklore, theology, philosophy, ethics, law, history of science, literature, and languages of all countries in which Islam is or has been present either as a major or an important way of life.

(15)   The first edition was begun in 1908 and completed in 1938. Ten years later, the Twenty-first International Congress of Orientalists resolved that a new edition of the encyclopedia was required to take account of advances in knowledge and to include
(20) subjects not covered previously. It asked the International Union of Academics to undertake a revision. Since 1979, an editorial committee under the auspices of the International Union of Academics has been engaged in preparing a revised edition that will
(25) provide more comprehensive and current information about the Islamic world in a form accessible to the general reader.

According to Bernard Lewis, Cleveland E. Dodge Emeritus Professor of Near Eastern Studies at
(30) Princeton University, "Much had happened in the world, particularly in the Islamic world since 1938. We needed a new start that would take account, first, of the changed condition of the Islamic world, second, of the vast amount of new information—new topics, new
(35) books, new problems—which had been brought to light, and third, new methodologies, particularly social science methods, which are almost totally missing from the earlier volumes of the first edition." Wolfhart Herinrichs, professor of Arabic in the Department of
(40) Near Eastern Languages and Civilization at Harvard University and current project director for the encyclopedia, notes that the revised edition will also include numerous articles written by scholars from the Middle Est and India. "That's a change vis-a-vis the
(45) first edition, which was very much a European-American enterprise."

Unlike the Jewish or Catholic encyclopedias, the Islamic encyclopedia is not written as a guide for those who press Islam as a religion, although religious topics
(50) are included. "We are not producing an Islamic encyclopedia in that sense," Lewis explains. "That is something which, of course, only the Muslims can do. Our aim is a work of independent scholarship. Some

of our authors are Muslims; some are not. They are
(55) not chosen by faith or creed but by their qualifications."

But there remains the small definitional problem with respect to the meaning of the word *Islam.* Lewis points to the encyclopedia's use of the word in at least
(60) two different senses, "first, to mean the religion itself and its subsequent development; and second, as the equivalent of Christendom, not Christianity." Although in the Western world, *Christianity* is the name of a religion and *Christendom* is the name of the
(65) civilization that arose under the aegis of that religion, there is no such differentiation in the Islamic world. "Unfortunately," he says, "we use the word *Islam*— and so do the Muslims—to mean these two different things. If, for example you say Christian art, it will be
(70) assumed that you mean religious art," he explains. "You wouldn't call a Rembrandt or a Picasso Christian art, even though the artists were Christians. On the other hand, if you say Islamic art, you are understood to mean any kind of art that was produced in the
(75) Islamic civilization even if it is in no sense religious." Studying Islam in the same way that one studies Greek or Roman or European history is comparative recent, says Lewis. Therefore, the amount of accepted or agreed knowledge—which is what encyclopedias are
(80) supposed to contain—is comparatively small. "If you want to write something on a period of American history," he explains, "you have a vast pool of secondary literature on which to draw, and a fair amount of it is generally agreed. That is not the case
(85) in most fields of Islamic studies. These are young disciplines, relatively undeveloped."

Normally, an encyclopedia article is a summary of what is known. Where a subject is important and either very little or no work has been done before, the
(90) encyclopedia article can itself become a piece of original research. Many articles in the new edition are, in themselves, major works of scholarship covering such topics as irrigation, agriculture, warfare, art, languages and literatures, taxation, Islamic law, and marriage and
(95) divorce. The entry for *kissa,* (in modern Arabic, used to designate the novel) for example, provides a 22-page exploration of the genre that begins with a discussion of modern Arabic literature and includes information about Turkish, Persian, Urdu, Malaysian, Indonesian, Swahili,
(100) and Judeo-Arabic and Judeo-Berber forms of the short story and novel. Pointing out the European origins of the novel in Arabic and that, indeed, the first one was written in Paris by an Egyptian in 1914—*Zaynab,* by Haykal— the article goes on to explain that throughout its sixty-
(105) year existence Arabic fiction has had to cope with two basic problems: the first, whether to use a dialect or *fusha,* the "pure" written form of Arabic; the second, how to treat a central theme in many of the novels, which is the

relationship of the Arabic novel to Europe, "the master,
(110) in both senses of the word, pedagogic and colonialist."
The first edition of the encyclopedia was much more
literary, philosophical and religious in its scope, says
Lewis, and although the editorial committee has not
abandoned any of these subjects, many others have been
(115) added. An article on constitutions is one example. "There
was no article on constitutions in the earlier edition
because there were no constitutions, excepts perhaps in
two states," says Lewis. "At the same time of the first
edition, there were the Ottoman Empire and Iran with
(120) most of the rest of the Muslim world under various
European imperial regimes. Now there are more than
forty independent Muslim states, most of which have
constitutions. A comprehensive article on constitution
making and constitutional law in the Islamic world is
(125) something new."

Some articles are almost entirely original,
particularly those dealing with social and economic
history; because not very much was covered on these
topics in the past. Also, certain ideas were not
(130) examined. The revised edition, for example, includes
an article on freedom. "In 1908 people just didn't think
of that as a subject for an encyclopedia article," Lewis
points out. "We don't try to keep up to date. We're
producing a work of reference that we hope will stay
(135) on the self in the reference room for at least a half
century and perhaps longer." For that reason,
contributors are asked to write in such a way that their
articles will shed light on, rather than be outdated by,
the events recounted in tomorrow's newspaper."

15. The *Encyclopedia of Islam* can be used:

   A. as a comprehensive guide to understanding political events in the Middle East.
   B. as a compendium of information on Islamic religious laws.
   C. to understand the Islamic world from 1908 to 1938.
   D. to research events in the Middle East since 1938.

16. According to the passage information, the next edition of the Islamic encyclopedia will **not** provide one of the following:

   A. topics on irrigation, agriculture, and warfare.
   B. a discussion of the novel in modern Arabic literature.
   C. the development of constitutional law in parts of the Muslim world.
   D. an article on the effects of the Christian crusades in medieval Jerusalem.

17. One of the changes expected in the forthcoming edition of the Islamic encyclopedia is:

   A. including Middle Eastern and Indian scholars.
   B. including both Middle Eastern and Christian scholars.
   C. limiting contributions by American and European scholars.
   D. limiting the contributions from non-Islamic scholars.

18. The passage explains that the meaning of the word *Islam* is used:

   A. in the Islamic world to separate religious meaning and secular meaning.
   B. by Christians to differentiate between Christianity and Islam as religions.
   C. to identify followers of Mohammed.
   D. to refer to both the religion and the Islamic culture.

19. Regarding an interest in studying Islam in the same manner as studying Roman or European history by using the Islamic encyclopedia, the author asserts that:

   A. there will be a fair amount of information to research.
   B. the accepted knowledge found will be sizeable.
   C. information is slight since this discipline is still new.
   D. few scholars have written sufficient articles on the religion.

20. The novel *Zaynab,* published in 1914 by an Egyptian writer, is cited in the passage as evidence that:

   A. Muslim writers are acknowledged in the Islamic Encyclopedia.
   B. even an article of original research on Arabic literature is important enough to be included in the encyclopedia.
   C. very few Arabic writings will be included in the revised edition.
   D. the revised edition will have extensive scholarly articles on works written by expatriate Muslims.

21. Which statement best sums up the passage?

    A. The revised edition will attempt to have scholarly research written primarily by Middle Eastern writers.

    B. The revised edition will reflect current information about the Islamic world that is accessible to major scholars.

    C. The revised edition will offer thorough and current information about the Islamic world, along with topics not covered previously.

    D. The revised edition should be seen as a useful work of reference that covers additional areas not provided in the original.

Passage IV (Questions 22–29)

At an international conference in Europe in the early 1870s, the young, Harvard-educated scientist Charles Peirce astounded geodetic experts with his discovery of a flaw in standard pendulum experiments
(5) and soon won broader respect for other scientific achievements. In 1877, the noted British mathematician and philosopher W.K. Clifford remarked, "Charles Peirce is the greatest living logician, the second man since Aristotle who has added
(10) to the subject something material"—the other, for Clifford, being George Boole, a pioneer in modern logic. Widely regarded as brilliant, Charles Sanders Peirce spun a legacy of ideas that left his mark on a dozen disciplines. Most notably, he was the father of
(15) American pragmatism. If Peirce had done nothing more than originate the method of pragmatism, his place in the history of American philosophy would be secure. But his importance extends as well to his work in logic, the philosophy of science, mathematics, and
(20) semiotics, which is equally original and philosophically significant. He was a prolific writer whose work appeared in publications ranging from dictionaries and encyclopedias to popular journals like *The Nation* and *Popular Science Monthly*. By the end
(25) of his life, however, Peirce already suffered the obscurity that would shadow his intellectual legacy for decades. At his death, in Milford, Pennsylvania, he was isolated, forgotten by his contemporaries, and dependent on the generous support of his loyal friend
(30) William James.

Today, a growing number of scholars regard Peirce as America's most original and versatile thinker. The surge of interest in Peirce is fueled in part by the growing popularity of semiotics—analyzing the nature
(35) of signs and symbols in everyday language to "decode" culture and its communications. Researchers in fields as diverse as law, art, political science, drama, marketing, and animal communication have made semiotics a hotbed of academic interest. Indiana
(40) University-Purdue University at Indianapolis has become the primary center for Peirce studies. Scholars from around the world have visited the university to consult the extensive Peirce collection. Although Peirce's published writings total more than 10,000
(45) pages, and several collections have appeared since his death, the bulk of his work remains unpublished. So far, researchers have tracked down more than 90,000 unpublished manuscript pages on file at Harvard and other repositories. Many of these manuscripts will be
(50) included in the *Writings of Charles Peirce: A Chronological Edition* in which three volumes of the projected thirty have been published.

Each volume of the new edition includes a historical introduction, and *Volume I* sketches the
(55) rigorous intellectual tutoring Peirce received under his famous mathematician father. The boy showed a fascination for puzzles, mathematical games, and code languages. By the age of twelve, he was devouring his brother's logic textbook and working seriously at
(60) chemistry, for which he later earned his degree at Harvard. His early encounter with logic and fundamental questions of scientific inquiry shaped the course of his life's thought. Despite his scientific and mathematical achievements, Peirce always referred to
(65) himself as a logician. As one scholar notes, Peirce's initial concern as a logician was with the forms of language, which led him eventually to view logic as lying within a philosophical framework he named "semeiotic," his preferred spelling. Starting from the
(70) claim that all thought is in signs, he developed a tradic sign theory, consisting of sign, referent, and interpreter, that he explored in nearly all his later work.

Peirce originated pragmatism as a method for determining the meaning of ideas or intellectual
(75) conceptions, and he insisted that this meaning resides in its conceivable effects. To conceive of what a thing is, then, is to conceive of what effects it could have. Pragmatically, for example, motion is as motion does or might do. Peirce formulated his pragmatic rule as
(80) follows: in order to ascertain the meaning of an intellectual conception, one should consider what practical consequences might conceivably result by necessity from the truth of that conception; and the sum of those consequences will constitute the entire
(85) meaning of the conception. The complexity and scope of Peirce's ideas makes his thought difficult to grasp even for those who come eagerly to the task. His writing is sometimes obscure and technical, and he often uses diagrams, symbols, and mathematical
(90) equations. He even coined neologism to make conceptual distinctions when existing words failed. For

example, years after Peirce had originated the term "pragmatism" to signify a method for logically determining the meaning of concepts, William James (95) began using the term as a label for his own theory, in which the truth of an idea is construed as its usefulness in addressing human problems. Consequently, Peirce, somewhat indignant, coined the term "pragmatism" to distinguish his logically grounded method from (100) James's psychologically grounded one.

During his lifetime, Peirce never developed large readership. He wasn't a popular writer like William James, who always wrote in a beautiful, pleasing style, which may help explain why James, and not Peirce, (105) is more commonly associated with pragmatism. Peirce's personality may have also helped seal his fate. Although he enjoyed the patronage of some of America's most influential men of science, he had a careless regard for manners that made him something (110) of an *enfant terrible* in the halls of academia. Still, Peirce lectured for a while at Harvard and Johns Hopkins but was never able to secure the academic career that presumably would have provided greater institutional support for his work. Instead, he earned (115) his livelihood for thirty years at the U.S. Coast and Geodetic Survey, before retiring to the country, where he continued his philosophical pursuits at the expense of financial prudence and died, impoverished, of cancer. He left no single published work that provides (120) a coherent introduction to his ideas. Indeed he published only a single monograph in his lifetime, a scientific treatise based on astronomical observations made while he worked at the Harvard Observatory. Yet, his total extant writings, both published and (125) unpublished, are an extraordinarily rich, if sometimes rough, gold mine. A significant part in the new critical edition will enable scholars to read in a single chronological order the most important portion of Peirce's philosophical and logical writings as well as (130) those scientific and mathematical papers that shed light on the development of his thought.

22. According to the passage, the public's lack of recognition for Charles Peirce's contributions to science during his lifetime was due to:

    A. Peirce's fierce determination not to publish his writings for mere profit.

    B. the complexity of his writings being unintelligible to the general public.

    C. Pierce's disinterest in developing a writing style to attract interested readers and his personal behavior in the academic community.

    D. Pierce's single-minded concern with developing the field of American philosophy.

23. Regarding Peirce's method in determining what ideas or intellectual conceptions mean, which of the following best paraphrases his philosophy?

    A. To understand what something is and to understand that it has always existed

    B. To perceive something is to also understand its composition

    C. To perceive something exists and to accept its existence

    D. To realize what something is and to realize its possible effects

24. The description of Peirce as an *enfant terrible* strongly suggests that:

    A. he was clearly acknowledged as a man of great intellect.

    B. he was greatly respected by many important scientists of his time.

    C. despite his brilliant mind, his behavior among colleagues was not well regarded.

    D. his philosophy of pragmatism was highly regarded by logicians of the period.

25. Which of the following statements strongly *challenges* one of the assertions made about Peirce's writings?

    A. The complexity of Peirce's ideas baffled even enthusiastic learners.

    B. Much of his writing incorporated technical and unknown terminology.

    C. His philosophical framework relied strongly on using symbols, mathematical equations, and diagrams.

    D. The bulk of Peirce's writings were published before his death and any unpublished manuscripts were destroyed by his family.

26. The author infers that Charles Peirce's remarkable brilliance, his scientific and mathematical achievements, and his creation of American pragmaticism earned him after death:

    A. an enviable academic career with public respect and acknowledgment of his achievements.

    B. international fame as America's leading advocate of pragmaticism.

    C. disregard for his accomplishments and oblivion by the public.

D. ranking in the National American Academy of Sciences.

27. According to the passage, Peirce's development of American pragmatism and his work in logic also influenced the philosophies of which of the following fields?

    A. Political Science, Mathematics, and Humanities

    B. Political Science, Philosophy, and Journalism

    C. Political Science, Animal Communication, and Law

    D. Political Science, Cultural Studies, and Communications

28. Which of the following statements would most likely describe the author's attitude toward Charles Peirce?

    A. A bright mind and an obnoxious personality does not ensure permanent fame.

    B. Geniuses are never appreciated.

    C. It's best to depend on the loyalty of a few friends when the world ignores your scientific accomplishments.

    D. Here is an individual whose immeasurable contributions to science and logic have earned him recognition.

29. The author views present-day interest in Peirce among scholars as due to:

    A. the discovery of Peirce's 90,000 unpublished pages relating his theories.

    B. the efforts of several notable scientists collaborating their research on Peirce's accomplishments.

    C. current analysis of semiotics that apply to divergent fields of academic study.

    D. a sympathetic view of Peirce as an unacknowledged genius.

Passage V (Questions 30–36)

Quantum field theory, as developed by P.A.M. Dirac and his successors, gives a basic framework for understanding the forces of physics in fundamental terms. Nonetheless, this approach leads to a problem:
(5) Quantities that should have well-defined values calculate as finite values. This is true even in electromagnetic theory, where efforts to overcome this difficulty have led to several Nobel prizes.

In electromagnetism, the problem took the form
(10) of a paradox. The mass of the electron, known from experiment to be $9.11 \times 10\text{-}28$ gram, was calculated as having an infinite value. The resolution took form in the realization that the electron mass actually had two components, one of which would be complete arbi-
(15) trary; nothing whatever could be said concerning its value. Physicists thus were free to assign it the value of negative infinity. When added to the positive infinity of the other component, the result could be set equal to the observed total. This approach to the problem led
(20) to subtle theoretical predictions that were verified by experiment.

Related procedures, however, do not work when applied to a quantum field theory of gravity. Here, the infinities cannot be removed by assigning even such
(25) strange values as negative infinity to one or a few quantities. The University of Texas's Steven Weinberg notes that such a procedure would lead to a theory involving an infinite number of quantities. "If you had to do that, you'd have to say that we know very little
(30) about gravity," he adds.

Lacking a suitable quantum theory, physicists have nevertheless tried to nibble around the edges of the problem. The most widely studied approach has been the string theory, which holds that the fundamen-
(35) tal entities of physics are strings—short lengths or loops. They can vibrate in a number of ways, and the models of vibration correspond to particles such as quarks or electrons. Other quantum theories, such as those dealing with the strong force or the electron weak
(40) force, are merely approximations of this more fundamental theory, which are valid at low energies. As Weinberg notes, string theories incorporate gravity "in a very satisfying and believable way. Always these theories contain a massless particle that has just the
(45) right properties to play the role of the graviton. String theories not only incorporate gravity; they predict the existence of gravity." That's remarkable, Weinberg says, because no other theory predicts from first principles that gravity should exist. Further, string theo-
(50) ries lead to a formalism where "the bugbear of infinities doesn't arise."

The problem is that string theories have not yet led to concepts of physics that match observation. "Nobody knows how to solve these theories to get quanti-
(55) tative predictions," Weinberg adds. The forces in these theories are so strong as to invalidate "our favorite computational tools." Important questions may be answered by strings, but "we don't know how to read the answers." The quest for a proper quantum gravity,
(60) then, has produced little of actual use in physics. Quantum field theory remains bedeviled by the problem of infinities. String theory avoids the infinities, but also avoids contact with the world of observations and of

calculable results. Approaches based on pure math-
(65) ematics leave out the gravitons. And for lack of quantum gravity, the most significant issues in cosmology
also remain without solution.

30. According to the passage, which of the following is **not** considered an issue in a quantum field theory of gravity?

   A. The string theory
   B. The role of gravitons
   C. Infinities
   D. Protons

31. String theory is useful to physicists according to the article because it predicts one of the
following:

   A. quarks.
   B. the mass of electrons.
   C. neutrinos.
   D. gravity.

32. A major weakness of string theory is that it:

   A. avoids the infinites.
   B. avoids contact with the world of observation and mathematical calculation.
   C. seems to create infinites for electrons that
are unexplainable.
   D. creates contradiction with other parts of
quantum theory.

33. The passage states that in electromagnetism:

   A. infinites can be assigned negative or positive values.
   B. infinites cannot be removed by assigning
negative infinities to quantities.
   C. subtle theoretical predictions often were
not verified by experiment.
   D. subtle theoretical predictions were infre-
quently verified by experiment.

34. In studying a quantum field theory of gravity, scientists:

   A. are able to work with quantities of well-
defined values.
   B. can freely assign values of positive and
negative infinities to components.
   C. have an approach where results do not
match observation.
   D. utilize the procedure of observations to
test their theoretical predictions.

35. The passage indicates that its author would
agree with which of the following statements?

   A. Quantum field theory of gravity poses
insolvable problems for physicists.
   B. Although physicists have not discovered
a suitable theory, the string theory approach has been used widely.
   C. The string theory approach has become
the most reliable method of using finite
values.
   D. Physicists realize that using string theories are problematic in studying proper
quantum gravity.

36. Which statement in the passage best sums up
the discussion of using string theories?

   A. The theories are devoid of infinites making it difficult for scientists to use computational tools.
   B. The theories are based on infinites that
are not successfully verified with theoretical predictions.
   C. The paradox of the theories both incor-
porating gravity and predicting its existence.
   D. The theories are not based on infinities,
observations, and foreseeable results.

Passage VI (Questions 37–43)

   Visitors to the Vatican are awed by the beauty
of the glorious paintings and its magnificent
architecture. For many scholars, however, the
Vatican's treasure includes not only its works of art
(5) but also the rare documents housed in its archives. The
nearly five miles of correspondence and registers that
fill the shelves of the Vatican archives record both the
signal events that seem to define European civilization
and the background against which they stand out. The
(10) list of texts relating to eminent individuals or decisive
moments in the last 1,100 years of Western history is
rivaled by few archives anywhere. The proceedings of
Galileo's trial over his belief in a heliocentric solar
system, petitions of the English lords urging the Pope
(15) to accept Henry VIII's marriage to Catherine of
Aragon: These are among the crown jewels in the
Vatican's collection.

   The resources of the archives, however, are much
broader than any list of its most famous manuscripts can
(20) suggest. The Vatican has been no mere repository of
important papers, but an active shaper of social,
intellectual, and political history on an ecumenical scale.
The archival record of its involvement in spiritual and

mundane affairs reaches beyond the institutional history
(25) of the church into every domain of human activity. Even
the early history of urban planning is well represented,
the changing shape of Rome having been of constant
interest to the popes.

Francis Blouin, an archivist at the University of
(30) Michigan's Bentley Library, is constructing a
computerized database for the archives, which he calls
an extraordinary resource for studying "the history of the
discovery of knowledge." The collection contains not
only material vital for understanding the conflicts between
(35) orthodoxy and the dawning scientific view of the heavens
but also an abundance of texts recounting European
exploration of this world as well. Among the most
impressive documents from the Age of Discovery is Pope
Alexander VI's bull *Inter Cetera* of 1493, which arbitrates
(40) between Spanish and Portuguese claims to the lands just
visited by Columbus. Less celebrated, but perhaps more
useful for current research, is the correspondence of the
Propaganda Fide, which forms a continuous account of
Catholic evangelism worldwide from 1470 to the present.
(45) This material, says Blouin, can be invaluable to scholars
tracing the dynamics of cross-cultural interaction and the
development of colonialism. No less important is the part
played by the Vatican in shaping Europe's sense of its
Greek and Roman past. In the eighteenth century, for
(50) example, the papacy commissioned archaeological
excavations and amassed large collections of ancient art.
Papal communications also played an important role in
fostering the use of classical forms in new works.
According to Blouin, the record of the Vatican's activities
(55) in this area holds valuable information for art historians,
who are only beginning to understand the social and
institutional context of neoclassicism.

The archives are not, however, just the private
textual preserve of historical characters the stature of
(60) popes, explorers, and artists. Blouin is quick to point
out that they contain a surprising wealth of information
on social life in the seventeenth and eighteenth
centuries. For example, petitions for papal benefices,
the ecclesiastical equivalent of grant proposals, provide
(65) detailed information about the petitioner that historians
can use to reconstruct social relations of status and
obligation. Given the growing interest in social history,
this is a vein in the Vatican collection that scholars are
likely to mine with increasing thoroughness.
(70) The archives are open to any serious scholar. A
real hindrance researchers confront is the 1,300
indexes. Some are first-rate works of archival
scholarship, but many are outdated and incomplete.
Aside from tracing the footnotes of others and using
(75) specialized subject guides, these indexes serve as the
only points of entry into the archives' vast holdings.
The indexes, essentially lists of the contents of record

series, are currently not organized into any readily
apparent system. A scholar new to the archives must
(80) pore through a list of indexes to find those that are
most promising. More problematic, many of the
archives' holdings are not listed in any index or
Vatican guide. To find these texts, the scholar has to
rely on luck or the advice of the staff.
(85) The University of Michigan's database will
remedy this situation by providing an automated
overview of the complete archives. Each series of
related documents will have its own bibliographic
record in the database, which will contain more than
(90) 2,500 entries. When it is completed, scholars on this
side of the Atlantic will be able to review the entire
archive through the Research Libraries Information
Network before leaving for Rome. To make this
ancient repository "user friendly," the database will be
(95) structured according to modern archival methods like
those used in state and national archives in the United
States. The organizing principle behind modern
archives is the grouping of documents according to the
bureaucratic structure of the institution that generated
(100) them. Because the Vatican is one of the earliest modern
bureaucracies, its collection lends itself well to this
approach, which will allow anyone with general
knowledge of the church's administrative history to
home in on the records that are most likely to be
(105) valuable for his or her research.

37. The passage indicates the author sees the
Vatican's archives as valuable resources:

   A. second to the its architectural wonders
   and magnificent art collections.
   B. that reflect the diversity of influences the
   church has wielded in its history.
   C. for scholars researching significant
   events in European history.
   D. whose vast holdings will be modernized
   with automated databases for serious
   scholars.

38. The *Inter Cetera of 1493* and the *Propaganda
Fide* are cited in the passage as evidence that:

   A. the Catholic Church's mission to Chris-
   tianize the known world of the time were
   at first documented.
   B. evidence for Spain and Portugal's territorial claims to the New World was pre-
   served in the Vatican.
   C. information on Columbus's voyages to
   the New World and the eventual mission
   of the Church to spread Christianity were
   housed in the archives.

D. valuable documents on Columbus's explorations in the New World and materials on the church's mission to spread world-wide Catholicism are among the records in the archives.

39. Passage information indicates that any serious scholar interested in research by going through the Vatican's archives would **not** find information on which of the following?

A. The architectural design of various monuments in ancient Rome

B. Correspondence of 1519 between the Spanish conquistador, Hernan Cortez and the Aztec emperor, Montezuma

C. Various collections of Greek art financed by the church

D. Records of information kept on individuals seeking grant proposals from the church in the 1600s

40. According to the passage, the Vatican's system of access for scholars today is:

A. a cumbersome and outdated system.

B. one of the best modern database systems created in Europe

C. in the process of being automated.

D. a database currently patterned after modern archival methods used in the U.S.

41. Regarding the availability of the archives to scholars, the author asserts that the archives:

A. are open to scholars genuinely interested in only European history and art.

B. will provide information on any church correspondence with non-European countries such as China and Japan.

C. are shelved underground so that access is limited.

D. are not adequately organized for easy access.

42. The author infers that most visitors to the Vatican would **not** be aware of:

A. its beautiful art collections.

B. its vast archives stretching almost five miles.

C. its religious significance.

D. its impressive architectural designs.

43. Which of the following statements most strongly *challenges* the assertions made in the passage?

A. The Vatican continues to inspire and lead its followers in the 21st century.

B. The Vatican is also an important repository of rare documents and manuscripts recording European social, historical, and political affairs.

C. The Vatican was involved in preserving ancient Greek and Roman influences in European art.

D. The Vatican's archives are readily accessible to serious scholars.

Passage VII (Questions 44–50)

In a previously unexplored area of Serce Limani Bay on the southern coast of Turkey, an ancient shipwreck—a medieval ship, it was to be learned, presumably sunk in a storm a thousand years ago. *(5)* Researchers excavated the wreck with teams of divers bringing up glass, pottery, rusted iron objects, and the wooden remains of the hull. Ship specialist J. Richard Steffy and archaeologist Frederick van Doorninck, both from the Institute of Nautical Archaeology at *(10)* Texas A&M University, reconstructed and studied the pieces, which had been removed to the Bodrum Museum of Underwater Archaeology inside the medieval castle of Saint Peter overlooking the harbor in Bodrum, Turkey.

(15) The Serce Limani ship is a "one-of-a-kind ship," says Steffy. Its design fills a void in scholars' understanding of the transition from ancient to modern forms of ship construction. "Ancient ships were essentially built as planking shells with the planking *(20)* determining the shape of the hull," he says. "Mode naval architecture is just the opposite. First the keel is laid, then the framework is built on top of the keel, and then planks are fastened to it."

The Serce Limani ship is the earliest example *(25)* found of this "frame first" construction. Evidence suggests that it was probably a commercial ship, a two-masted, 37-ton lateener characterized by a triangular sail lashed to a tilted spar attached to a low mast. When it sank in 1025 A.D., the ship was carrying an odd *(30)* cargo—more than half a million pieces of broken glass. Roughly two tons of this cullet consisted of raw glass destined to be re-melted and fashioned into glassware. The remaining ton consisted of glassware that appear to have been damaged in a fire, and a *(35)* variety of waste produced during the manufacture of glassware. This part of the cargo was evidently smashed so as to take up as little space as possible; it was estimated 10,000 vessels and some 200 vessel types. Secondary cargoes were in glass artifacts, *(40)* ceramics, amhoras of wine, and tools for fishing and shipboard repairs.

The conservation and reconstruction offer scholars valuable new insights into eleventh-century Mediterranean watercraft. "The Serce Limani wreck *(45)* represents an undocumented ship type from a period and area in which comparatively little is known about maritime matters," says Steffy. Specializing in the technological aspects of wreck remains, Steffy examines the construction of ships to learn about *(50)* building materials and techniques. "The study of a ship's structure and contents is usually a study of the best technology and innovation that a society has to offer," he says. Steffy also examines ships' cargoes to draw inferences about the economies and politics of a *(55)* period. "By studying just one ship in detail," he points out, "we can learn a great deal about the material culture, commercial practices, and even the political atmosphere of the time." Steffy originally believed the ship was of Islamic origin. However, as scholars *(60)* examined artifacts more closely, the origin of the ship and its crew became less evident. Equipment and coins found on the ship have both Islamic (Arabic) and Byzantine (Greek) characteristics. The amphoras are inscribed with Greek letters or monograms, indicating *(65)* that they were produced for or owned by individuals with Greek names. The discovery also sheds light on shipboard life. Artifacts indicate that those aboard played chess in the stern and played backgammon amidships. Tools for shipboard repairs included wood *(70)* chisels, drill bits, a claw hammer, and a sail-repair kit. Recovered fishing equipment included lead weights, fornets, some with Greek religious inscriptions; line fragments from nets; and bronze netting needles. The ship was also well supplied with defensive weapons. *(75)* A dozen swords, one with an elaborately decorated bronze hilt, and lances and some sixty javelins were recovered.

According to van Doorninck, who specializes in the study of amphoras and anchors of the Byzantine *(80)* period, one of the most valuable artifacts found on the ship was the cache of eight iron Y-shaped anchors. "These anchors have added a great deal of knowledge about medieval metallurgy and the evolution of iron anchors," says van Doorninck. Because medieval *(85)* anchors are the largest surviving iron objects of the period, they are useful in tracing the history of iron-making technologies. Anchors shaped like Ys were unknown until the mid-1970s, when finds were documented in the waters of the Aeolian Islands, *(90)* Bulgaria, Cyprus, Israel, Sicily and Turkey. "Previous research held that this sort of anchor did not exist," says van Doorninck. "Originally, some scholars even

denied that the Y-shaped objects were anchors. After careful examination, we have come to the conclusion *(95)* that they are, in fact, very good anchors, obviously the product of much practical experience."

In examining the clues offered by the Serce Linmani in the transition from shell-first to frame-first forms of hull construction, researchers found that the *(100)* vessel combines both techniques. By combining excavated evidence with experiments on research models, it was found that the keel, stem, sternpost, and ten frame midships were erected first. The shape of the hull was dictated by a series of proportions based on *(105)* the vessels' beam, or width, and simple angles. Then the boulders began fastening belts of planks along the bottom, adding more frames in the hull's ends to stiffen the planking as construction progressed. Ship specialists conclude that skeletal, or frame-first, *(110)* building evolved in the Mediterranean area out of the earlier Graeco-Roman shell construction method. This development eventually led to the building of larger, faster, more specialized ships that enabled Europe to explore and colonize other parts of the world.

44. The discovery of the Serce Limani ship built in the eleventh century provided:

  A. valuable artifacts revealing the wealth of passengers aboard.
  B. knowledge that the ship was built for war against marauders of that time.
  C. maps of the ship's extensive journeys through the Mediterranean Sea.
  D. information on the physical construction of the ship.

45. The transition that took place in ship building in the eleventh century was:

  A. from frame first to shell first.
  B. from shell first to frame first.
  C. from shell first to building the shell and the frame at the same time.
  D. None of the above

46. Studying this ship's cargo does not offer one of the following:

  A. A society's technology and innovations
  B. A society's economy and politics
  C. A society's commercial practices
  D. A society's use of transportation

47. The presence of the iron Y-shaped anchors on the Serce Limani indicated to scholars:

    A. that anchors were beginning to be built of iron during the medieval period.

    B. that anchors were so valuable it was common practice to put extra pieces in the ship's cargo.

    C. that the shape of the anchors was considered to be good luck.

    D. that the anchor was a well thought out and reliable design.

48. According to the author, one major reason that this ship's discovery was important was that:

    A. it filled a major void in the development of ship building techniques.

    B. the ship was filled with valuable relics from the past.

    C. the ship was one of the largest ancient ships ever discovered.

    D. an enormous amount of hither to unknown information about the lives of sailors was discovered.

49. It would be reasonable to infer from the discovery of a number of defensive weapons on the ship that:

    A. the ship was a war ship.

    B. the ship was a cargo ship operating during a time of war.

    C. commercial ships in the eleventh century were subject to attack and needed to be able to defend themselves.

    D. that people of this time carried weapons for decoration and not necessarily for defense.

50. Information in the article indicates which one of the following must be true?

    A. The Serce Limani provides modern ship specialists with valuable evidence of the type of ship construction in the early medieval period.

    B. The discovery of the Serce Limani demonstrates that commerce existed between countries along the Mediterranean.

    C. The presence of defensive weapons on the Serce Limani indicates that it was clearly a fine example of an early medieval warship.

    D. The cargo materials on the Serce Limani provide scholars with first-hand artifacts unknown in the modern world.

Passage VIII (Questions 51–57)

Astronomers of the late nineteenth century needed more accurate star maps and catalogues of stellar positions for use in their observations and computations. The *Carte du Ciel,* or Astrographic
(5) Catalog, was the first program to map the entire sky homogeneously from the North Pole to the South Pole. Since banal geometry prevents access to the whole sky from any non equatorial site, the concept assumes an international effort. Such a project can be, and has
(10) since been, undertaken with only two observatories, one in the Northern Hemisphere, another in the southern. The *Carte du Ciel* was too grand an idea for that. The photographic fidelity achieved in the early 1880s at the Paris Observatory by the brothers Paul and
(15) Prosper Henry permitted their director, Admiral Ernest B. Mouchez, to dream of a completeness previously unthinkable. He proposed to chart all of the stars down to eleventh magnitude, a brightness level a hundredth as bright as that visible to the naked eye. This
(20) represents several million stars, over ten times as many as recorded in previous catalogues.

Such an undertaking exceeded the technical and fiscal capacities of any pair of observatories of the period. Mouchez conceived an audacious plan. Major
(25) observatories all over the world would be asked to participate, each to be assigned a unique zone of declination—the celestial equivalent of terrestrial latitude—and each to bear its share of the cost. Invitations were issued for an organizational meeting in Paris. It was
(30) held April 16 through 27, 1887, but not everyone came. The most notable absentee was Harvard's William C. Pickering. Indeed, apparently no American astronomer was there, although Benjamin A. Goule's Cordoba (Argentina) Observatory later signed on. The Americans
(35) would not participate directly in the *Carte du Ciel,* because Pickering intended to organize a purely made-in-U.S.A. version, using the Harvard substation at Arequipa, Peru. The wisdom of Mouchez's approach was vividly underscored by Pickering's failure, apparently
(40) caused by funding problems.

Virtually every aspect of the program represented an important innovation. Holographic uniformity was achieved by equipping all participating observatories with identical telescopes and imposing
(45) identical procedures. The Henry brothers invented the first astronomical optical system color-corrected for the blue wavelength to which the photographic emulsions were most sensitive. Paris telescope maker Paul

Gautier produced 18 copies of their prototype, one for
(50) each of the collaborators. Special measuring machines
were constructed. To permit precise measurements in
the event of emulsion creep, each plate was pre-
exposed with a rectangular grid containing five-
millimeter intervals and having a positional accuracy
(55) of only two to three micrometers. The plate fields were
overlapped by 50 percent in both axes so that each star
appeared in the central zone of at least one plate. To
aid in separating real images from the numerous
photographic defects, each "catalogue" plate was
(60) exposed twice with a slight offset, and each "map"
plate three times in a triangular pattern.

The observations began in 1891. World War I
interrupted the work at most sites, but Algiers finished
its zone in 1915. Although all of the sky was
(65) eventually photographed uniformly, the *Carte du Ciel*
was never really finished. Some of the original 18
observatories abandoned their zones unfinished; for
example, the Santiago zone became the Hyderabad
zone. In many places, the work dragged on and on. The
(70) last catalogue was published as recently as 1964. The
quality of the positions varied from one institution to
another. Roughly half of the charts were never
published.

Nonetheless, the project was a success on two
(75) counts. Even with their flaws, the maps and catalogues
represent a major astronomical resource that is still
important. Perhaps even more important than the
scientific merit of Admiral Mouchez's *chef d'oeuvre*,
however, is that the survey established a model for
(80) global scientific collaboration and coordination that has
been followed with much success ever since. The
International Astronomical Union, organized in 1922,
and the International Geophysical Year (1957–58) are
good examples. According to Harvard astronomer and
(85) historian Owen Gingerich, the American
nonparticipation was, in a perverse way, advantageous
to American astronomy. *Carte du Ciel* astronomy was
labor-intensive and costly, occupying most of the
sources of the participating observatories. Several
(90) ruined themselves, both scientifically and financially.
Meanwhile, their American counterparts were free to
improve instrumentation and to attack new problems
in observational astrophysics where they became
preeminent.

51. According to the article, the successful
completion of the Astrographic Catalog
project was due to:

A. the international cooperation among participating countries.

B. the absence of scientific competition
among participating countries.

C. the continuing financial support of major participating countries.

D. the strong, determined leadership of Admiral Mouchez, the project's director.

52. In the article, the author states the project as
"an audacious plan," in reference to:

A. its goal to chart all of the stars in the
heavens.

B. not including the sponsorship of the
United States.

C. relying on European and South American
powers to support it.

D. involving major observatories to also pay
for its own finances.

53. Regarding the project's approach, the author
asserts that major observatories were:

A. given their choice of celestial zones to
chart.

B. assigned designated celestial zones.

C. given opportunities to trade celestial
zones with cooperating observatories.

D. often forced to withdraw from the project
due to financial problems.

54. The author observes that photographic innovations flourished in the project among participating observatories primarily due to:

A. each being equipped with specialized
cameras.

B. each being given limitless time to complete its observations.

C. each being provided with the same telescopes and following the same procedures.

D. each receiving the same financial back-
ing from its host country.

55. Which of the following would **not** be a plausible explanation for the length of completion
time for the Astrographic Catalog project?

A. A few observatories gave up finishing the
project.

B. World War II permanently ended participation among several observatories.

C. Some observatories were financially unable to continue.

D. For many observatories the work lagged
behind schedule.

56. The passage implies that the U.S. chose not to participate in the undertaking because:

    A. the project was conceived by a well-known French astronomer.

    B. most participating countries were anti-American.

    C. the government believed its share of the cost would be excessive.

    D. the leading American astronomer planned to develop an American version of the project.

57. Which of the following statements best sums up the article's conclusion?

    A. The scientific cooperation of participating countries created two well-known organizations—The International Astronomical Union and the International Geophysical Year.

    B. The Astrographic Catalog project provided an important resource for astronomy and developed a standard for international scientific cooperation and organization.

    C. The Astrographic Catalog project created finite celestial maps and catalogues for astronomers and a model for an international network of sciences and humanities.

    D. The lack of American participation was clearly detrimental to the completion of the project and was the major reason the project was not fully successful.

Passage IX (Questions 58–65)

On a quiet country road in Monroe County in southeast Michigan, one of the state's Centennial farms can be found, designated as such because it has been owned by the same family for more than one hundred
(5) years. The stone farmhouse was built by Theophilus and Roxanna Osgood, who left western New York State in the middle-1830s to farm 160 acres in Michigan territory. For ten years, they lived in a primitive wooden house until they could afford to build
(10) a proper house in a provincial Greek Revival style, using the construction they remembered from back home, coursed cobblestone. The Osgoods painstakingly collected cobblestones, three to four inches in size, from nearby Stony Ridge and had a
(15) local mechanic lay them in regular horizontal courses in the walls of their new house.

Forty known surviving farmhouses of coursed cobblestone construction, built between 1829 and the 1870s, embellish the landscape of southern Michigan.
(20) The cobblestones were a legacy of the Ice Age, polished, rounded, and deposited by glaciers, and were used in houses from upper New York State to Wisconsin, wherever the stones were common. Sometimes the builders selected cobblestones of all one
(25) color; other times the stones were set in herringbone patterns or just in straight courses. These houses, made of local materials by local people, eloquently evoke the histories of their builders and occupants. "Vernacular buildings like the cobblestone houses are important,"
(30) says Kathryn Bishop Eckert, acting state historic preservation officer for Michigan. "They are close to the land, the place, and the people."

Eckert describes cobblestone houses in *Buildings of Michigan*, the first complete architectural history of
(35) the state. It is one of the first volumes in *Buildings of the United States*, a major series under the editorial direction of the Society of Architectural Historians in Philadelphia. When completed, this project will be the first comprehensive, state by state architectural survey
(40) and guide to the built environment of the United States. The story of Michigan architecture begins with the arrival of nomadic Paleo-Indians more than 12,000 years ago, to a half-frozen land still in the grip of the Ice Age. The wigwams, longhouses, and lodges of the
(45) native peoples have disappeared. The Norton burial mounds west of Grand Rapids survive as one of the few visible reminders of the times before the Europeans arrived. French and English traders, soldiers, and missionaries followed the water route
(50) from Canada in the seventeenth and eighteenth centuries, and constructed forts, trading posts, and houses. In territorial days, especially after the completion of the Erie Canal in 1825, settlers such as the Osgoods left worn-out farms in western New York
(55) State and New England for fertile farmland in southern Michigan, building in the style that they remembered from the East. Nineteenth-century entrepreneurs were quick to discover the cornucopia of resources left by the Ice Age. Besides the rich soil in the southern part
(60) of the state, there were lakes large and small, rivers, minerals, and countless acres of pine and hardwood forests. From around 1830 to 1910, logging was a principal Michigan industry. "Michiganians love wood," Eckert says. "We have wood houses of all
(65) kinds, from elaborate Queen Anne mansions of the lumber barons to the simple log houses of the trappers and traders."

One of the mansions was built in Traverse City in 1891 for a prosperous lumberman, Perry Hannah
(70) and his wife. Noted Grand Rapids architect William G. Robinson designed the Queen Anne house, which has gables, turrets, a generous wraparound porch, and

more than forty rooms. Queen Anne houses can be found throughout the United States, but the *(75)* imaginative use of wood in the Hannah house unmistakably connects to the Michigan lumber industry. The house is ornamented with intricately carved and decorated wood inside and out; every room is paneled in a different hardwood. "This lavish use *(80)* of wood," Eckert suggests, "identifies the house equally with the pine and hardwood forests of Michigan, and with Hannah, whose life was shaped and sustained by that forest."

Stone, rather than wood, was the natural building *(85)* material for the rocky terrain of the Upper Peninsula. The mining industry—copper and iron—that dominated the Upper Peninsula created specialized building types. The buildings were designed by company engineers and were constructed of mine- *(90)* waste rock, brick, and Lake Superior red sandstone rubble. Many of these buildings are still used, although not for their original purposes.

Michigan's geography, another gift of the Ice Age, offers miles of wild shoreline along the Great *(95)* Lakes, many rivers, and thousands of inland lakes. From the late nineteenth century, mid-westerners have enjoyed their holidays at Michigan resorts. Mackinac Island, for instance, has splendid "cottages" built by the affluent, while simple cabins for working-class *(100)* vacationers can be found on the state's shoreline, rivers, and lakes. The Grand Hotel, prominently sited on a high bluff overlooking the Straits of Mackinac was constructed of local white pine by Michigan architect-builder, Charles W. Caskey.

(105) Michigan has many special architectural elements. For instance, because of its long shoreline, Michigan has more lighthouses than any other state in the union. Bay City was the home of the Alladin Company, one of the most prolific manufacturers of mail-order houses from the *(110)* end of World War I through the 1920s. Homeowners across the country ordered bungalows, Queen Anne, American foursquare, and colonial revival houses from the firm, whose catalogue even offered plans for industrial towns, complete with stores, churches, schools, *(115)* warehouses, hotels and dwellings. The William W. Maier house is the ultimate expression of Michiganians' fascination with wood: Maier developed a technique for siding the exterior walls of buildings with concrete shaped in the form of logs. The chimneys of his house resemble *(120)* tree trunks—all in concrete. Eckert remarks, "We even love imitation logs. You can find Perma-Log houses in the middle of a forest, sometimes as a facing over a real log house."

The Buildings of the United States Series, which *(125)* includes Michigan, will represent each state by a single volume. Introductory material in each volume will discuss the development of the state and its

architectural history, lacing it in a national and international context. It is hoped that the series of *(130)* complete architectural histories of each state will help prevent destruction of the national's architectural treasures by fostering a deep appreciation of their beauty and historic importance.

58. The statement that best summarizes the passage is:

   A. Houses in Michigan were built with ingenious architectural styles.
   B. Many buildings in Michigan reflected the use of local and natural materials.
   C. Most buildings in Michigan were built with a mixture of cobblestones and wood.
   D. Michigan is proud of its architectural development.

59. Which of the following would most likely describe the references to the Hannah mansion and the Maier home?

   A. The wealthy class in Michigan built homes with stone as the primary material.
   B. It was typical of the well-to-do in Michigan to have lavish surroundings in local forests.
   C. Most of the rich home owners in Michigan preferred using local architects to design their homes.
   D. Both buildings reflect the owners' preference for Michigan's local lumber.

60. The passage indicates that the author would **not** agree with which of the following statements?

   A. Michigan's rich natural resources influenced architectural development in the state.
   B. Local forests of pine and hardwood were common sources for building constructions.
   C. Copper, iron and marble were the types of stones used in buildings in Michigan's Upper Peninsula.
   D. Michigan's forests were so abundant that a company in the state specialized in mail-order homes made of Michigan wood.

61. The author sees Michigan's natural abundance of forests as a likely explanation for:

   A. the popular use of wood for all types of homes.

   B. the strong environmental consciousness of its citizens.

   C. the major attraction for people living in the state.

   D. the preference for an alternative heating system in homes.

62. According to the passage, which of the following is **not** representative of Michigan's natural resources?

   A. A vast shoreline with numerous rivers and inland lakes

   B. Fertile soil

   C. Minerals such as copper and iron

   D. Burial mounds of native peoples

63. The author asserts that Michiganians' use of wood in building construction in even a resort such as Mackinac Island reflects:

   A. that the interest extended to vacation homes for the wealthy and working-class.

   B. that the interest was limited only to that region.

   C. that most of the state's citizens permitted only the use of local wood.

   D. that only local white pine was the preferred choice of material.

64. The author is primarily concerned with demonstrating that Michigan:

   A. is a popular vacation place due to its natural waterways.

   B. offers numerous forests and wildlife.

   C. has abundant forests and minerals.

   D. developed an architectural style influenced by its use of natural sources.

65. The inclusion of *Buildings of Michigan* primarily underscores the article's emphasis on:

   A. the importance of exploiting natural materials in the building industry.

   B. the conservation history of the state's natural resources.

   C. Michigan's own unique architectural history.

   D. pointing out the European-copied styles of building.

END OF TEST 1.

IF YOU FINISH BEFORE THE TIME IS UP, YOU MAY CHECK YOUR WORK ON THIS TEST ONLY.

PHYSICAL SCIENCES

Time: 100 Minutes
Questions 66–142

Directions: This test contains 77 questions. Most of the questions consist of a descriptive passage followed by a group of questions related to the passage. For these questions, study the passage carefully and then choose the best answer to each question in the group. Some questions in this test stand alone. These questions are independent of any passage and independent of each other. For these questions, too, you must select the one best answer. Indicate all your answers by blackening the corresponding circles on your answer sheet.

A periodic table is provided at the beginning of this book. You may consult it whenever you wish.

Passage I (Questions 66–69)

The figure below shows a cylinder, which is closed by a freely-moving piston of negligible mass.

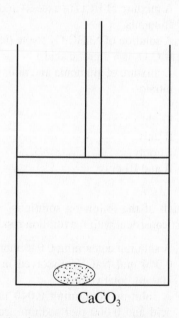

CaCO₃

(a) At the start of an experiment, a sample of $CaCO_3$ (molar mass = 100.0 g/mol) weighing 10.0 g is placed in the cylinder, which also contains 224 mL of nitrogen gas. The temperature inside the cylinder is $0°C$ and the external pressure is 1.00 atm.

(b) The cylinder and its contents are heated to a temperature of 500 K. (The external pressure is unchanged.) At that temperature, the following reaction goes to completion:

(Reaction 1) $CaCO_3(s) \rightarrow CaO(s) + CO_2(g)$

(c) Finally, the cylinder and its contents are cooled to $0°C$.

66. What is the mass of solid remaining in the cylinder at the end of part (b)?

   A. 0.0 g
   B. 5.6 g
   C. 6.4 g
   D. 11.2 g

67. What is the volume of gas in the cylinder at the end of part (b)?

   A. 2.46 L
   B. 4.10 L
   C. 4.51 L
   D. 5.10 L

68. Find the work (in units of L atm) for the process described in (b).

   A. –4.51 L atm
   B. –4.29 L atm
   C. 4.29 L atm
   D. 4.51 L atm

69. Find P_{CO2}, the partial pressure of $CO_2(g)$, at 500 K.

   A. 0.10 atm
   B. 0.91 atm
   C. 1.00 atm
   D. 1.83 atm

Passage II (Questions 70–75)

A solution is prepared by dissolving 1 or more unknown substances in 100 mL of water. A chemist makes the following measurements of the solution:

(1) The pH of the solution is 4.73.

(2) (a) A titration of a 10.00-mL sample using 0.100 M NaOH resulted in a gradual increase in pH, followed by a sudden rise in pH after 40.0 mL of base had been added.

(b) A titration of a second 10.00-mL sample using 0.100 M HNO_3 also resulted in a gradual decrease in pH, followed by a sudden drop in pH after 60.0 mL of acid had been added.

(3) The osmotic pressure of the solution was the same as that of a 0.800 M NaCl solution.

(4) When a drop of the solution was tested in a flame, it showed an intense yellow color.

70. Noting the acidic pH, (and ignoring the other information) a student wonders whether the substance might be a strong acid. What would the concentration of a strong acid need to be in order to show the pH that is reported in (1)?

A. 1.9×10^{-5} M
B. 0.002 M
C. 0.473 M
D. 2.7 M

71. What is $[H^+]$ in a solution that is 0.10 M in formic acid ($K_a = 1.8 \times 10^{-4}$) and 0.30 M in sodium formate?

A. 6.0×10^{-5} M
B. 4.4×10^{-4} M
C. 0.10 M
D. 0.40 M

72. Which of the tests reported can suggest a specific element that is present in the unknown substance?

A. (1)
B. (2)
C. (3)
D. (4)

73. How does the osmotic pressure of 0.10 M sucrose(aq) compare to that of 0.10 M $NaNO_3$(aq)? (Assume the temperature of each to be 25.0 °C.)

A. The osmotic pressure in the sucrose solution is equal to that in the sodium nitrate solution.
B. The osmotic pressure in the sucrose solution is equal to one-half of that in the sodium nitrate solution.
C. The osmotic pressure is zero in the sucrose solution but is greater than zero in the sodium nitrate solution.
D. The osmotic pressure in the sucrose solution is equal to twice the osmotic pressure in the sodium nitrate solution.

74. The unknown solution produced an endpoint when strong acid was added *and* in separate trial when strong base was added. Which of the following substances or mixtures would give such a result?

I. A mixture of HCl (in excess) and ammonia
II. A solution of $NaHC_2O_2$.(Note that $H_2C_2O_4$ is a diprotic acid.)
III. A mixture of ammonia and ammonium nitrate

A. I only
B. II only
C. III only
D. II and III only

75. Which of the following solutions would be most consistent with the titration results in (2)?

A. A solution containing 0.040 mol HCl and 0.060 mol NaOH, dissolved in water to 100 mL total volume.
B. A solution containing 0.040 mol acetic acid and 0.060 mol sodium acetate, dissolved in water to 100 mL total volume.
C. A solution containing 0.040 mol $NaHC_2O_2$. (Note that HC_2O_2 is a diprotic acid.)
D. A solution containing 0.060 mol acetic acid and 0.040 mol sodium acetate, dissolved in water to 100 mL total volume.

Passage III (Questions 76–81)

The following is a summary of information relating to the properties of water in its different states:

Specific heat of $H_2O(s)$ = 2.03 J/g °C
Specific heat of $H_2O(l)$ = 4.18 J/g °C
Specific heat of $H_2O(g)$ = 2.05 J/g °C
Molar enthalpy of fusion = 6.02 kJ/mol
Molar enthalpy of vaporization = 40.7 kJ/mol
Density of $H_2O(l)$ at 25 °C = 0.997 g/cm³
Density of $H_2O(s)$ at 25 °C = 0.917 g/cm³
Vapor pressure of water at various temperatures:

T (°C)	$P_{vap(torr)}$
30	31.8
85	433.6
90	527.8
95	633.0
100	760.0

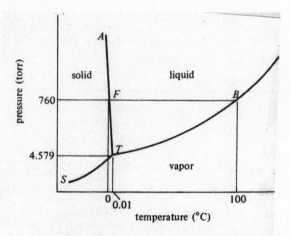

76. A glass bottle filled with water was sealed and put into a freezer overnight; in the morning it was found to have cracked. Which of the data given at the beginning of the passage would best explain this result?

   A. The specific heat values for the solid and liquid phases of water
   B. The large positive value for the molar heat of fusion of water
   C. The densities of the solid and liquid phases of water
   D. The slope of the liquid/vapor boundary of the phase diagram for water

77. A beaker contains 100 g of water at 30.0 °C. After 1 hour in a cool room, the water's temperature has dropped to 24.0 °C. How much heat was lost to the surroundings?

   A. 4.18 J
   B. 418 J
   C. 2.5 kJ
   D. 12.5 kJ

78. Using the information at the beginning of the passage, estimate the strength of the hydrogen bonds in liquid water.

   A. 4.18 J/g °C
   B. 41.4 J/mol °C
   C. 6.02 kJ/mol
   D. 40.7 kJ/mol

79. Use the information at the beginning of the passage to predict the change, if any, in the freezing point of water, as the pressure is increased from 1 atm to 50 atm.

   A. At 50 atm, the freezing point will be less than 0 °C.
   B. At 50 atm, the freezing point will be greater than 0 °C.
   C. At 50 atm, the freezing point will remain equal to 0 °C.
   D. Cannot be determined from the information given.

80. A solution is prepared by mixing an unknown mass of LiCl (MM = 42.39 g/mol) with 180 g of water. The vapor pressure of water above the solution is found to be 31.2 torr at 30.0 °C. Find the mass of LiCl in the solution.

   A. 4.1 g
   B. 8.2 g
   C. 11.6 g
   D. 14.4 g

81. A student performed the following experiment: She heated a flask containing 200 mL of pure water to boiling, allowed it to boil for 5 minutes, then sealed the top. She then cooled the flask by holding it under running tap water for 10 seconds. When she removed it from the running water, keeping the seal intact, she saw that the water inside was boiling again.

Which of the following is the best explanation of the students' observations?

A. Cooling the flask lowered the air pressure inside. But since the boiling point dropped as the pressure above the liquid dropped, the water could boil at a reduced pressure.

B. After 5 minutes of boiling, the water vapor would have swept most of the air out of the flask. Cooling the sealed flask caused some of the vapor inside to condense, lowering the overall pressure. But since the boiling point dropped as the pressure above the liquid dropped, the water could boil at a reduced pressure.

C. As the temperature of the liquid dropped below 100 °C, more of the air above the surface was able to dissolve in the water, thus lowering the pressure above the liquid and allowing the water to boil at a reduced pressure.

D. As the temperature of the flask was reduced, water vapor condensed, releasing heat, which was absorbed by the rest of the liquid and caused it to boil.

Passage IV (Questions 82–87)

The "Born-Haber Cycle" is a means of explaining the stability of ionic solids by graphically depicting the thermodynamic steps involved in the formation of the crystal. The example below illustrates this process for LiCl:

Reactions:

(1) $Li(s) + 1/2\ Cl_2(g) \rightarrow LiCl(s)$ $\Delta H_{formation} = -409$ kJ
(2) $Li(s) \rightarrow Li(g)$ $\Delta H_{sublimation} = 161$ kJ
(3) $Li(g) \rightarrow Li^+(g)\ +\ e^-$ $\Delta H_{ionization} = 520$ kJ
(4) $Cl_2(g) \rightarrow 2Cl(g)$ $\Delta H_{dissociation} = 240$ kJ
(5) $Cl(g) + e^- \rightarrow Cl^-(g)$ $\Delta H_{electron\ affinity} = -349$ kJ
(6) $Li^+(g)\ + Cl^-(g) \rightarrow LiCl(s)$ $\Delta H_{crystal\ lattice\ energy} = ?$

Graphical representation (enthalpies in kJ). Any reaction above can be represented by a pair of levels in the diagram. For example, reaction (2), which is endothermic by 161 kJ, has its reactant, Li(s), listed at the level labelled "0", and its product, Li(g), listed at the level labelled "161". (The chlorine species is also listed but is unchanged in the two levels.) By examining the entire diagram, we can discover relationships among all of the equations. In particular, we can determine the value of $\Delta H_{crystal\ lattice\ energy}$.

801	_____	$Li^+(g) + Cl(g) + e^-$
[3]	_____	$Li^+(g) + Cl^-(g)$
[2]	_____	$Li(g) + Cl(g)$
161	_____	$Li(g) + 1/2Cl_2(g)$
0	_____	$Li(s) + 1/2Cl_2(g)$
[1]	_____	$LiCl(s)$

82. What is the enthalpy change when 0.25 mole of Li(g) is ionized?

A. −87.3 kJ
B. 130 kJ
C. 161 kJ
D. 520 kJ

83. Which of the following are endothermic processes?

I. the sublimation of Li(s)
II. the formation of $Cl^-(g)$ from Cl(g)
III. the creation of LiCl(s) from the gas-phase ions

A. I only
B. II only
C. III only
D. I and II only

84. What value should be placed in "[2]" on the left side of the diagram?

A. 120
B. 240
C. 281
D. 401

85. What is the enthalpy change for the reaction

$$Li(g) + 1/2\ Cl_2(g) \rightarrow Li^+(g) + e^- + Cl(g)$$

   A. 240 kJ
   B. 520 kJ
   C. 640 kJ
   D. 801 kJ

86. Of the enthalpies listed, which is the major contributor to the stability of crystalline silver chloride?

   A. $\Delta H_{formation}$
   B. $\Delta H_{dissociation}$
   C. $\Delta H_{electron\ affinity}$
   D. $\Delta H_{crystal\ lattice\ energy}$

Passage V (Questions 88–93)

Atomic absorption

Modern chemical analysis relies on atomic absorption spectroscopy as a key tool for determining the composition of samples containing metals. The method relies on the following facts: optical absorption lines of gas-phase metals are narrow in wavelength, absorption spectra are highly distinctive, and light sources can be made to produce light of just the right wavelength for a particular metal atom.

The diagram below shows the basic features of the spectrometer. The light source uses a "hollow cathode lamp" that contains the metal under study; this ensures that the emitted light will be of the precise wavelength that can be absorbed by the atom. The dissolved sample is sprayed into a flame whose temperature (from 1700–3150 °C) is high enough to produce gaseous atoms of the metallic sample. The light passes through the flame, where some of it is absorbed. The light then passes through a monochromator, which eliminates light of all but the wavelength of interest, and the light intensity is measured by a photodector. Comparison with a "blank" reading allows the experimenter to determine the fraction of light absorbed by the sample and, using suitable calibration, to determine the concentration of the target element. The sensitivity of the method can reach parts-per-billion.

Detector

Power supply   Lamp   Burner   Monochromator

The following "calibration curve" gives typical values for a series of standard solutions of magnesium, measured at 285.2 nm.

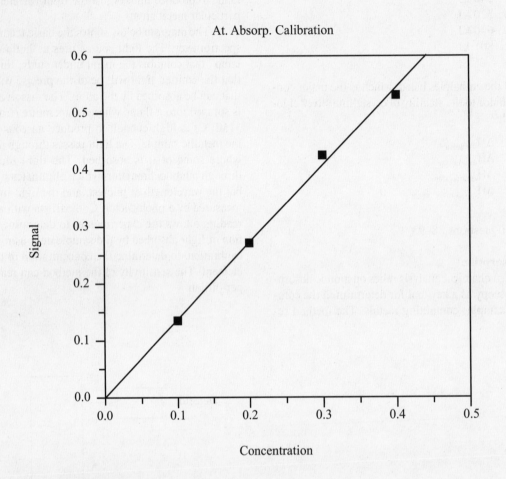

At. Absorp. Calibration

We can understand the way atomic absorption works at the atomic level by considering the following (partial) energy-level diagram for the neutral magnesium atom.

Energy
(kJ/mol)

0
−107 _____ 5s
−136   _____ 4p
−181   _____ 3d
−215 _____ 4s
−317   _____ 3p

−738 _____ 3s

87. Sodium vapor displays strong absorption of light whose wavelength is 589 nm. What is the frequency of this light?

    A. $3.90 \times 10^{-31} s^{-1}$
    B. $5.89 \times 10^{-9} s^{-1}$
    C. $5.09 \times 10^{5} s^{-1}$
    D. $5.09 \times 10^{14} s^{-1}$

88. When magnesium atoms are heated in an intense flame, some are ionized. A strong transition in the Mg^{2+} absorption spectrum involves photons with an energy of 7.10×10^{-19} J. Find the wavelength of the photons absorbed in this transition.

    A. 280 nm
    B. 359 nm
    C. 567 nm
    D. 654 nm

89. Judging from the diagram, what is the lowest-energy transition from the ground state of magnesium?

    A. $3s \rightarrow 3p$
    B. $3p \rightarrow 4s$
    C. $4s \rightarrow 4p$
    D. $4p \rightarrow 4d$

90. Transitions in atoms such as magnesium obey a *selection rule* that stipulates that $l = \pm 1$, where l is the angular momentum quantum number. Following this rule, which of the following transitions on the chart would be expected to observed?

    I. $4s \rightarrow 5s$
    II. $3p \rightarrow 4d$
    III. $3s \rightarrow 5p$

    A. I only
    B. II only
    C. III only
    D. II and III only

91. The first ionization energy of sodium is 496 kJ/mol. A transition from the 3s orbital to the 3p orbital occurs with the absorption of a photon at 590 nm. Estimate the ionization energy of sodium from its 3p excited state.

    A. 203 kJ/mol
    B. 317 kJ/mol
    C. 421 kJ/mol
    D. 496 kJ/mol

92. An analyst uses the calibration curve shown on page 256 to determine the concentration of an unknown magnesium solution. If the value of the detector signal is 0.510, find the concentration of the magnesium in parts per million (ppm).

    A. 1.49 ppm
    B. 1.70 ppm
    C. 1.82 ppm
    D. 1.91 ppm

Passage VI (Questions 94–97)

In the Kjeldahl method of nitrogen analysis, the nitrogen in a protein or another biological molecule is converted to ammonium nitrate, which is in turn converted to ammonia. The ammonia is distilled into a vessel containing a known amount of strong acid, which is present in excess. After the ammonia reacts, the remaining acid is titrated with standardized sodium hydroxide.

93. Give the hybridization of the nitrogen in the ammonium ion, NH_4^+.

    A. sp^2
    B. sp^3
    C. sp^4
    D. sp^3d

94. Which of the following processes is most important in determining the pH of a 0.10 M solution of $NH_3(aq)$?

    A. Weak acid dissociation
    B. Disproportionation
    C. Buffer action
    D. Weak base hydrolysis

95. A solution of $NH_3(aq)$ is known to be approximately 0.1 M. If a chemist wishes to determine the quantity of $NH_3(aq)$ in solution by direct titration with 0.100 M HCl, which of the following indicators would be best? (Note that K_b for ammonia is 1.8×10^{-5})

    A. Methyl orange (pH 3.2 – 4.4)
    B. Ethyl red (pH 4.0 – 5.8)
    C. Cresol red (pH 7.0 – 8.8)
    D. Alizarin yellow (pH 10.1 – 12.0)

96. In one Kjeldahl analysis, a sample of protein weighing 1.20 g yields a quantity of ammonia which is reacted with 40.0 mL of 0.500 M HCl. After the reaction, the remaining acid is titrated with 0.250 M NaOH, and an endpoint occurs after 25.20 mL. Find the percentage of nitrogen in the protein sample.

- **A.** 0.19%
- **B.** 6.30%
- **C.** 13.7%
- **D.** 16.0%

Passage VII (Questions 96–100)

In the photoelectric effect, photons strike the surface of a photoemissive material. If the photon has sufficient energy, an electron, called a photoelectron, is ejected. There is a one to one correspondence between the photon and the ejected electron: One photon in produces one electron out.

The photon must have a certain threshold energy for a photoelectron to be ejected.

    I. A photon with energy below this value will not cause an electron to be ejected.

    II. A photon with this minimum energy will eject an electron that has approximately zero kinetic energy.

    III. A photon with energy above this value will eject an electron that has kinetic energy.

    IV. The energy threshold required depends on the identity of the photoemissive material and is called the work function, _.

    V. The relationship among the energy of the photon $h\nu_0$, the work function of the material, Φ, and the kinetic energy of the ejected electron E_K is given by:

$$E_K = h\nu_0 - \Phi$$

where h is Planck's constant, $h = 4.2 \times 10^{-15}$ eV s (electron volt seconds), and ν_0 is the frequency of the photon.

97. What is a reasonable estimated threshold frequency of a metal with a work function of 2.5 eV?

- **A.** $1.7 \times 10^{-15}\ s^{-1}$
- **B.** $1.0 \times 10^{-14}\ s^{-1}$
- **C.** $4.5 \times 10^{14}\ s^{-1}$
- **D.** $6.0 \times 10^{14}\ s^{-1}$

98. Photoelectrons are emitted from a metal surface when it is exposed to monochromatic light of a particular wavelength. Which statement is true if the intensity of the monochromatic light is decreased to half its original value?

    I. Fewer photoelectrons are emitted

    II. The same number of photoelectrons are emitted

    III. The kinetic energy of the emitted photoelectrons is less

    IV. The kinetic energy of the emitted photoelectrons remains the same

- **A.** I and III
- **B.** I and IV
- **C.** II and III
- **D.** II and IV

99. The plot of kinetic energy of photoelectrons versus frequency of impinging photons for a particular photoemissive metal is shown below. Which of the values below is a good estimate of the work function of the metal?

- **A.** 0.7 eV
- **B.** 1.3 eV
- **C.** 3.0 eV
- **D.** 5.0 eV

ν_0, 10^{14} Hz

100. A photoelectron is emitted from a given metal when it is struck by a photon with a frequency greater than 1.4×10^{15} Hz. What is the kinetic energy of ejected electrons if the metal is struck by light with a frequency of 1.8×10^{15} Hz?

- **A.** 2.1 eV
- **B.** 5.9 eV
- **C.** 7.6 eV
- **D.** 10 eV

101. A photoemissive material is struck by dim yellow light but no photoelectrons are ejected. Which of the following changes could produce ejection of photoelectrons?

    A. Increase the brightness of the yellow light.
    B. Replace the yellow light with red light.
    C. Use light with a shorter wavelength.
    D. Use light with a lower frequency.

Passage VIII (Questions 101–106)

I. Germanium, Ge, a common semiconductor element has four valence electrons per atom, and in the solid state, forms four covalent bonds with adjacent Ge atoms.

In N-type semiconductors the semiconductor is "doped" with an element that has more valence electrons. These extra "free" electrons are the charge carriers.

In P-type semiconductors the semiconductor is "doped" with an element that has fewer valence electrons. The "holes" due to the missing electrons are the charge carriers.

II. The simplest semiconductor device is a diode. In the standard symbol

the arrow points from a P-type semiconductor to an N-type semiconductor. The interface between two semiconductors is called a P-N junction. When an electron from the N-type side migrates into a hole in the P-type side it forms a covalent bond and is no longer free to move. The N-type side loses an electron and gains a hole. The P-type side loses a hole and gains an electron. As a result, the N-type side develops a net positive charge and the P-type side a net negative charge creating an *electric field barrier* that prevents further migration of charge across the junction.

In a process called *biasing*, applying a potential difference across the P-N junction modifies the strength of the electric field barrier.

In *forward biasing*, the N-type side is connected to the negative terminal of a battery and the P-type side to the positive terminal. The free electrons and holes both migrate towards the junction and towards each other. The *electric field barrier* is reduced.

The opposite connections are used in *reverse biasing*. The free electrons and holes do not cross the junction. Instead they migrate away from the junction in opposite directions and the *electric field barrier* is increased.

102. What is formed if a germanium crystal is doped with the group IIIA element boron, B?

    A. N-type semiconductor
    B. P-type semiconductor
    C. Negatively charged semiconductor
    D. Positively charged semiconductor

103. For current to flow a diode must be:

    A. Forward biased
    B. Reverse biased
    C. Operated at high temperature
    D. Connected to a source of small potential difference

104. Which statement is valid for the flow of charge between points A and B of the following circuit?

    I. Holes flow from A to B
    II. Holes flow from B to A
    III. Electrons flow from A to B
    IV. Electrons flow from B to A

    A. I and IV
    B. II and III
    C. III only
    D. IV only

105. A given circuit consists of a P-type semiconductor in series with a battery. Which statement is most valid?

    A. The holes flow only toward the positive terminal of the battery.

    B. The holes flow only toward the negative terminal of the battery.

    C. The holes flow equally towards both terminals of the battery.

    D. The holes do not move, and current is due to the flow of electrons only.

106. Which statement is most valid for the following circuit?

    A. Current increases because the *electric field barrier* increases.

    B. Current increases because the *electric field barrier* decreases.

    C. Current decreases because the *electric field barrier* increases.

    D. Current decreases because the *electric field barrier* decreases.

107. In which of the following circuits is current most likely to flow?

A.

B.

C.

D.

Passage IX (Questions 108–113)

Elasticity is an inherent property of a material that describes the material's response to a deforming external force and its ability to return to its original dimensions once the external force is removed. Stress and strain characterize the elasticity of a material.

Tensile, or longitudinal, stress is defined as a force that causes a linear deformation in the dimensions or shape of the body. The stress is generally expressed as force per unit area, S = F/ **A.** If stress is described as force per unit area, then stress is the same as the elongation caused by the stress.

Tensile strain, ε, measures the amount of deformation produced by the stress. It is the ratio of the change in length to the original length, ε = ΔL/L. Strain depends on the molecular structure of the material and is independent of the material's shape.

For elastic materials like muscles strain initially increases in proportion to the stress applied to the material. The proportionality constant is called the Young's modulus, Y, of the material. Within this region, if the distorting force is removed the material recovers and returns to its original dimensions.

Y = stress/strain

In an experiment to examine elasticity in muscles, muscle fiber bundles are simulated by elastic bands. All bands are identical in composition and diameter. Three systems are set up as follows:

Summary of Results:

System	Number of elastic bands	Length of each band band	Cross sectional area of each	Force applied	Change in length/band
1	1	L	A	F	ΔL
2	1	L	2A	F	ΔL/2
3	1	2L	A	F	2ΔL
4	2	L	A	2F	ΔL

108. A muscle of length L and cross-sectional area A is stretched a distance ΔL by a force F. What force is needed to stretch the muscle the same distance, ΔL, if the muscle's length is cut in half?

   A. F/2
   B. F
   C. 2F
   D. 4F

109. A muscle sample is stretched a certain length ΔL when a 1.5 kg mass is suspended from it. When an additional 0.5 kg mass is added the muscle stretches an additional 0.4 cm. How far did the original 1.5 kg mass stretch the muscle?

   A. 0.6 cm
   B. 1.2 cm
   C. 1.6 cm
   D. 2.0 cm

110. The stress produced by a mass, m, supported by a muscle is independent of:

   A. the acceleration due to gravity
   B. the density of the muscle
   C. the diameter of the muscle
   D. the length of the muscle

111. A band of muscle stretches a distance ΔL under a force F. If the length of the muscle is doubled and the diameter of the muscle is also doubled, by how much would the same load F stretch the muscle?

   A. Half as much, ΔL/2
   B. The same amount, L
   C. Twice as much, 2ΔL
   D. Four times as much, 4ΔL

112. In an experiment, elastic bands A and B are of equal length, L = 0.50 m, and equal cross-sectional area, A = 80×10^{-4} m^2. Band A requires 40 N to elongate it 0.08 m. Band B requires 80 N to produce the same strain. If the Young/s modulus for the material in band A is 6.25×10^4 N/m^2, what is the value of Y for the material in *band B*?

   A. 3.12×10^4 N/m^2
   B. 6.25×10^4 N/m^2
   C. 1.25×10^5 N/m^2
   D. 1.25×10^6 N/m^2

113. What is the percent change in length for a 2.0 m elastic band with cross-sectional area 2×10^{-6} m^2, and Young's modulus 2×10^{10} N/m^2 when subjected to a stress of 200 N?

   A. 0.050%
   B. 0.50%
   C. 5.0%
   D. 50.0%

Passage X (Questions 114–119)

When the source of a wave and the receiver or observer of the wave are in motion relative to each other, the frequency perceived by the observer will be different from the frequency actually produced by the source. This apparent change in frequency is called the Doppler Effect.

For mechanical waves such as sound waves, the shift between source and observed frequencies is described by the general formula:

$$f_o = f_s[(v + v_o)/(v - v_s)]$$

Where v, v_s, and v_o are, respectively, the speed of the wave in the given medium, the speed of the wave source and the speed of the wave observer. f_s and f_o are, respectively, the frequencies produced by the source and perceived by the observer.

The sign for v_s and v_o depend on the direction of their motions. By convention, the observer's velocity is positive if the observer is moving toward the source and negative if moving away. Similarly the velocity of the source is positive if moving toward the observer and negative if moving away.

For electromagnetic waves, the shift is described by: $f_o = f_s[(1 + v/c)/(1 - v/c)]^{1/2}$ where c = 3.00×10^8 m/s is the speed of light and v is the relative velocity between the source and the observer. v is negative if they are moving apart and positive if they are moving toward each other.

114. Which equation best describes the case of a wave source approaching a stationary observer?

   A. $f_o = f_s[(v)/(v - v_s)]$
   B. $f_o = f_s[(v)/(v + v_s)]$
   C. $f_o = f_s[(v + v_o)/(v)]$
   D. $f_o = f_s[(v - v_o)/(v)]$

115. Which equation best describes the case of an observer approaching a stationary wave source?

A. $f_o = f_s[(v)/(v - v_s)]$
B. $f_o = f_s[(v)/(v + v_s)]$
C. $f_o = f_s[(v + v_o)/(v)]$
D. $f_o = f_s[(v - v_o)/(v)]$

116. Which equation best describes the case of both the source and the observer moving in the same direction?

A. $f_o = f_s[(v + v_o)/(v - v_s)]$
B. $f_o = f_s[(v + v_o)/(v + v_s)]$
C. $f_o = f_s[(v - v_o)/(v + v_s)]$
D. $f_o = f_s[(v - v_o)/(v - v_s)]$

117. Which equation best describes the case of the source and the observer both moving away from each other?

A. $f_o = f_s[(v + v_o)/(v - v_s)]$
B. $f_o = f_s[(v + v_o)/(v + v_s)]$
C. $f_o = f_s[(v - v_o)/(v + v_s)]$
D. $f_o = f_s[(v - v_o)/(v - v_s)]$

118. A radio station transmits at a frequency of 90 MHz. A man listening to the station's classical music broadcast on his car radio drives toward the broadcast tower at a speed of 25 m/s. Which statements are most valid?

The observed frequency:
1. increases noticeably
2. doesn't change noticeably
3. decreases noticeably

The observed frequency is best calculated using:

I. $f_o = f_s[(v + v_o)/(v)]$
II. $f_o = f_s[(v - v_o)/(v)]$
III. $f_o = f_s[(1 + v/c)/(1 - v/c)]^{1/2}$

A. 1 and II
B. 2 and I
C. 2 and III
D. 3 and III

119. The Doppler Effect is used to show that the universe is expanding. Which statement is valid?

A. Observed wavelengths from space are shifted toward the blue end of the spectrum.
B. Observed wavelengths from space are shifted toward the red end of the spectrum.
C. Observed frequencies from space are higher than the emitted frequencies.
D. Observed wavelengths from space are shorter than the emitted wavelengths

Passage XI (Questions 120–124)

The 1966 sci-fi movie *Fantastic Voyage* presented the adventures of a group of U.S. scientists who, along with a submarine, are miniaturized to microscopic proportions and injected into the blood stream of a Russian defector who is dying from a blood clot on the brain. The mission is to reach the brain, dissolve the clot with the submarine's laser, and get out before the miniaturization process starts to reverse. Whew!

While the movie showed the ship being attacked by white blood cells as if it were an antigen, it ignored questions about physical, and physiological, consequences related to the size change.

Scaling is a tool used in science and engineering to determine the effect of size on function.

For each dimension of interest a scaling factor lambda, λ, is determined.

$$\text{Scaling factor} = \lambda = d'/d$$

Where d' is a given dimension of some object and d is the similar dimension of a second object. Both objects have the same shape and differ only in relative size. Any dimension can be used to determine the scaling factor provided the same dimension is used for both objects.

$$\begin{aligned}
&\text{Length, L, scales as :} && \text{L'/L} = \lambda \\
&\text{Area, A, scales as:} && \text{A'/A} = \lambda^2 \\
&\quad \text{because } A = L \times L \\
&\text{Volume, V, scales as:} && \text{V'/V} = \lambda^3 \\
&\quad \text{because } V = A \times L = L \times L \times L
\end{aligned}$$

Volume can also be defined as mass over density.

Object I consists of two cubes. Each cube is 1 unit per side, u. Object II is scaled up by a factor of 3.

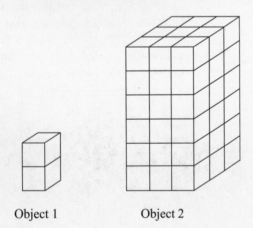

Object 1   Object 2

Property	Object I	Object II	Scaling factor
Length (= width)	1 u	3 u	λ 3(1)
Height	2 u	6 u	λ 3(2)
Area (height × length)	2 u2	18 u2	$\lambda2$ 32(2)
Volume (area × width)	2 u3	54 u3	$\lambda3$ 33(2)

120. Two men, A and B, have similarly shaped bodies and identical body densities. Man A weighs 686 N (70 kg) and man B weighs 784 N (80 kg). What is the scaling factor, _, of man B compared with man A?

    A. 0.87
    B. 1.05
    C. 1.14
    D. 1.48

121. What is the surface area of Object II in the passage if its center column of cubes is removed?

    A. 48 u2
    B. 84 u2
    C. 96 u2
    D. 112 u2

122. The strength of muscle is proportional to its cross-sectional area. If a 90 kg person can lift a 300 N weight with his forearm, what is the approximate weight a 60 kg person should be able to lift?

    A. 100 N
    B. 150 N
    C. 200 N
    D. 250 N

123. The drag of air on a body falling through the atmosphere can eventually balance the body's weight. At that point the body stops accelerating and falls with a constant velocity called the terminal speed, vT, given by:

$$vT = (2w/CD\_A)1/2$$

where w is the weight, CD is the drag coefficient, _ is the air density, and A is the cross-sectional area of the falling body. What is the scaling factor for terminal speed for two objects with the same drag coefficient?

A. _1/2
B. _
C. _2
D. _3

124. An architect wishes to test the stability of the design of a building prior to construction. The material used to construct a building can support a maximum weight per unit area of 7.5×10^4 N/cm^2 without collapsing. If the model is 1/1000th the size of the building, the material it's constructed from should be able to support a maximum weight per unit area of:

A. 150 N/cm^2
B. 75 N/cm^2
C. 1.5×10^4 N/cm^2
D. 7.5×10^4 N/cm^2

125. Before constructing a dam a model is created. The dimensions of the model scale at 1/1000th the proposed dam. The model is designed to fill with water in 1/100th the time it will take to fill the reservoir behind the proposed dam. If the reservoir is expected to fill at a rate of 10,000 m^3/hr, at what rate should the model be filled?

A. $10-1$ m^3/hr
B. $10-2$ m^3/hr
C. $10-3$ m^3/hr
D. $10-4$ m^3/hr

Questions 126–139 are independent of any passage and independent of each other.

126. Use the partial list of reduction potentials below to determine which of the questions that follow are true.

$MnO_4\text{-}(aq) + 8H^+ (aq) + 5e^- \Leftrightarrow Mn^{2+}(aq) + 4H_2O$ (1.51 v)

$Cl_2(g) + 2e^- \Leftrightarrow 2Cl^-(aq)$ (1.36 v)

$PbSO_4(s) + 2e^- \Leftrightarrow Pb(s) + SO_4^{2-}(aq)$ (–0.36)

   I. $Cl_2(g)$ is a better oxidizing agent than $PbSO_4(s)$.
   II. $MnO_4\text{-}(aq)$ will become a stronger oxidizing agent as the pH is lowered.
   III. $Mn^{2+}(aq)$ will react spontaneously with $Cl^-(aq)$.

A. I only
B. II only
C. III only
D. I and II only

127. Which of the following procedures would increase the solubility of a sample of 5.0 g $Fe(OH)_3(s)$ added to 500 mL of water?

A. Adding 1.0 M NaOH(aq)
B. Adding 1.0 M $HNO_3(aq)$
C. Adding $Fe(NO_3)(aq)$
D. Adding additional $Fe(OH)_3(s)$

128. The vapor pressure of water at 30.0 °C is 0.00419 atm. Find the mass of water that will fill a room at this temperature, if water vapor is in equilibrium with liquid. The room dimensions are 4.0m × 4.0m × 3.5m.

A. 0.170 g
B. 170 g
C. 189 g
D. 1.70 kg

129. A sample containing 10.0 mL of 1.15 M $Cr(NO_3)_3(aq)$ is diluted to 25.00 mL with water and mixed. Then 1.00 mL of the resulting solution is diluted to 50.00 mL. What is the final concentration of the $Cr(NO_3)_3(aq)$?

A. 0.000920 M
B. 0.0092 M
C. 0.0460 M
D. 0.460 M

130. Which (if any) of the following gas-phase molecules have the same molecular geometry?

  I. H_2O
  II. CO_2
  III. I_3^-

A. I and II
B. I and III
C. II and III
D. none; they are all different

131. When a chemist studies the decomposition reaction

$$N_2O_5(g) \rightarrow 2NO_2(g) + 1/2\ O_2(g)$$

she finds that the time needed to drop to one-fifth of the original reactant pressure is 4.77×10^4 s, regardless of the value of the initial pressure. What does she conclude about the order of the reaction and the half-life?

A. 0th-order, 1.91×10^5 s
B. 1st-order, 1.91×10^4 s
C. 1st-order, 2.06×10^4 s
D. 2nd-order, 8.56×10^4 s

132. A 100 gram lead ball at the end of a 2.00 meter string is swung in a horizontal circle. What is the centripetal acceleration if the ball sweeps through an angle of 12 radians in 4 seconds?

A. 6 m/s^2
B. 18 m/s^2
C. 48 m/s^2
D. 300 m/s^2

133. What is the value of the single capacitor equivalent to the three capacitors in the following circuit?

A. 2F
B. 3F
C. 5F
D. 8F

134. Two tuning forks are vibrating at 222 Hz and 258 Hz, respectively. How many beats per second are produced by the interference of the acoustical waves?

A. 480 Hz
B. 240 Hz
C. 36 Hz
D. 18 Hz

135. Two masses, M_A and M_B, where M_B is greater than M_A, are suspended over a massless, frictionless pulley. Which relationship below gives the downward acceleration of M_B?

A. gM_AM_B
B. g
C. $g(M_A - M_B)/(M_A + M_B)$
D. $g(M_AM_B)/(M_A + M_B)$

136. The dimensions of the foot of a 90 kg man standing still on a hard surfaced floor are 30 cm × 8 cm. The pressure exerted by the man on the floor is approximately:

A. 3.68 N/m^2
B. $1.88 \times 10^3 \text{ N/m}^2$
C. $36.8 \times 10^3 \text{ N/m}^2$
D. $18.4 \times 10^3 \text{ N/m}^2$

137. The radius of curvature of a concave mirror is given by r = 2f, where f is the focal length. An object is placed 10 cm in front of a mirror with a 60 cm radius of curvature. What is the image distance?

A. −10 cm
B. −15 cm
C. 6 cm
D. 50 cm

138. An ideal gas at 1.5 atm pressure is heated from 100 °C to 200 °C at constant volume. The resulting pressure is:

A. More than twice the original pressure
B. Twice the original
C. Less than twice the original
D. Half the original

139. Blocks A and B, with mass 6.0 kg and 3.0 kg, respectively are connected by a massless spring and rest on a frictionless horizontal surface. The blocks are pushed together, held at rest for a moment, and then released. Block A moves with a velocity of 8 m/s to the right. What is the velocity of block B?

A. 4.0 m/s to the right
B. 4.0 m/s to the left
C. 16 m/s to the right
D. 16 m/s to the left

140. Which of the following statements is/are valid for the transition of an electron in a Bohr atom from a given orbital to one of larger radius?

  I. The total energy of the atom increases
 II. The energy of the electron remains the same
 III. The force acting on the electron decrease

A. I and II
B. I only
C. I and III
D. III only

141. Which of the following is an excited-state configuration? (All are neutral atoms.)

A. $[\text{Ne}]\, 3s^2 3p^4$
B. $[\text{Ar}]4s^2 3d^6$
C. $[\text{Ar}]4s^1 3d^6$
D. $[\text{Ar}]4s^2 3d^{10} 4p^1$

142. When 25.00 mL of 0.415 M HCl reacts with 26.00 mL of 0.456 M NaOH in an insulated calorimeter, the temperature of the solution rises from 22.0 deg C to 25.2 deg C. Use this information to determine ΔH for the reaction

$$HCl(aq) + NaOH(a) \longrightarrow NaCl(aq) + H_2O$$

(Assume that the density of the solution is 1.00 g/L and that the specific heat of the solution is 4.18 J/g deg.)

A. 660 J
B. −660 J
C. 58 kJ
D. −58 kJ

WRITING SAMPLE

Time: 60 Minutes
2 Essays

Directions: This test consists of two parts. You will have 30 minutes to complete each part. During the first 30 minutes, you may work on Part 1 only. During the second 30 minutes, you may work on Part 2 only. You will have three pages for each essay answer, but you do not have to fill all three pages. Be sure to write legibly; illegible essays will not be scored.

Part 1

Consider this statement:

Those who live by the sword die by the sword.

Write a unified essay in which you perform the following tasks. Explain what you think the above statement means. Describe a specific situation in which those who live by the sword do NOT die by the sword. Discuss what you think determines whether or not death is the outcome for those who use the sword.

DO NOT START THE NEXT TOPIC UNTIL THE TIME IS UP.

Part 2

Consider this statement:

All things come to those who wait.

Write a unified essay in which you perform the following tasks. Explain what you think the above statement means. Describe a specific situation in which all things DO NOT come to those who wait OR all things come to those who DO NOT wait. Discuss what you think determines whether things come to those who wait and whether things do not come to those who wait.

END OF SECTION 3.

DO NOT RETURN TO PART 1.

BIOLOGICAL SCIENCES

Time: 100 Minutes
Questions 143–219

Directions: This test contains 77 questions. Most of the questions consist of a descriptive passage followed by a group of questions related to the passage. For these questions, study the passage carefully and then choose the best answer to each question in the group. Some questions in this test stand alone. These questions are independent of any passage and independent of each other. For these questions, too, you must select the one best answer. Indicate all your answers by blackening the corresponding circles on your answer sheet.

A periodic table is provided at the beginning of the book. You may consult it whenever you wish.

Passage I (Questions 143–149)

Various changes in volume, pressure, and electrical activity take place concurrently, each time the heart undergoes the sequence of atrial and ventricular systole (contraction) and diastole (relaxation). The accompanying figure depicts many of the changes that occur in the heart during the cardiac cycle.

Changes that occur in the heart during a cardiac cycle.

143. Papillary muscles and chordae tendinae are structures in the ventricles that allow the tricuspid and bicuspid valves to close properly and, additionally, prevent them from opening in the wrong direction. Which event in the cardiac cycle most likely contributes to the sound made when these A-V valves close?

    A. Atrial systole
    B. Atrial diastole
    C. Ventricular systole
    D. Ventricular diastole

144. End-diastolic volume (EDV) is the amount of blood in the ventricles after filling during diastole. Approximately how much blood represents EDV in the figure?

    A. 80–100 ml
    B. 100–120 ml
    C. 120–140 ml
    D. 140–160 ml

145. If end-systolic volume (ESV) is the amount of blood remaining in the ventricle after contracting, what term represents the *difference* between EDV and ESV?

    A. Heart rate
    B. Stroke volume
    C. Cardiac output
    D. Pulse pressure

146. The figure shows that pressure in the aorta is highest during ventricular systole. Assuming that blood pressure decreases as the distance from the left ventricle increases, where would you expect blood pressure to be lowest?

    A. Pulmonary arteries
    B. Pulmonary veins
    C. Vena cavae
    D. Systemic capillaries

147. Based on the figure, which of the following takes place as pressure in the ventricles decreases?

    A. The ventricles fill.
    B. The semilunar valves close.
    C. Both A and B
    D. Neither A nor B

148. What is the approximate heart rate (beats/minute) of the individual represented in the figure?

    A. 80–85 bpm
    B. 75–80 bpm
    C. 70–75 bpm
    D. 65–70 bpm.

149. The term "afterload" refers to the level of resistance that must be overcome in order for the ventricles to eject blood into the arteries. What is the expected result of an increase in afterload?

    A. Increased ESV and decreased stroke volume
    B. Increased ESV and increased stroke volume
    C. Decreased ESV and decreased stroke volume
    D. Decreased ESV and increased stroke volume

Passage II (Questions 150–156)

In humans, visual signals begin at the receptors (rods and cones) in the retina. The neural pathway then leaves the eyes via the optic nerves, continues along the optic tracts to the lateral geniculate bodies in the thalamus, and ends in the occipital lobes of the cortex. Along the way, connections are made with the superior colliculi in the midbrain.

150. According to the figure, which of the following statements is correct?

A. Signals from the **entire** visual field of the right eye go to the left occipital lobe.

B. Signals from the **entire** visual field of the left eye go to the left occipital lobe.

C. Signals from the **right** visual field of both eyes go to the left occipital lobe.

D. Signals from the **right** visual field of both eyes go to the right occipital lobe.

151. The superior colliculi are associated with somatic and autonomic motor signals that control specific eye muscles. Which of the following autonomic motor activities are most likely to be regulated by these signals?

A. Contraction and relaxation of the smooth muscles in the iris that control the amount of light entering the pupil.

B. Contraction and relaxation of the extrinsic eye muscles that move the eye left, right, up, down, etc.

C. Both A and B

D. Neither A nor B

152. The region of the retina where the optic nerve leaves the eye contains the central retinal artery and vein, but no rods or cones. What will happen when light strikes this region of the retina?

A. It will go unnoticed.

B. Signals along the optic nerve will stop at the optic chiasma.

C. The brain will be able to perceive color, but not black, white and shades of gray.

D. The brain will be able to perceive black, white and shades of gray, but not color.

153. Which area of the brain is **not** part of the visual pathway?

A. Brain stem

B. Diencephalon

C. Cerebrum

D. None of the above

154. When one looks directly at an object, the image of that object is focussed on the fovea centralis, a region in the center of the macula lutea, which contains no rods, but where the concentration of cones is highest. When directly viewing a distant star at night, it appears blurry or it cannot be seen at all. Yet, when viewed from the side, the same star can be seen clearly. What is the best explanation for this phenomenon?

A. The shape of the lens cannot be adjusted precisely enough when viewing such distant objects.

B. Cones require bright light to function, while rods require dim light.

C. At night, the cones are significantly more responsive than the rods.

D. The smooth muscles that control the size of the pupil cannot be regulated precisely enough in dim light.

155. Which statement about the visual pathway is most accurate concerning a "split-brain" individual who has had his corpus callosum cut?

A. Each eye would only send signals to the same side of the cerebrum.

B. Each eye would only send signals to the opposite side of the cerebrum.

C. Each eye would continue sending signals to both sides of the cerebrum as before.

D. Signals arriving at the lateral geniculate bodies would be the same, but they would not be able to reach the cerebrum.

156. A color-blind man (color-blindness is a sex-linked recessive trait) and his wife, who is a homozygous dominant individual, produce a daughter. What is the probability that she will be color-blind?

A. 0%

B. 25%

C. 50%

D. 100%

Passage III (Questions 157–163)

The accompanying chart summarizes the digestion and absorption of carbohydrates, lipids, and proteins in the human digestive tract, as well as some of the control mechanisms that help regulate these processes. Utilize information in the chart and your related knowledge about digestive systems to answer the following questions.

A Summary of Some Chemical Events of Digestion

(a)   (b)   (c)

157. Digestion is completed in the small intestine. How many different organs make enzymes that contribute to the digestion of proteins?

    A. One
    B. Two
    C. Three
    D. Four

158. Which groups of molecules require ATP for the absorption of their digestive end-products?

    A. Carbohydrates and lipids
    B. Carbohydrates and proteins
    C. Lipids and proteins
    D. Carbohydrates, lipids, and proteins

159. According to the chart, which of the following contributes to the regulation of stomach activity?

    A. Neurons
    B. Endocrine secretions from the stomach and small intestine
    C. Exocrine secretions from the stomach
    D. All of the above

160. Which of the following statements is true?

    A. All digestive end-products are absorbed into the blood.
    B. The digestion of carbohydrates is completed by intestinal enzymes.
    C. The liver plays no role in the processes summarized in the chart.
    D. After digestion is completed, all digestive end-products pass across the intestinal mucosa and enter the body fluids.

161. The intestinal hormone, secretin, stimulates the pancreas to release sodium bicarbonate into the duodenum. Which of the following statements best explains the function of sodium bicarbonate?

    A. Enzymes are pH specific.
    B. The buffering system in the blood plasma must be maintained.
    C. Bicarbonate ions are involved in the transport of carbon dioxide in the plasma during the chloride shift.
    D. All of the above

162. Intrinsic factor is a substance produced by the same gastric cells (parietal cells) that make hydrochloric acid. It binds to vitamin B12 so that this important vitamin, needed for nucleic acid synthesis, can be absorbed across the intestinal mucosa. Which symptom would be associated with a vitamin B12 deficiency?

    A. Muscle weakness
    B. Skeletal deterioration
    C. Red blood cell deficiency
    D. CNS disturbances

163. Through which organ will nutrients pass first after being absorbed into the capillaries of the small intestine?

    A. Heart
    B. Liver
    C. Lungs
    D. Large intestine

Passage IV (Questions 164–169)

The skin is a highly complex organ with functions that include protection, detecting changes in the environment, and various aspects of homeostatic regulation. It ranges in thickness from approximately 0.5mm (eyelids) to 6mm (soles of the feet). Its numerous accessory structures work as coordinated units in what is described as an integrated organ system, the integumentary system.

The Skin

164. Which structures are **not** regulated by autonomic neurons?

    A. Eccrine glands
    B. Arrector pili muscles
    C. Dermal blood vessels
    D. Touch receptors

165. Which skin components are **not** involved with maintaining body temperature?

    A. Eccrine glands
    B. Sebaceous glands
    C. Dermal blood vessels
    D. Hypodermis

166. Where would the most cells undergoing mitosis be found?

    A. Stratum corneum
    B. Stratum granulosum
    C. Stratum spinosum
    D. Stratum basale

167. Malignant melanoma, the most dangerous form of skin cancer, arises from melanocytes, which can metastasize (spread to other parts of the body) rapidly if the condition is not diagnosed and treated early. In which specific region would such cancerous cells originate?

    A. Stratum corneum
    B. Stratum granulosum
    C. Stratum basale
    D. Dermis

168. Which of the following would most likely be influenced by sex hormones?

    A. Sebaceous glands and apocrine glands
    B. Sebaceous glands and eccrine glands
    C. Apocrine glands and eccrine glands
    D. Sebaceous glands, apocrine glands, and eccrine glands

169. Which structures of the skin do not develop from ectoderm?

    A. Glands of the dermis
    B. Blood vessels of the dermis
    C. Receptors of the dermis
    D. All of the above

Passage V (Questions 170–175)

Archaebacteria are prokaryotic organisms that are as different from all other prokaryotes (eubacteria) as they are from eukaryotes. Archaebacteria differ from other organisms in such basic cellular and molecular characteristics, that a debate has arisen as to whether these organisms belong in their own kingdom, separate from other forms of life. Differences have been found in their ribosomes, plasma membranes, cell walls, and metabolic activities. Archaebacteria have been found in amazingly diverse habitats including: (1) anaerobic environments in sewage and swamps (methanogens), (2) hot and/or acidic environments such as deep-sea vents, volcanic regions and hot sulfur springs (thermoacidophiles), and (3) extreme salt environments (halobacteria).

170. If archaebacteria were placed in their own kingdom, how many kingdoms would there be?

    A. Three
    B. Four
    C. Five
    D. Six

171. Certain halobacteria are photosynthetic under anaerobic conditions. When their membrane-bound pigment absorbs light, protons are forced to the opposite side of the cell membrane. Then, as the protons return, ATP is made. To which process is this pattern of ion flow similar?

    A. Troponin-tropomyosin binding
    B. Glucose reabsorption
    C. Chemiosmosis
    D. Hormonal activation of target cells

172. The cell walls of archaebacteria are made of pure protein in some species, pure carbohydrate, or glycoproteins. However, they are never composed of the molecule found in eubacterial cell walls called:

    A. cellulose.
    B. chitin.
    C. peptidoglycan.
    D. phospholipid.

173. The characteristics of the genetic material in archaebacteria and eubacteria are very similar. Which of the following **would not** be found in these cells?

   A. Paired chromosomes
   B. DNA with histone proteins
   C. Mitochondrial DNA
   D. All of the above

174. Why is it that the same antibiotics often do not work on both eubacteria and archaebacteria?

   A. Differences in ribosomes
   B. Differences in plasma membranes
   C. Differences in cell walls
   D. All of the above

175. Which statement is **not true** about drug resistance in microbes?

   A. Microbes can become drug-resistant due to a mutation.
   B. Viruses are susceptible to most antibiotics because the antibiotics interfere with the host cell's normal functions.
   C. Drug-resistant microbes usually become the dominant species in environments that contain that anti-microbial agent.
   D. In humans, many adverse reactions to broad-spectrum drugs are due to the fact that the microbes normally living inside the body are killed by these drugs.

Passage VI (Questions 176–181)

The autonomic nervous system is responsible for regulating the body's involuntary effectors (smooth muscle cells, cardiac muscle cells, and a variety of gland cells). The two branches of the autonomic nervous system, the parasympathetic and sympathetic divisions, dominate in different situations. The parasympathetic is active under ordinary "everyday" conditions, while the sympathetic prepares the body for intense physical activity and energy expenditure, stress, emergencies, or, what is often summarized as "fight-or-flight" conditions. Visceral organs respond differently to parasympathetic and sympathetic stimulation, in part, because the two divisions release different neurotransmitters at their neuro-effector junctions. Acetylcholine is released at parasympathetic neuro-effector junctions (cholinergic transmission), while sympathetic neurons release norepinephrine onto effectors (adrenergic transmission). The figure below summarizes some of the differences between the two divisions of the autonomic nervous system.

Aspects of the Autonomic Nervous System

176. One major difference between the autonomic and somatic nervous systems involves the fact that:

   A. the number of motor neurons used to reach the effector is different.

   B. motor neurons directly leave the CNS in autonomic circuits only.

   C. neurotransmitters can be excitatory or inhibitory in the autonomic nervous system only.

   D. All of the above

177. Adrenergic receptor sites at autonomic synapses are classified as alpha and beta. This explains, in part, why:

   A. acetylcholine can have different effects at different synapses.

   B. norepinephrine can have different effects at different synapses.

   C. Both A and B

   D. Neither A nor B

178. When certain adrenergic receptors are stimulated, the enzyme adenylate cyclase is activated, leading to the formation of the "second messenger", cAMP. The cAMP then causes a change in response by the effector cell. This second messenger effect of cAMP can also be seen in:

   A. sensory neuron – interneuron interactions.

   B. hormone – target cell interactions.

   C. cell-to-cell recognition during embryological development.

   D. All of the above

179. One of the sympathetic post-ganglionic neurons in the figure is causing the release of norepinephrine and epinephrine directly into the bloodstream. In which specific visceral effector is this post-ganglionic neuron located?

   A. Hypothalamus

   B. SA node

   C. Smooth muscle of the small intestine

   D. Adrenal medulla

180. Parasympathetic neurons leave the CNS directly from the brain and from the sacral region of the spinal cord, while sympathetic neurons leave the CNS from the thoracic and lumbar regions of the spinal cord. In which of the following structures would most neurons be found that regulate our visceral effectors during normal "everyday" activities?

   A. Spinal nerve T – 1

   B. Spinal nerve L – 1

   C. Vagus nerve

   D. Spinal nerve S – 4

181. Which of the following statements is true about the autonomic nervous system?

   A. Sympathetic circuits have long pre-ganglionic neurons and ganglia near the effectors.

   B. Parasympathetic circuits have short pre-ganglionic neurons and ganglia near the effectors.

   C. Parasympathetic circuits have long pre-ganglionic neurons and ganglia near the spinal cord.

   D. Sympathetic circuits have short pre-ganglionic neurons and ganglia near the spinal cord.

Passage VII (Questions 182–187)

Successful human reproduction involves the flawless production of gametes in the male and female gonads, the fortuitous meeting of those gametes within the female tract to ensure fertilization, and a 40-week nurturing period during which time the developing offspring is supported and sustained within the female's body. The figure below depicts the secondary oocyte leaving the ovarian follicle during ovulation and some of the changes taking place as it makes its way into the fallopian tubes and uterus during the early stages of development.

Early Stages of Human Development

182. The ovulated secondary oocyte is surrounded by numerous follicular cells forming the corona radiata. Between the corona radiata and the oocyte is a region called the zona pellucida, which will be penetrated by a single sperm cell. The structure most responsible for helping the sperm break through the zona pellucida is the:

A. flagellum.
B. midpiece (neck).
C. acrosome.
D. nucleus.

183. If the sperm that successfully fertilizes the oocyte carries the sex-linked gene for color-blindness, and the mother has normal color vision, which of the following can be stated with certainty?

A. The child will be a color-blind boy.
B. The child will not be a color-blind girl.
C. The child will be a girl who is a carrier for color-blindness.
D. None of the above

184. What term is used to describe the developmental phenomenon taking place between the zygote and blastocyst stages?

A. Meiosis
B. Gestation
C. Cleavage
D. Differentiation

185. What is the source of hormones that maintain the preparedness of the uterine lining during the early stages leading up to the blastocyst?

A. Hypothalamus
B. Anterior pituitary gland
C. Corpus luteum
D. Morula

186. Where is the hormone produced that is responsible for the uterine contractions leading to parturition?

A. hypothalamus
B. anterior pituitary gland
C. posterior pituitary gland
D. ovary

187. If the developing embryo is Rh-positive and the mother is Rh-negative, what will occur when bloods from both come in contact during childbirth?

A. Anti-Rh antibodies will be produced by the mother's immune system, endangering the new-born child.
B. Anti-Rh antibodies will be produced by the mother's immune system for approximately one month, and then will no longer be produced.
C. The new-born will begin making anti-Rh antibodies.
D. None of the above

Passage VIII (Questions 188–192)

Haloalkenes are produced when hydrogen halides (HX) react with alkenes (I) or by the addition of a halide salt and a strong acid like phosphoric acid (II).

$$\text{I } CH_3CH=CH_2 \, HBr \longrightarrow \underset{\underset{Br}{|}}{CH_3CHCH_3}$$

$$\underset{HAc}{}$$

The mechanism for both I and II involves the protonation of the alkene to form a carbocation followed by the addition of the halide ion.

188. According to Markovnikov's Rule, the electrophilic addition of HBr to 1-butene would yield mostly:

A. 1-bromobutene.
B. 2-butene.
C. 2-bromobutane.
D. 1,2-dibromobutane.

189. Reactions that follow Markovnikov's Rule are said to proceed with Markovnikov orientation, while those that do not are said to proceed with anti-Markovnikov orientation. The addition of HBr to 3,3,3-trifluoropropene proceeds with anti-Markovnikov orientation. The most likely explanation is:

   A. A carbanion is formed in the rate-determining step.

   B. $H_2\overset{+}{C}\text{-}CH_2\text{-}CF_3$ is the more stable carbocation.

   C. A bromonium cation adds to the alkene.

   D. The reaction violates mechanistic principles.

190. Hydrogen chloride adds to 3,3-dimethyl-1-butene to give 2-chloro-2,3-dimethylbutane (44% yield) and 2-chloro-2,2-dimethylbutane (37% yield). The best explanation is:

   A. a rearrangement to form a more stable carbocation occurs.

   B. a methide shift occurs.

   C. both A and B are correct.

   D. a different mechanism applies.

191. The addition of hydrogen iodide to 2-butene yields:

   A. a racemic 2-iodobutane solution.

   B. only the R enantiomer.

   C. only the S enantiomer.

   D. 3-butene.

192. Which statement is true concerning the two carbocations formed by the protonation of 2-methylpropene?

   A. The activation energy associated with the primary carbocation intermediate is less than the activation energy associated with the tertiary carbocation.

   B. The rate constant for the formation of the tertiary carbocation is less than the rate constant for the formation of the primary carbocation.

   C. The activation energy and the rate constant associated with the formation of the primary carbocation is greater.

   D. The activation energy is greater for the formation of the primary carbocation but its rate constant is less.

Passage IX (Questions 193–198)

The functional derivatives of carboxylic acids are the acid chlorides, anhydrides, amides, and esters. These derivatives like carboxylic acids all contain the acyl group

$$\underset{(R\text{–}C\text{–}X)}{\overset{\overset{\textstyle O}{\|}}{}}$$

and typically undergo nucleophilic substitution in which –OH, –Cl, –OOCR, –NH$_2$, or –OR' is replaced by some other basic group.

193. Aldehydes and ketones also contain the acyl group but they typically undergo addition reactions. The explanation for this difference is:

   A. the carbon of the carbonyl group in aldehydes and ketones is more electronegative than in the derivatives of carboxylic acids.

   B. the carbonyl carbon of carboxylic acid groups is sterically hindered.

   C. the X groups of the carboxylic acid derivatives are weaker bases than the hydride ion ($: H^-$) or alkide ion ($: R^-$) and are thus better leaving groups.

   D. the carbonyl carbon of aldehydes and ketones is sp^3 hybridized while the carbonyl of carboxylic acid derivatives has sp^2 hybridization.

194. The first step in nucleophilic acyl substitution reactions involves the formation of a tetrahedral intermediate:

$$R\overset{\overset{\textstyle O}{\|}}{-}C\text{-}X + :Z \longrightarrow R\overset{\overset{\textstyle O^-}{\|}}{-}\underset{\underset{\textstyle X}{|}}{C}\text{-}Z$$

The rate of this reaction is increased by:

   A. electron-withdrawing groups that stabilize the negative charge.

   B. the presence of bulky groups.

   C. Both A and B

   D. a neutral solution.

195. Nucleophilic substitution occurs much more readily at an acyl carbon than at a saturated carbon because:

    A. nucleophilic attack on a tetrahedral alkyl carbon gives rise to a crowded transition state.

    B. a pentavalent carbon is unstable.

    C. attachment of a nucleophile to a carbonyl carbon involves the breaking of a weak π bond.

    D. All of the above

196. The alcoholysis (cleavage by an alcohol) of an ester is called:

    A. acid hydrolysis.

    B. transesterification.

    C. hydrogenolysis.

    D. basic hydrolysis.

197. Mineral acids speed up esterification as well as the hydrolysis of esters. The best explanation is:

    A. there is a tetrahedral intermediate.

    B. the carbonyl carbon is protonated so that it is more susceptible to attack by a nucleophile.

    C. it gives rise to a better leaving group.

    D. the proton causes cleavage to occur between the oxygen and the acyl group.

198. Isotopic exchange experiments indicate that the greatest fraction of the tetrahedral intermediate that goes on to form product in the hydrolysis of carboxylic acid derivatives follows the sequence

acid chloride > acid anhydride > ester > amide

Which of the following is probably the most important factor?

    A. The nature of the solvent

    B. The acidity of the solution

    C. The basicity of the leaving group

    D. The basicity of the solution

Passage X (Questions 199–204)

    Starch, cellulose, and glycogen are all made of (+)-glucose, making it the most abundant monosaccharide in nature. The first structure proposed for D-(+)- glucose, a pentahydroxy aldehyde was

199. Experimental data which were inconsistent with this structure include:

    A. D-(+)- Glucose does not form a bisulfite addition product.

    B. D-(+)-Glucose undergoes osazone formation.

    C. D-(+)- Glucose exists in two isomeric forms which undergo mutarotation.

    D. Both A and C

200. Aldehydes react with alcohols to form acetals according to

$$H-C=O \xrightarrow{CH_3OH/H+} H-C-OCH_3 \xrightarrow{CH_3OH/H+} H-C-OCH_3$$
$$\qquad\qquad\qquad\quad OH \qquad\qquad\qquad OCH_3$$

When D-(+)-glucose is treated with methanol and HCl, only one –CH$_3$ group is added although the product has the properties of a full acetal. The best explanation is that:

    A. glucose is not a pentahydroxy aldehyde.

    B. glucose is not optically active.

    C. glucose has a cyclic structure.

    D. glucose exists in two isomeric forms.

201. Which of the following most closely describes glucose in aqueous solution?

   A. A straight chain structure that is in equilibrium with a cyclic structure

   B. Two planar cyclic diastereomers differing in configuration about C-1

   C. A six membered, puckered, pyranose ring

   D. A six membered pyranose ring in a chair conformation

202. β-D-(+)-glucose is the most abundant isomer of naturally occurring glucose because:

   A. it is not stable.

   B. every bulky group occupies an equatorial position in the chair conformation.

   C. most of the bulky groups occupy equatorial positions in the chair conformation.

   D. Both A and B

203. Both cellulose and starch are made up of chains of D-glucose units joined by:

   A. double bonds.

   B. an ether linkage.

   C. C-1.

   D. glycosidic linkage.

204. D-glucose and D-mannose are examples of:

   A. stereoisomers.

   B. epimers.

   C. ketohexoses.

   D. fats.

Questions 205–216 are independent of any passage and of each other.

205. How many nucleotides are present in the mRNA molecule that codes for a protein containing fifty amino acids immediately after translation is completed?

   A. 50

   B. 53

   C. 150

   D. 153

206. After drinking sea-water, in which direction will water tend to flow between a person's tissues and her blood?

   A. Water will move from tissues to blood.

   B. Water will move from blood to tissues.

   C. There will be an equal flow of water in both directions.

   D. No flow of water will occur in either direction.

207. Osteoclasts are cells in the inner lining of long bones with functions that include the breakdown of bone tissue in order to raise blood calcium levels. Which hormone is most likely to speed up the activation of these cells?

   A. Growth hormone

   B. Calcitonin

   C. Parathyroid hormone

   D. Progesterone.

208. When the lower arm is flexed to lift a piece of chalk, less work is done by the biceps brachii muscle than when the lower arm is flexed to lift a heavy weight. This is due to:

   A. differences in the strength of each muscle cell's contraction.

   B. differences in the number of muscle cells contracting.

   C. Both A and B

   D. Neither A nor B

209. Which of the following would not involve an autonomic nervous system circuit?

   A. Motor signals to speed up muscle contractions in the stomach during a meal.
   B. Motor signals to speed up contractions in leg muscles during exercise.
   C. Motor signals to the heart to speed up contractions during exercise.
   D. Motor signals to sweat glands to increase their activity during exercise.

210. Ataxia is a disturbance in balance and motor control, in which patients can exhibit unsteady and irregular patterns of movement when trying to sit, stand, walk or reach for objects. This condition most likely is due to malfunction in the:

   A. cerebrum.
   B. medulla oblongata.
   C. diencephalon.
   D. cerebellum.

211. Vibrations from sound waves appear to be stronger when they reach the oval window compared to when they leave the tympanum. What is the best explanation for this phenomenon?

   A. Vibrations from sound waves increase in amplitude as the distance they travel increases.
   B. Vibrations from sound waves are amplified by bones in the middle ear.
   C. Vibrations from sound waves are amplified after they have stimulated receptor cells in the cochlea.
   D. All of the above

212. Specific immune responses begin when specialized cells arrive at the site of infection, partially engulf the invading organism, and then "present" or "display" the foreign antigen of the invader for appropriate B-cells and T-cells to recognize. Which cells are most likely to "present" these foreign antigens?

   A. Neutrophils and lymphocytes
   B. Macrophages and lymphocytes
   C. Neutrophils and macrophages
   D. Neutrophils, lymphocytes and macrophages

213. Albinism is an autosomal recessive trait. What is the probability of parents who are both carriers having two children in a row with albinism?

   A. 1/2
   B. 1/4
   C. 1/8
   D. 1/16

214. The "hardening" and "whitening" of the albumin in egg-whites during cooking can serve as indirect evidence for which of the following:

   A. Transamination of non-essential amino acids.
   B. Substrate-level phosphorylation.
   C. Enzyme specificity.
   D. Radial cleavage in telolecithal eggs.

215. Renin and aldosterone control of sodium concentration involves which of the following?

   A. The macula densa
   B. The adrenal cortex
   C. Angiotensin
   D. All of the above

216. Given the structural formula for a compound we can determine:

   I. the absolute configuration of its stereoisomers.
   II. the direction of optical activity for each stereoisomer.
   III. if it has a meso form.
   A. I and II only
   B. All of the above.
   C. I and III only
   D. II only

217. In keto-enol tautomerism:

   A. the enol form is usually more stable.
   B. phenol is an exception.
   C. the keto form is usually more stable.
   D. B and C are both true.

218. Which of the following is correct?

    A. All amines react with acid chlorides to form amides.

    B. All peptides have amide linkages.

    C. Alkylation of a tertiary amine produces an amide.

    D. The alkylation of amines by alkyl halides is an electrophilic substitution reaction.

219. Phosphoglycerides differ from fats because:

    A. phosphoglycerides have only two acyl groups while fats have three.

    B. fats are esters while phosphoglycerides are acid anhydrides.

    C. fats can be hydrolyzed while phospholipids cannot.

    D. phosphoglycerides have R groups while fats do not.

PRACTICE EXAM IV ANSWER KEY

VERBAL REASONING		PHYSICAL SCIENCES		BIOLOGICAL SCIENCES	
1. D	45. B	66. B	110. D	143. C	187. D
2. B	46. D	67. C	111. A	144. D	188. C
3. C	47. D	68. B	112. C	145. B	189. B
4. D	48. A	69. B	113. B	146. C	190. C
5. C	49. C	70. A	114. A	147. C	191. A
6. A	50. A	71. A	115. C	148. B	192. D
7. B	51. A	72. D	116. B	149. A	193. C
8. D	52. D	73. B	117. C	150. C	194. A
9. A	53. B	74. D	118. C	151. A	195. D
10. D	54. C	75. B	119. B	152. A	196. B
11. D	55. B	76. C	120. B	153. D	197. B
12. D	56. D	77. C	121. D	154. B	198. C
13. C	57. B	78. D	122. C	155. C	199. D
14. B	58. B	79. A	123. A	156. A	200. C
15. C	59. D	80. A	124. B	157. C	201. D
16. D	60. C	81. B	125. C	158. D	202. B
17. A	61. A	82. B	126. D	159. D	203. D
18. D	62. D	83. A	127. B	160. B	204. B
19. C	63. A	84. A	128. A	161. A	205. D
20. B	64. D	85. C	129. B	162. C	206. A
21. D	65. C	86. D	130. C	163. B	207. C
22. C		87. D	131. C	164. D	208. B
23. D		88. A	132. B	165. B	209. B
24. C		89. A	133. A	166. D	210. D
25. D		90. D	134. C	167. C	211. B
26. C		91. A	135. C	168. A	212. C
27. C		92. A	136. D	169. B	213. D
28. D		93. B	137. B	170. D	214. C
29. C		94. D	138. C	171. C	215. D
30. D		95. B	139. D	172. C	216. C
31. D		96. D	140. C	173. D	217. B
32. B		97. D	141. D	174. D	218. B
33. A		98. B	142. C	175. B	219. A
34. C		99. B		176. A	
35. B		100. A		177. B	
36. D		101. C		178. B	
37. B		102. B		179. D	
38. D		103. A		180. C	
39. B		104. D		181. D	
40. C		105. B		182. C	
41. D		106. C		183. D	
42. B		107. B		184. C	
43. A		108. C		185. C	
44. D		109. B		186. A	

PRACTICE EXAM IV EXPLANATORY ANSWERS

Verbal Reasoning

1. **D** This is the best answer to the question, as the remaining answers do not respond to the point of Grant's "mystery" as a person. The answer is based on several statements: The last statement in paragraph 1 says "Yet despite such fame, his personality remains a riddle"; the first statement in paragraph 2 actually states "There's always been a mystery about Grant" and the last two statements in paragraph 5 say, "A failed bid for a third term, a plunge into financial ruin that left him penniless, the onset of the throat cancer that slowly and painfully killed him—all the outward facts of Grant's life are well documented. Yet Grant's personality remains intriguing."

2. **B** The answer is based on the inferences in the following statements in paragraph 2: "In battle, he's been called a butcher, a man of great luck, someone who really didn't win the Civil War but was simply on the scene when the Confederates finally were forced to abandon it. In terms of the presidency, he's been looked upon as a man who did too much and a man who did too little. On Reconstruction, for example, he was viewed as a man who pushed too hard for black civil rights and when he should have known better, and as a man who didn't do nearly enough."

3. **C** The answer is based on the following statement in paragraph 4: "One of the pleasures for Simon [the scholar] in his work with the Grant papers is the precision and grace of Grant's prose. Simon observes a direct correlation between Grant's literary ability and his capacity for leadership... 'The letter expressed exactly what Grant wanted with the greatest economy,' says Simon. 'It shows a man who is direct, clear-headed, and perhaps there's a glint of genius in his expressing things that others didn't see.'"

4. **D** The answer is based on paragraph 5 where choices A to C are actual events referred to during Grant's presidency while choice D is not an event included.

5. **C** The answer is given in the following statement in paragraph 5: "As both soldier and president, Grant helped shape the United States as a modern nation."

6. **A** The answer is based on understanding that one definition of the word "vertiginous" means rapid change, unstable, and inconstant, which is stated in the sentence.

7. **B** The answer is based on paragraph 3 and the following statement: "The volumes of the Grant papers have become the essential resource in modern studies of Grant."

8. **D** This is a reasonable assumption based on the first paragraph where the author describes Neanderthals as thoughtful with brains larger than modern humans. He also says in the same paragraph that their brains are no less impressive the those of the Cro-Magnon.

9. **A** The answer is based on the following statements in paragraph 2: "Molecular evidence indicates that they may have appeared a good deal earlier, as descendants of a prehistoric Eve who may have lived 250,000 years ago. That suggestion rests on analyses of samples of maternally inherited DNA from more than 2,000 individuals from all continents. The greatest DNA diversity, an index of more remote origins, occurs among the Africans, a conclusion supported by other genetic studies."

10. **D** The answer is based on the following statements in paragraph 3: "Even though they were strong, and intelligent, and knew their land intimately, the Neanderthals ultimately could not compete with the newcomers though for many thousands of years they did coexist. It is possible that an inability to adapt led to the ultimate extinction of the Neanderthals. Set in their ways, they may have continued to live as they had always done making the same tools century after century, hunting with the same jabbing weapons in close encounters with big game even after the newcomers had developed weapons that could be used from greater distances."

11. **D** Choices A, B, and C are presented as explanations while choice D is not a stated reason.

12. **D** Choices A, B, and C are all possible scientific theories, but there is no explanation for the extinction of the Neanderthals, and the author asserts in paragraph 4 the following statement: "All parties (scientists) agree a hundred percent on one thing, however—the need for further research is always a wise position for scientists to take."

13. **C** This answer is the best possible answer as the Neanderthals were unable to adapt as seen in the following statement in paragraph 3: "In a sense they may been too well adapted, inflexible and committed to traditional living patterns," suggesting that Cro-Magnon were prone to adaptability.

14. **B** The answer is based on the several scientific theories proposed by specialists in paragraph 4 as to the disappearance of the Neanderthals. There is no one accepted theory.

15. **C** The answer is based on the following statement in paragraph 1: "Islamic scholars have long had access to the *Encyclopedia of Islam*, which is widely recognized as the major research tool for the field with articles on topics related to history, geography, aspects of public and private life, people, dynasties and sects, art, archaeology, music, folklore, theology, philosophy, ethics, law, history of science, literature, and languages of all countries in which Islam is or has been present either as a major or an important way of life" and on the following statement in paragraph 2: "The first edition was begun in 1908 and completed in 1938."

16. **D** The answer is based on the following statement in paragraph 7: "Many new articles in the new edition are, in themselves, major works of scholarship covering such topics as irrigation, agriculture, warfare, art, languages and literature, taxation, Islamic law, and marriage and divorce."

17. **A** The answer is based on the following statement in paragraph 3: "Wolfhart Herinrichs, professor of Arabic in the Department of Near Eastern Languages and Civilization at Harvard University and current project director for the encyclopedia, notes that the revised edition will also include numerous articles written by scholars from the Middle East and India."

18. **D** The answer is based on the following statements in paragraph 5: "Although in the Western world, *Christianity* is the name of a religion and *Christendom* is the name of the civilization that arose under the aegis of that religion, there is no such differentiation in the Islamic world. "Unfortunately," he (Bernard Lewis) says, "we use the world *Islam*—and so do the Muslims—to mean these two different things. If, for example you say Christian art, it will be assumed that you mean religious art," he explains. "You wouldn't call a Rembrandt or a Picasso Christian art, even though the artists were Christians. On the other hand, if you say Islamic art, you are understood to mean any kind of art that was produced in the Islamic civilization even if it is in no sense religious.'"

19. **C** The answer is based on the following statement in paragraph 6: "that is not the case in most fields of Islamic studies. These are young disciplines, relatively underdeveloped."

20. **B** The answer is based on the following statements in paragraph 7: "Where a subject is important and either very little or no work has been done before, the encyclopedia article can itself become a piece of original research...The entry for *kissa*—in modern Arabic, used to designate the novel—for example, provides a 22-page exploration of the genre that begins with a discussion of modern Arabic literature and includes information about...forms of the short story and novel. Pointing out the European origins of the novel is Arabic and that, indeed the first one was written in Paris by an Egyptian in 1914—*Zaynab*, by Haykal...'"

21. **D** The answer is based on the following statements in paragraphs 8 and 9 respectively: 'The first edition of the encyclopedia was much more literary, philosophical, and religious in its scope,' says Lewis, 'and although the editorial committee has not abandoned any of these subjects, many others have been added' (paragraph 8). "...We're producing a work of reference that we hope will stay on the shelf in the reference room for at least a half century and perhaps longer" (paragraph 9).

22. **C** The answer is based on the following statements in paragraph 5: "During his lifetime,

Peirce never developed a large readership. He wasn't a popular writer like William James, who always wrote in a beautiful, pleasing style, which may help explain why James, and not Peirce, is more commonly associated with pragmatism. Peirce's personality may have also helped seal his fate. Although he enjoyed the patronage of some of America's most influential men of science, he had a careless regard for manners that made him something of an *enfant terrible* in the halls of academia."

23. **D** The answer is based on the following statements in paragraph 4: "Peirce originated pragmatism as a method for determining the meaning of ideas or intellectual conceptions, and he insisted that this meaning resides in its conceivable effects. To conceive of what a thing is, then, is to conceive of what effects it could have."

24. **C** The answer is based on understanding the definition of an *enfant terrible*, which is a person who causes trouble by making frank, bold remarks at the wrong times. In the following statement in paragraph 5: "Although he (Peirce) enjoyed the patronage of some of America's most influential men of science, he had a careless regard for manners that made him something of an *enfant terrible* in the halls of academia."

25. **D** The answer is based on this statement being the only false statement among the given statements and that it is challenged by the following statements in paragraph 2: "Although Peirce's published writings total more than 10,000 pages, and several collections have appeared since his death, the bulk of his work remains unpublished. So far, researchers have tracked down more than 90,000 unpublished manuscript pages on file at Harvard and other repositories."

26. **C** The answer is based on the following statements in paragraph 1: "By the end of his life, however, Peirce already suffered the obscurity that would shadow his intellectual legacy for decades. At his death, in Milford, Pennsylvania, he was isolated, forgotten by his contemporaries and dependent on the generous support of his loyal friend William James."

27. **C** The answer is based on the following statements in paragraph 2: "The surge of interest in Peirce is fueled in part by the growing popularity of semiotics—analyzing the nature of signs

and symbols in everyday language to "decode" culture and its communications. Researchers in fields as diverse as law, art, political science, drama, marketing, and animal communication have made semiotics a hotbed of academic interest."

28. **D** The answer is based on the overall tone of the article, which acknowledges Peirce's accomplishments as a logician and his development of American pragmatism.

29. **C** The answer is based on the following statements in paragraph 2: "Today, a growing number of scholars regard Peirce as America's most original and versatile thinker. The surge of interest in Peirce is fueled in part by the growing popularity of semiotics—analyzing the nature of signs and symbols in everyday language to "decode" culture and its communications."

30. **D** Choices A, B, and C are issues in quantum field theory of gravity according to the passage. Choice D is not an issue.

31. **D** The answer is based on the following statement in paragraph 4: "String theories not only incorporate gravity; they predict the existence of gravity."

32. **B** The answer is based on the following statements in paragraph 5: "The problem is that string theories have not yet led to concepts of physics that match observation. 'Nobody knows how to solve these theories to get quantitative predictions,' Weinberg adds. 'The forces in these theories are so strong as to invalidate 'our favorite computational tools.'"

33. **A** The answer is based on the following statements in paragraph 2: "The mass of the electron...was calculated as having an infinite value. The resolution took form in the realization that the electron mass actually had two components, one of which would be complete arbitrary; nothing whatever could be said concerning its value. Physicists thus were free to assign it the value of negative infinity. When added to the positive infinity of the other component, the result could be set equal to the observed total."

34. **C** The answer is based on the following statement in paragraph 5: "Quantum field theory remains bedeviled by the problem of infinities. String theory avoids the infinities, but also

avoids contact with the world of observations and of calculable results."

35. **B** The answer is based on the following statements in paragraph 3: "Lacking a suitable quantum theory, physicists have nevertheless tried to nibble around the edges of the problem. The most widely studied approach has been the string theory, which holds that the fundamental entities of physics are strings—short lengths or loops."

36. **D** The answer is based on the following statements in paragraph 5: "The problem is that string theories have not yet led to concepts of physics that match observations...String theory avoids the infinities, but also avoids contact with the world of observations and of calculable results."

37. **B** The answer is based on the following statement in paragraph 2: "The resources of the archives, however, are much broader than any list of its most famous manuscripts can suggest. The Vatican has been no mere repository of important papers, but an active shaper of social, intellectual, and political history on an ecumenical scale. The archival record of its involvement in spiritual and mundane affairs reaches beyond the institutional history of the church into every domain of human activity."

38. **D** The answer is based on the following statements in paragraph 3: "Among the most Impressive documents from the Age of Discovery is Pope Alexander VI's bull *Inter Cetera of 1493*, which arbitrates between Spanish and Portuguese claims to the lands just visited by Columbus. Less celebrated, but perhaps more useful for current research, is the correspondence of the *Propaganda Fide*, which forms a continuous account of Catholic evangelism worldwide from 1470 to the present."

39. **B** Choices A, C, and D are factual statements presented in the article, while choice B is not stated.

40. **C** The answer is based on the following statements in paragraph 7: "The University of Michigan's data base will remedy this situation by providing an automated overview of the complete archives. Each series of related documents

will have its own bibliographic record in the data base, which will contain more than 2,500 entries."

41. **D** The answer is based on the following statements in paragraph 6: "A real hindrance researchers confront is the 1,300 indexes. Some are first-rate works of archival scholarship, many are outdated and incomplete. Aside from tracing the footnotes of others and using specialized subject guides, these indexes serve as the only points of entry in the archives' vast holdings. The indexes, essentially lists of the contents of record series, are currently not organized into any readily apparent system."

42. **B** The answer is based on the inference of the third statement in paragraph 1: "Visitors to the Vatican are awed by the beauty of the glorious paintings and its magnificent architecture. For many scholars, however, the Vatican's previous treasure include not only its works of art but also the rare documents housed in its archives. *The nearly five miles of correspondence and registers that fill the shelves of the Vatican archives record both the signal events that seem to define European civilization and the background against which they stand out.*"

43. **A** Choices B, C, and D are stated in the article, while choice A is not presented.

44. **D** The answer is based on the following statements in paragraph 2 and 7: "Its design fills a void in scholars' understanding of the transition from ancient to modern forms of ship construction" in paragraph 2, and "Ship specialists conclude that skeletal, or frame-first, building evolved in the Mediterranean area out of the earlier Graeco-Roman shell construction method" in paragraph 7.

45. **B** The answer is based on the following statements in paragraphs 2 and 3: "Ancient ships were essentially built as planking shells with the planking determining the shape of the hull..." in paragraph 2, and "The Serce Limani ship is the earliest example found of this "frame first" construction" in paragraph 3.

46. **D** Choices A, B, C are presented in paragraph 4, while answer D is not stated.

47. **D** The answer is based on the following statements in paragraph 6: "Originally, some scholars even denied that the Y-shaped objects were anchors. After careful examination, we have come to the conclusion that they are, in fact, very good anchors, obviously the product of much practical experience."

48. **A** The answer is based on the following statements in paragraph 4: " 'The conservation and reconstruction offer scholars valuable new insights into eleventh-century Mediterranean watercraft. The Serce Limani wreck represents an undocumented ship-type from a period and area in which comparatively little is known about maritime matters,' says Steffy."

49. **C** The answer is based on the following statements in paragraph 5 that imply commercial ships were subject to possible attacks: "The ship was also well supplied with defensive weapons. A dozen swords, one with an elaborately decorated bronze hilt, and lances and some sixty javelins were recovered."

50. **A** This answer is the best possible answer based on the article's emphasis of the eleventh-century ship's physical construction.

51. **A** The answer is based on the following statements in paragraph 6: "Nonetheless, the project was a success on two counts...The survey established a model for global scientific collaboration and coordination that has been followed with much success ever since."

52. **D** The answer is based on the following statements in paragraph 3: "Such an undertaking exceeded the technical and fiscal capacities of any pair of observatories of the period. Mouchez conceived an audacious plan. Major observatories all over the world would be asked to participate, each assigned a unique zone of declination—the celestial equivalent of terrestrial latitude—and each to bear its share of the cost."

53. **B** The answer is based on the following statement in paragraph 3: "Major observatories all over the world would be asked to participate, each to be assigned a unique share of declination—the celestial equivalent of terrestrial latitude..."

54. **C** The answer is based on the following

statement in paragraph 4: "Holographic uniformity was achieved by equipping all participating observatories with identical telescopes and imposing identical procedures."

55. **B** Choices A, C, and D are stated as specific reasons, while choice B is not a stated reason.

56. **D** The answer is based on the following statements in paragraph 3: "The Americans would not participate directly in the *Carte du Ciel*, because Pickering intended to organize a purely Made-in-U.S.A. version, using the Harvard substation at Arequipa, Peru. The wisdom of Mouchez's approach was vividly underscored by Pickering's failure, apparently caused by funding problems."

57. **B** The answer is based on the following statements in paragraph 6: "Nonetheless, the project was a success on two counts. Even with their flaws, the maps and catalogues represent a major astronomical resource that is still important. Perhaps even more important than the scientific merit of Admiral Mouchez's *chef d'oeurve*, however, is that the survey established a model for global scientific collaboration and coordination that has been followed with much success ever since."

58. **B** The answer is based on the following statements in paragraphs 2 and 5: "Sometimes the builders selected cobblestones of all one color; other times, the stones were set in herringbone patterns or just in straight courses. These houses, made of local materials by local people, eloquently evoke the histories of their builders and their occupants" in paragraph 2, and 'Michiganians love wood,' Eckert says. We have wood houses of all kinds, from elaborate Queen Anne mansions of the lumber barons to the simple log houses of the trappers and traders" in paragraph 5.

59. **D** The answer is based on the following statements in paragraphs 3 and 5: "...but the imaginative use of wood in the Hannah house unmistakably connects to the Michigan lumber industry. The house is ornamented with intricately carved and decorated wood inside and out; every room is paneled in a different hardwood" in paragraph 3, and "The William W. Maier house is the ultimate expression of Michiganians' fascination with wood: Maier developed a technique for siding the exterior

walls of buildings with concrete shaped in the form of logs" in paragraph 5.

60. **C** Choices A, B, and D are accurate statements presented in the article, while choice C includes marble, which is not in the following statement in paragraph 7: "The mining industry—copper and iron—that dominated the Upper Peninsula created specialized building types."

61. **A** The answer is based on the following statements in paragraph 5: "Besides the rich soil in the southern part of the state, there were lakes large and small, rivers, minerals, and countless acres of pine and hardwood forests. From around 1830 to 1910, logging was a principal Michigan industry. 'Michiganians love wood,' Eckert says. We have wood houses of all kinds..."

62. **D** Chioces A, B, and C are stated in the article, while choice D is not stated at all as a reason.

63. **A** The answer is based on the following statement in paragraph 8: "Mackinac Island, for instance, has splendid "cottages" built by the affluent, while simple cabins for working-class vacationers can be found on the state's shoreline, rivers, and lakes."

64. **D** This answer is the best possible answer since the article emphasized how Michigan's use of its natural resources created the architectural styles of many buildings.

65. **C** The answer is based on the following statements in paragraph 10: "The Buildings of the United States Series, which includes Michigan, will represent each state by a single volume. Introductory material in each volume will discuss the development of the state and its architectural history, lacking it in a national and international context."

Physical Sciences

66. **B** The original mass of $CaCaO_3$ is 10.0 g, or 0.100 mole; the balanced equation implies that this will react to form 0.10 mole of CaO, or 5.6 g.

67. **C** The gas in the cylinder is a mixture of the 0.100 mol of $CO_2(g)$ formed in the reaction, together with the moles of nitrogen, which equals, at the STP conditions at the start of the problem,

$$224\text{mL N}_2 \times \frac{1\text{L}}{10^3\text{mL}} \times \frac{1\text{ mol}}{22.4\text{ L}} = 0.0100\text{ mol N}_2$$

When heated to 500 K, the gas mixture expands until the internal pressure equals the external pressure of 1.00 atm:

$$V = \frac{nRT}{P} = \frac{(0.110\text{ mol})(0.08206\text{ L atm/K mol})(500\text{ K})}{(1.00\text{ atm})} = 4.51\text{ L}$$

68. **B** For work, we use

$w = -P_{ext}\ \Delta V$

where $P_{ext} = 1.00$ atm and $\Delta V = V_{final} - V_{initial}$

   $= 4.51\text{ L} - 0.22\text{ L}$

   $= 4.29\text{ L}$

   $w = -P_{ext}\ \Delta V = -4.29\text{ Latm}$

(Had we been asked to calculate an answer in J, we would have used the conversion 1 L atm = 101.3 J/L atm. You can memorize this conversion factor, or derive it from the ratio of the gas constant R in the two common units.)

69. **B** The partial pressure of $CO_2(g)$ in the mixture is given by

$$P_{CO2} = X_{CO2}P_{tot}$$

$$= [(\text{moles } CO_2)/(\text{moles } CO_2 + \text{moles } N_2)](1 \text{ atm})$$

$$= [(0.100)/(1.10 \text{ mol})](1 \text{ atm})$$

$$= 0.91 \text{ atm}$$

70. **A** For a strong acid, $C_a = [H^+]$, and

$$[H^+] = 10^{-pH}$$

$$= 10^{-4.73}$$

$$= 1.9 \times 10^{-5} M$$

71. **A** This solution is a buffer, since it is a mixture of a strong acid and its conjugate base.

$$[H^+] = K_a \frac{[HFor]}{[For^-]}$$

$$= (1.8 \times 10^{-4}) \frac{(0.10M)}{(0.30M)}$$

$$= 6.0 \times 10^{-5} M$$

72. **D** A flame test is an elemental analysis test; here, the yellow color may indicate that sodium is present.

73. **B** Although the molarities are the same, the sodium nitrate dissociates completely, so it has twice the number of particles, hence twice the osmotic pressure.

74. **D** Ammonia, which is a weak base, would react with strong acid. Ammonium nitrate would dissociate completely to produce NH_4^+, the conjugate acid of ammonia; this acid would react with strong base.

In addition, a substance such as $NaHC_2O_4$, which dissociates to form $HC_2O_4^-(aq)$, reacts either with strong acid to form $H_2C_2O_4(aq)$, or with strong base to form $C_2O_4^{2-}(aq)$.

Choice I is not acceptable, since the product of excess HCl reacting with NH_3 would be NH_4^+ (a weak acid) and the remaining strong acid. This mixture would show an endpoint when strong base was added, but not strong acid.

75. **B** A 10.0-mL sample of this solution would contain 0.0040 mol (4.00 mmol) of acetic acid, which would react with 40.0 mL of 0.100 M NaOH. The sample would also contain 0.0060 mol (6.00 mmol) of acetate ion from sodium acetate, which would react with 60.0 mL of 0.100 M HNO_3.

76. **C** Since liquid water is denser than ice (an unusual property), the ice will occupy a larger volume than the original liquid. If the bottle is sealed, then the expansion will crack the glass.

77. **C** Use the specific heat of liquid water:

heat = $(100 \text{ g})(4.18 \text{ J/g }^\circ C)(-6.0 ^\circ C)$

= -2.5 kJ, or "2.5 J lost" to the surroundings

78. **D** Hydrogen bonds are the chief intermolecular force in liquid water; these must be overcome as the liquid vaporizes. The enthalpy of vaporization is a measure of the combined strength of the hydrogen bonds in one mole of water.

79. **A** Values of T and P that correspond to freezing must lie on the liquid-solid boundary of the phase diagram for water. Because of the negative slope of this boundary, an increase in pressure leads to a lower temperature.

80. **A** This problem in vapor-pressure lowering due to a nonvolatile solute calls for Raoult's Law:

$$P_{solution} = X_{solvent}P^\circ,$$

where $X_{solvent}$ is the mole fraction of solvent *particles*, and P° is the vapor pressure of pure solvent at the temperature specified (found from the vapor pressure chart at the start of the passage).

$$X_{solvent} = P_{solution}/P^\circ$$

$$= 31.2 \text{ torr}/31.8 \text{ torr}$$

$$= 0.981$$

But, $X_{solvent} = n_{solvent}/(n_{solvent} + 2n_{solute})$

where $n_{solvent} = 180 \text{ g } H_2O /(18.0 \text{ g/mol}) = 10.0 \text{ mol}$

and we have inserted the factor of "2" to indicate that each mole of LiCl produces 2 ions.

$0.981 = 10.0$ mol $/ (10.0$ mol $+ 2n_{solute})$

$n_{solute} = 0.097$ mole

mass of solute $= (0.097$ mole$)(42.39$ g/mol $)$

$= 4.1$ g

81. **B** Since the vapor pressure of water drops dramatically as the temperature is lowered below $100°C$ (see table), this solution is the most reasonable. Choice A, which relies on Charles' Law, would not produce as large an effect.

82. **B** Refer to the equations at the start of the passage for enthalpy of ionization.

$\Delta H = (0.25$ mol$)(520$ kJ/mol$)$

$= 130$ kJ

83. **A** While sublimation of the metal requires heat, the formation of $Cl^-(g)$ from neutral $Cl(g)$ is exothermic, as is the formation of $LiCl(s)$ from $Li^+(g)$ and $Cl^-(g)$.

84. **A** When we go up on the diagram from the level at 161 kJ to that at [2], the only change is the dissociation of 1/2 mole of $Cl_2(g)$. From Eq. 4, the enthalpy change for this process equals $1/2(240$ kJ$) = 120$ kJ.

85. **C** On the chart, this reaction corresponds to the difference between the level at 801 kJ and that at 161 kJ, which is 640 kJ. We can also use Hess's law with reactions 2, 3, and 4; in fact, the diagram is a summary of the results of Hess's law calculations.

86. **D** The crystal lattice energy is the largest exothermic term in the cycle, greater than the heat of formation, choice A, or the electron affinity, choice C. Choice B, the dissociation energy, is endothermic, so it detracts from the overall stability.

87. **D** $\nu = c/\lambda$

$= (3.00 \times 10^8 \text{ m/s}^2) / (589 \times 10^{-9} \text{ m})$

$= 5.09 \times 10^{14} \text{ s}^{-1}$

88. **A** $E = \dfrac{hc}{\lambda}$

$\lambda = \dfrac{hc}{E}$

$= \dfrac{(6.63 \times 10^{-34} \text{ J s})(3.00 \times 10^8 \text{ m/s})}{7.10 \times 10^{-19} \text{ J}}$

$= 280$ nm

89. **A** Since the ground state has electrons in the 3s level but not the 3p or above, the lowest-energy transition from the ground state must originate in the 3s level.

90. **D** I is not allowed, since l doesn't change. Note that there is no restriction on n; therefore, III is allowed, since although n increases by 2, l only increases by 1.

91. **A** First determine 3.37×10^{-19} J /atom for the 3s→3p transition:

$\Delta E = hc/ \lambda = (6.63 \times 10^{-34}$ J s$)(3.00 \times 108$ m/s$)/ (590$ nm $\times 1$ nm$/10^{-9}$ m$)$

$= 3.37 \times 10^{-19}$ J /atom

$(3.37 \times 10^{-19}$ J/atom$)(1$ kJ$/10^3$ J$)$
$(6.02 \times 10^{23}$ atoms/mol$)$

$= 203$ kJ/mol

Now we use the fact that the first IE (496 kJ/mol) is from the 3s orbital to the "zero" of energy, while the IE requested (a smaller number) is from the 3p orbital to the zero of energy. Thus

IE (from 3p) = IE (from 3s) $- \Delta E$ (3s $\rightarrow$ 3p)

$= 496$ kJ/mol $- 203$ kJ/mol

$= 293$ kJ/mol

92. **A** Locate 0.510 on the *y*-axis, follow over to the calibration curve, then look down to find concentration on the *x*-axis.

93. **B** The ammonium ion requires 4 equivalent bonds, which it can form by using its 2s orbital and all three of its 2p orbitals. (Choice C is impossible, since there are not four 2p orbitals available.)

94. **D** $NH_3(aq)$ is a weak base, so its principal reaction in solution is hydrolysis:

$$NH_3(aq) + H2O \Leftrightarrow NH_4^+(aq) + OH^-(aq)$$

95. **B** At the equivalence point, the solution will be $NH_4^+(aq)$ of approximately 0.05 M, since approximately equal volume of reacting solutions will be needed, and each was about 0.1 M. We use an approximate result for weak acids:

$$[H^+(aq)] = (C_a K_a)^{1/2}$$

To calculate K_a, we use

$$K_a = (1.00 \times 10^{-14})/(1.8 \times 10^{-5})$$

$$= 5.6 \times 10^{-10} M$$

$$[H^+(aq)] = [(0.050)(5.6 \times 10^{-10})]^{1/2}$$

$$= 5.2 \times 10^{-10} M$$

$$pH = 5.3$$

96. **D** mmol NaOH used in final titration = (25.2 mL)(0.250 M) = 6.30 mmol

Therefore the amount of HCl used up

= (40.0 mL)(0.500 M) – 6.30 mmol

= 13.7 mmol

= mmol of NH_3 in sample = mmol N in sample

mass of N = (0.0137 mol)(14.0 g/mol)

$$= 0.192 \text{ g}$$

$$\%N = \frac{0.192 \text{ g}}{1.20 \text{ g}} \times 100\% = 16.0\%$$

97. **D** At the threshold frequency the kinetic energy of the photoelectron is approximately zero.

$$E_K = 0 = h\nu_o - \Phi \text{ and } h\nu_o = \Phi/h =$$

$$2.5 \text{ eV}/4.2 \times 10^{-15} \text{ eV s}$$

This can be estimated as $\sim 2./4 \times 10^{-15} \sim 0.5 \times 10^{15} \text{ s}^{-1}$. Since the numerator was rounded down more than the denominator the estimate is a lower bound and we expect the actual value to be higher. Choice D is the best fit to this estimate.

98. **B** Intensity decreases as the number of photons emitted per unit time decreases. Since each photon is responsible for ejected one electron, the number of ejected photoelectrons must also decrease. The energy of the photon depends only on its frequency (or wavelength). Since this doesn't change the kinetic energy imparted to each photoelectron is the same since all monochromatic photons have the same frequency.

99. **B** From the graph, you can see the threshold frequency. Since the kinetic energy of the photoelectron is approximately zero at this value the work function can be found from the threshold frequency:

$$E_K = 0 = h\nu_0 - \Phi \text{ and } \Phi = h\nu_0 = \_ =$$

$$(4.2 \times 10^{-15} \text{ eV s})(3.0 \times 10^{14} \text{ s}^{-1}) = 1.26 \text{ eV}$$

100. **A** The kinetic energy acquired by the ejected electron equals the difference between the amount of energy provided by the photon and the amount of energy needed to overcome the work function. The difference in frequency:

$$1.8 \times 10^{15} \text{ Hz} - 1.4 \times 10^{15} \text{ Hz} = 0.4 \times 10^{15} \text{ Hz}.$$

The corresponding energy in E = hν =

$$(4.2 \times 10^{-15} \text{ eV s})(0.4 \times 10^{15} \text{ s}^{-1}) = 2.1 \text{ eV}$$

101. **C** You need to remember the relationship between frequency, wavelength, and energy of light:

$$E = h\nu = hc/\lambda$$

Energy and frequency are directly proportional while energy and wavelength are inversely proportional. To produce photoemission the photon energy must be increased to the threshold value for the material. The shorter the wavelength the greater the energy. The other three choices correspond to lowering the energy of the photons.

102. **B** Boron has three valence electrons and can only form three covalent bonds with surrounding Ge atoms. Therefore, one of the four valence electrons on a neighboring Ge atom is missing an electron to bond with. This missing electron is called a *hole*. It provides holes and forms P-type semiconductor. Choices C and D are eliminated since single semiconductors are electronically neutral. Separation of charge requires contact between N-type and P-type semiconductors.

103. **A** Section II describes forward biasing as reducing the *electric field barrier* which would increase current.

104. **D** The section of the circuit between A and B is outside of the semiconductor so it contains no moving holes, only electrons. This eliminates any choices containing I and II. Remember that current flows from the + battery terminal to the – battery terminal but that electron flow is in the opposite direction.

105. **B** Holes act as positive charge carriers and are attracted to the negative terminal of the battery.

106. **C** This is a reverse-biased diode so the connection will increase the electric field barrier and decrease the current flow.

107. **B** In each of the circuits current is flowing clockwise and electrons are flowing counter-clockwise. Now consider the biasing for each diode in a given circuit. A reverse-bias diode will stop the flow of current. Choice B is the only choice where both diodes are forward-biased.

108. **C** Based on the passage, if the length is cut in half, the same force would produce half the elongation. Therefore, to produce the same elongation the applied force must be doubled.

109. **B** Since Y = stress/strain, the relationship between the stress and the elongation is given is:

$$YA/L = constant = F_1/\Delta L_1 = F_2/\Delta L_2$$

The value of Young's modulus, the cross-sectional area of the muscle and its original length are constant for both cases. In case 1, $\Delta L_1 = x$ and F_1 is due to 1.5 kg. In case 2, $\Delta L_2 = x + 0.4$ cm and F_2 is a force due to 1.5 kg + 0.5 kg = 2.0 kg. Therefore: $1.5/x = 2.0/(x+.4)$ $0.5x = 0.6$ cm $x = 1.2$ cm

110. **D** Stress = Force/area. Force depends on g as well as mass, and area depends on diameter, so choices A and C are eliminated. Choice B is eliminated because density depends on mass. Stress is independent of the length of the material being stressed.

111. **A** The force and Young's modulus are constant, therefore for the two cases:

$$F/Y = constant = A_1 \Delta L_1 / L_1 = A_2 \Delta L_2 / L_2$$

Where

$A_1 = \pi(d/2)^2 = \pi d^2/4$ and $A_2 = \pi(2d/2)^2 = \pi d^2$

$L_1 = L$ and $L_2 = 2L$

$A_1 \Delta L_1 / L_1 = A_2 \Delta L_2 / L_2$ becomes $\pi d^2 \Delta L_1 / 4L = \pi d^2 \Delta L_2 / 2L$

And, therefore: $\Delta L_2 = \Delta L_1 / 2$

112. **C** $(\Delta L/L)A = F/Y$. Since $(\Delta L/L)A$ is the same for both band A and band B, then: $F_A/Y_A = F_B/Y_B$. The value of Young's modulus and the applied force are directly proportional. Since F doubles in value, Y doubles in value.

113. **B** $\Delta L/L \times 100\%$ is the percent change in length.

$(\Delta L/L) \times 100\% = (F/YA) \times 100\% =$

$(200 \text{ N})/(2 \times 10^{10} \text{ N/m}^2)(2 \times 10^{-6} \text{ m}^2) \times 100\%$
$= (0.5 \times 10^{-2}) \times 100\% = 0.5\%$

114. **A** Since the observer is stationary, $v_o = 0$. The source is moving toward the observer and, therefore, carries a positive sign. The general formula reduces to:

$$f_o = f_s[(v + v_o)/(v - v_s)] = f_s[(v + 0)/(v - (+ v_s))]$$
$$= f_s[v/(v - v_s)]$$

115. **C** Since the wave source is stationary, $v_s = 0$. The observer is moving towards the source and, therefore, carries a positive sign. The general formula reduces to:

$$f_o = f_s[(v + v_o)/(v - v_s)] =$$

$$f_s[(v + (+ v_o))/(v - 0)] = f_s[(v + v_o)/v]$$

116. **B** The observer is moving towards the source so v_o is positive. The source is moving away from the observer so v_s is negarive. The general formula reduces to:

$$f_o = f_s[(v + (+v_o)/(v - (-v_s)] =$$

$$f_s[(v + v_o)/(v + v_s)]$$

117. **C** The observer is moving away from the source so v_o is negative. The source is moving away from the observer so v_s is also negative. The general formula reduces to:

$$f_o = f_s[(v + (- v_o)/(v - (- v_s)] =$$

$$f_s[(v - v_o)/(v + v_s)]$$

118. **C** Radio waves are electromagnetic waves so only III is valid. This eliminates choices A and B. Since the speed of the car, v, is negligible compared to the speed of light, c, the v/c term is essentially zero and equation III reduces to:

$$f_o = f_s[(1 + 0)/(1 - 0)]^{1/2} \sim f_s$$

119. **B** Since the universe is expanding the observer on Earth and the source in space are moving apart. The frequency becomes lower. Frequency and wavelength are inversely related. The lower the frequency the longer the corresponding wavelength. Red light is lower in energy, has a longer wavelength and a lower frequency than blue light. As an aside choices A and D are equivalent.

120. **B** This question is a bit tricky. Since density is constant mass (and weight) is proportional to volume and, therefore, equals the scaling factor cubed. So, the answer is NOT C.

$$m'/m = \lambda^3, \lambda^3 = (80kg/70kg) =$$

$$(784N/686N) = (1.14)$$

therefore, $\lambda = (1.14)^{1/3} = 1.05$

An aside: Estimating the cube root of 1.14. The value must be greater than 1, but not by very much. Try cubing 1.1. Squaring 1.1 gives 1.21 so cubing will give a slightly larger number. Therefore $(1.14)^{1/3}$ must be greater than 1.0 but less than 1.1.

121. **D** The original object has four sides, each with 18 squares plus two sides with 9 squares each for a total surface area of 90 u^2. If the center column of 6 cubes is remove, the resulting object has four outer sides of 18 squares plus 2 outer sides of 8 squares plus four inner sides of 6 squares: 72 + 16 + 24 = 112 u^2.

122. **C** Mass and weight both scale as λ^3, therefore we don't need to know the actual value of λ:

$$m'/m = \lambda^3 = m'g/mg = \lambda^3$$

$$(60kg/90kg) = (x N/300 N) = 0.667$$
$$x N = 200 N$$

123. **A** The scaling factor is the ratio of terminal speed for the two objects, v_T and v'_T respectively. This gives:

$$v'_T / v_T = (2w'/C_D\rho A')^{1/2}/(2w/C_D\rho A)^{1/2} =$$

$$(w'A/wA')^{1/2} = ([w'/w][A/A'])^{1/2} =$$

$$([\lambda^3][1/\lambda^2])^{1/2} = \lambda^{1/2}$$

because weight scales as the third power and area scales as the second power.

124. **B** The model scales as 10^{-3}.

$$7.5 \times 10^4 \text{ N/m}^2 \times 10^{-3} = 75 \times 10^4 \text{ N/m}^2.$$

125. **C** Rate of flow =

Volume to be filled/time it takes to fill:

$Q = V/t$

The time scale factor is $\_ = t_{model} / t_{dam} = 10^{-2}$ and the volume scale factor is λ^3.

For the model this becomes:

$Q_{model} = V_{model}/t_{model} = \lambda^3 V_{dam} / \_ t_{dam} = Q_{dam}$

$Q_{model} = (10^{-3})^3 (10^4 \ m^3/hr)/(10^{-2}) = 10^{-3} \ m^3/hr.$

126. **D** I is true because $Cl_2(g)$ has a higher potential to be reduced than does $PbSO_4(s)$; thus $Cl_2(g)$ is a better oxidizing agent.

II is true because lower pH increases $[H^+]$, driving the reaction to the right by Le Chatelier's Principle (optionally, the Nernst Eqn. gives the same result.)

III is false; these species cannot react by the equations given because each is fully reduced. (It is true, however, that $MnO_4^-(aq)$ will react with $Cl^-(aq)$.)

127. **B** We want to drive the following reaction to the right:

$Fe(OH)_3(s) \Leftrightarrow Fe^{3+}(aq) + 3OH^-(aq)$

By adding a strong acid that will react with $OH^-(aq)$, we eliminate hydroxide ion from the right side, causing a shift to the right and increasing solubility. Adding $OH^-(aq)$ (as in A) or $Fe^{3+}(aq)$ (as in C) will drive the reaction to the left. Choice D is not effectual, since as long as there is sufficient solid to establish equilibrium, the actual amount does not matter.

128. **A** Vol of room = $(4.0 \ m)^2 \times (3.5m) = 56 \ m^3$

To convert to liters (in order to use the ideal gas law), you can use the identity of mL with cm^3:

$1 \ m = 10^2 \ cm$

$1 \ m^3 = 10^6 \ cm^3$

$= 10^6 \ mL$

$= 10^6 \ mL \times (1 \ L/10^3 \ mL)$

$= 10^3 \ L$

So V= $5.6 \times 10^4 \ L$

$n = PV/RT$

$= (0.00419 \ atm)(5.6 \times 10^4 \ L) \ / \ (0.08206 \ L \ atm/ \ K \ mol)(303 \ K)$

$= 9.4 \ mol \ water \ vapor$

mass of water = $(9.4 \ mol)(18.0 \ g/mol)$

$= 170 \ g \ water$

129. **B** The concentration after the first dilution is

$C_2 = C_1(V_1/V_2)$

$= (1.15 \ M)(10.00 \ mL/25.00 \ mL)$

$= 0.460 \ M$

After the second dilution the concentration is

$C3 = C_2(V_2/V_3)$

$= (0.460 \ M)(1.00 \ mL/50.00 \ mL)$

$= 0.00920 \ M$

130. **C** CO_2 and I_3^- are linear molecules, while H_2O is bent.

131. **C** Since the time to drop by one-fifth is independent of the initial pressure of $N_2O_5(g)$, we must have first-order kinetics. Use the integrated rate law:

$$\ln\left(N/N_O\right) = -kt$$

$$k = \frac{-\ln\left(N/N_O\right)}{t}$$

$$= -\ln\left(1/5\right)/\left(4.77 \times 10^4 s\right)$$

$$= 3.37 \times 10^{-5} s^{-1}$$

$$t_{\frac{1}{2}} = 0.693/k$$

$$= 2.06 \times 10^4 s$$

(Is the 1/2-life equal to 2/5 of the "1/5-life", as in choice B? No, although the result is close.)

132. **B** The mass of the ball is not relevant to the question. For circular motion: $a_c = \omega^2 r$ where ω is the angular velocity and r is the radius of the circular path. In linear motion the distance traveled is the product of velocity and time, $x = vt$. In circular motion the distance traveled is the angle swept out and is equal to the product of the angular velocity and time:

$$\theta = \omega t.$$

For this problem:

$$\omega = \theta/\tau = 12 \text{ rad}/4 \text{ s} = 3s^{-1} \text{ and}$$

$$a_c = \omega^2 r = (3s^{-1})^2 (2 \text{ cm}) = 18 \text{ cm/s}$$

133. **A** Replace the two capacitors in parallel with an equivalent capacitor:

$$C_{AB} = C_A + C_B = 2F + 2F = 4 \text{ F}$$

Next replace the two capacitors now in series with one equivalent capacitor:

$$1/C_{ABC} = 1/C_{AB} + 1/C_C = 1/4F + 1/4F = 1/2F$$

Therefore, $C_{ABC} = 2F$

134. **C** Beats/s equal the difference between the two frequencies:

$$f_{beat} = |f_2 - f_1| = |258-222| = 18 \text{ Hz}$$

135. **C** Look at the free body diagrams for each mass:

The tension, T, on the pulley is always upward and the acceleration due to gravity, g, is always downward. The acceleration of M_A is upward and that of M_B is downward. All motion is parallel to the *y*-axis.

From Newton's 2nd Law, $\Sigma F_x = 0$ and $\Sigma F_y = m_{total}a$

For M_A: $T - M_A g = M_A a$

For M_B: $T - M_B g = -M_B a$

Eliminate the tension, T, between the two equations and solve for the acceleration, a:

$$M_A g + M_A a = M_B g - M_B a$$

$$M_A a + M_B a = M_B g - M_A g$$

$$a(M_A + M_B) = g(M_B - M_A)$$

$$a = g(M_B - M_A)/(M_B + M_A)$$

136. **D** P=F/A. There are three things to consider in solving this problem. First, the force the man exerts is his weight, mg. Next, the dimensions of the foot should be changed from centimeters to meters. And finally, the man stands on two feet so his weight is distributed over twice the area of one of his feet.

$P = mg/2(\text{length} \times \text{width}) =$

$(90 \text{ kg})(9.8 \text{ m/s}^2)/2(0.30 \text{ m} \times 0.08 \text{ m}) =$

$882N/0.048 \text{ m}^2 = 18.4 \times 10^3 \text{ N/m}^2$

137. **B** Since r = 2f, the mirror equation becomes $1/o + 1/i = 1/f = 2/r$, where o and i are the object and image distances from the mirror surface respectively.

$1/i = 2/r – 1/o = 2/60 \text{ cm} – 1/10 \text{ cm} =$

$(20 – 60)/600 \text{ cm} = –40/600 \text{ cm}$

$i = –600 \text{ cm}/40 = –15 \text{ cm}$

138. **C** At constant volume, the pressure of an ideal gas sample is proportional to its absolute temperature in degrees Kelvin:

$P_1/T_1 = P_2/T_2$

While the temperature is doubled on the Celsius scale (100 °C to 200 °C), on the Kelvin scale it increases by less than a factor of two (373 K to 473 K).

139. **D** This is a conservation of momentum problem where the blocks are recoiling. Since the blocks are moving in opposite directions block B must move to the left. This eliminates choices A and C immediately.

$m_A v_A = –m_B v_B$

The negative sign maintains the validity of the equal sign since v_A and v_B are in opposite directions.

$(6.0 \text{ kg})(8 \text{ m/s}) = –(3.0 \text{ kg})v_B$
$v_B = –16 \text{ m/s} = 16 \text{ m/s}$ to the left

140. **C** An electron moving into a higher orbital (larger radius) must absorb energy. This supports statement I and eliminates statement II. From Coulomb's law, the force between the electron and the nucleus of the atom varies inversely with the square of the distance between them. As the radius increases, the force decreases. This supports statement III.

141. **C** The number of electrons in this configuration fits neutral Mn, but its configuration is $[Ar]4s^2 3d^5$. Therefore this must be an excited state. (This example might be confused with Cr, which achieves a half-filled d^5 configuration by promoting a 4s electron, resulting in $[Ar]4s^1 3d^5$. But no such promotion is needed to give Mn 5 electrons in the 3d orbital.)

142. **D** First determine the limiting reactant:

mol HCl = (.025 L)(0.415 mol/L) = 0.0117 mol

mol NaOH = (.026 L)(0.456 mol/L) = 0.0119 mol

HCl is the limiting reactant.

Now calculate the heat generated in the calorimeter using 0.0117 mol of HCl,

$q_{\text{calorimeter}}$ = (mass solution)(sp. heat)ΔT

$= (51.0 \text{ g})(4.18 \text{J/deg g})(3.1 \text{ deg})$

$= 682 \text{ J}$

But the heat gained by the calorimeter must have been *released* from the reaction:

$q_{\text{reaction}} = –q_{\text{calorimeter}} = –682 \text{ J}$

This result is not ΔH, because it does not refer to the 1 mol of HCl implied by the balanced reaction; there was only 0.0117 mol used. So,

ΔH = –(1 mol)(682 J/ 0.0117 mol) = –58 kJ

Biological Sciences

143. **C** The A-V valves **open** while blood passes from the atria to the ventricles. This occurs while the ventricles are relaxed (ventricular diastole) and are filling with blood. The A-V valves **close** when the ventricles contract (ventricular systole) and ventricular pressure is increasing, making the 1st sound (LUBB) associated with the cardiac cycle. Although atrial diastole, (choice B) also occurs at more or less the same time, this event does not contribute to the sound made by the closing A-V valves.

144. **D** The graph representing "ventricular volume" indicates that EDV is approximately 150ml. A common error would be Choice A (80–100 ml) if the reader mistakenly refers to the upper graph. However, this number refers to 80–100 mmHg in aortic pressure.

145. **B** If EDV is the amount of blood present after ventricular filling, and ESV is the amount remaining after contraction, the difference must be the amount of blood **pumped out** by the ventricle *during* contraction. This amount is stroke volume. Cardiac output (choice C) is heart rate × stroke volume. Pulse pressure (choice D) is systolic pressure – diastolic pressure.

146. **C** Blood in the superior and inferior vena cavae has returned from all parts of the body. It is as far as it can be from the left ventricle's "original push" into the systemic circulation. The blood pressure in the vena cavae is approximately zero!

147. **C** As pressure in the ventricles drops, their volume increases and they fill up. Since pressure from the ventricles no longer is enough to propel blood in the aorta and pulmonary artery forward, it momentarily "backs up" and forces the aortic and pulmonary semi-lunar valves to close.

148. **B** Based on the time line in the figure (top), one complete cardiac cycle takes approximately 0.77 seconds. Therefore, in 60 seconds, the heart rate would be approximately 78 bpm.

149. **A** If there is greater impedance to the ejection of blood from the ventricles (greater afterload), less blood will be ejected (decreased stroke volume), and more blood will remain in the ventricles after contraction (increased ESV).

150. **C** The figure shows that signals from the *right* visual field of each eye reach *the left half of the retina* and then proceed to the *left* occipital lobe (left dashed line from the left eye and left solid line from the right eye).

151. **A** The oculomotor nerve (cranial nerve III) originates in the midbrain and controls a number of activities including contraction of the smooth muscles of the iris, the smooth muscles of the ciliary bodies (for adjusting the lens for near and distant vision), and four of the six extrinsic eye muscles. However, since the question refers to *autonomic* motor activities contractions of the extrinsic eye muscles (skeletal muscles) cannot be included. They are voluntary muscles controlled by *somatic* motor neurons.

152. **A** Since there are no receptors (rods and cones) at the optic disc or "blind spot" to detect light, no signals along the visual pathway will be initiated and no visual image will be formed by the occipital lobe.

153. **D.** All choices are regions of the brain that *are* part of the visual pathway. The superior colliculi of the midbrain are part of the brain stem, the lateral geniculate bodies of the thalamus are in the diencephalon, and the occipital lobes are part of the cerebral cortex.

154. **B.** When viewed directly, the image of the star is focussed on the cones in the fovea. However, cones require bright light to function (not available at night). When viewed at an angle, the image is focussed on the an area peripheral to the macula lutea, stimulating rods which are sensitive enough to respond in dim light. The shape of the lens (choice A) and the size of the pupil (choice D) **can** be regulated under these conditions.

155. **C.** The corpus callosum is a tract which connects the two cerebral hemispheres. The crossing of the optic nerves (optic chiasma) and the lateral geniculate bodies (diencephalon) are "below" the corpus callosum. Therefore, the pathways **to** the cerebrum will not be affected by cutting this tract. However, once signals arrive at the cerbrum, one hemisphere will not

be able to "know" what the other hemisphere is "seeing" (Nobel prize-winning research with such "split brain" individuals contributed greatly to the discovery of the details of the visual pathway).

156. **A** All daughters will inherit the father's X chromosome carrying the recessive color-blind allele. However, daughters must have *both X chromosomes* with the color-blind allele in order to be color-blind. Since the mother is a *homozygous dominant* individual, each daughter must also receive a "normal" X chromosome as well.

157. **C.** The stomach produces pepsin, the pancreas contributes trypsin, chymotrypsin, and carboxypeptidase, and the small intestine itself releases aminopeptidase and dipeptidase.

158. **D.** Absorption can be defined as the passage of materials across epithelial membranes and into body fluids. The chart indicates that the active process of cotransport is needed to absorb monosaccharides and amino acids from the lumen of the small intestine across the intestinal mucosa, and that active processes (exocytosis and cotransport) are used to move lipids and amino acids, respectively, into the body fluids.

159. **D.** "Anticipation" of food must involve thought and, therefore, neurons. The stomach's smooth muscles and secretory cells are regulated, in part, by the autonomic nervous system. In addition, the stomach's own gastrin, intestinal gastrin, and GIP are hormones that contribute to gastric control. Finally, HCl is secreted by parietal cells directly into the gastric lumen to activate pepsinogen to pepsin.

160. **B.** The intestinal enzymes maltase, sucrase, and lactase complete the digestion of disaccharides to monosaccharides. Choice A is not correct because lipids are absorbed into the lacteals of the lymphatic system, not directly into the blood. Choice C is not correct because the liver makes bile. Choice D is not correct because the end-products of lipid digestion, mono-glycerides and fatty acids, must first be *recombined* into larger triglycerides before passing into the lymphatic fluid in the form of chylomicrons.

161. **A** The enzymes at work in the small intestine function best at a slightly alkaline pH. Sodium bicarbonate helps neutralize the acidic chyme entering from the stomach. Although both Choices B and C are correct statements, they have nothing to do with the sodium bicarbonate released by the pancreas in this context. Here, sodium bicarbonate goes to work in the lumen of the small intestine, not the bloodstream.

162. **C** Since vitamin B12 is needed for nucleic acid synthesis, highly mitotic areas such as the red bone marrow are affected by a deficiency (pernicious anemia can result).

163. **B** Nutrients absorbed into the blood capillaries will travel to the liver via the hepatic portal system. The liver's responsibilities include storage, conversion, detoxification and distribution of these molecules.

164. **D** Touch receptors detect changes due to mechanical forces exerted on the skin, and, together with their sensory neurons, are components of the somatic nervous system. Eccrine glands, arrector pili muscles (smooth muscles), and the smooth muscles in the walls of dermal blood vessels are all involuntary effectors innervated by motor neurons of the autonomic nervous system.

165. **B** Sebaceous glands release the oily secretion, sebum, into hair follicles, which helps prevent hair and the surface of the epidermis from drying out. Eccrine glands (through their release of sweat), dermal blood vessels (through vasodilation when body temperature is too high and vasoconstriction when body temperature is too low), and the hypodermis (through the insulating properties of adipose tissue) all directly contribute to thermo-regulation.

166. **D** The stratum basale (stratum germinativum) rests on the non-living basement membrane separating the epidermis from the dermis. It is here that mitosis takes place to produce new cells, while older cells are pushed closer to the surface. Although some mitotic activity takes place in the stratum spinosum, choice C, most occurs in the stratum basale.

167. **C** The stratum basale is also the site of melanocytes, the melanin-producing cells in which melanoma arises. The dark appearance of the stratum granulosum, choice B is due to an accumulation of the protein, keratin, which helps "waterproof" the skin.

168. **A** The secretory activities of both sebaceous glands and apocrine glands are influenced by sex hormones. Excessive sebaceous secretions starting at puberty can lead to blocked sebaceous ducts, subsequent bacterial infections, and the associated symptoms of acne. Apocrine glands, found primarily in the axillary and pubic regions, begin secreting odorous sweat at puberty (it may serve as a sex attractant!).

169. **B** Blood vessels and all components of the cardiovascular system arise from mesoderm.

170. **D** The present system of classification includes five kingdoms: Prokaryota (Monera), Protista, Fungi, Plantae, and Animalia.

171. **C** Proton gradients form the basis of chemiosmotic ATP synthesis in both cellular respiration and eukaryotic photosynthesis. The other choices refer to processes that utilize ATP already available (It was synthesized earlier by chemiosmosis!).

172. **C.** Peptidoglycan is the material found in bacterial cell walls. Cellulose (choice A) is found in plant cell walls, chitin (choice B) is often found in the cell walls of fungi, and phospholipids are important components of plasma membranes.

173. **D** All choices represent characteristics of genetic material in eukaryotes only.

174. **D** Antibiotics are designed to affect bacterial protein synthesis along their ribosomes, the permeability of bacterial membranes, and the osmotic fragility of their peptidoglycan walls. Since these cellular components have structural/molecular differences in the Archaebacteria, the antibiotics that are successful in fighting eubacterial infections may not work at all against archaebacterial cells.

175. **B** Most antibiotics are *ineffective* against viruses because it is difficult to damage the virus without damaging the host cell that the virus has entered. Choice C is correct because individuals *without resistance are the first to be eliminated*, while those *with resistance are the last to be eliminated*.

176. **A** Autonomic circuits always involve *two* neurons from CNS to involuntary effectors (pre-ganglionic and post-ganglionic neurons), compared to one somatic motor neuron used to reach the voluntary effectors. Motor neurons carry impulses from CNS to effectors in both somatic and autonomic circuits. Similarly, both circuits can carry excitatory and inhibitory signals.

177. **B** Adrenergic receptor sites respond to norepinephrine and epinephrine (beta receptors in the heart lead to increased heart rate and increased force of contraction; alpha receptors on the secretory cells of the digestive system decrease activity). Cholinergic receptors responding to acetylcholine are classified as either muscarinic or nicotinic.

178 **B** cAMP is an important "second messenger" for many hormones whose receptor sites are on the cell membranes of their target cells. cAMP can lead to the opening of ion channels, the activation of enzymes, etc. in target cells.

179. **D** The adrenal medulla is a target of the sympathetic nervous system. When stimulated, it releases norepinephrine and epinephrine into the blood to reinforce sympathetic effects throughout the body.

180. **C** The vagus nerve carries parasympathetic motor signals to most involuntary effectors in the thoracic and abdominopelvic cavities (heart, air passageways, digestive organs, spleen, etc.). The names of spinal nerves are based on their adjacent vertebrae as they pass out of the spinal cord. Since T – 1 and L – 1 would contain sympathetic circuits, they would not regulate visceral effectors during "everyday" activities. S – 4 would contain parasympathetic neurons, but they help regulate a relatively small percentage of our abdominopelvic effectors.

181. **D** Sympathetic circuits have short pre-ganglionic neurons with ganglia near the spinal cord, while parasympathetic circuits have long pre-ganglionic neurons with ganglia near the effectors.

182. **C** The acrosome, within the head of the sperm cell, contains small amounts of the enzyme, hyaluronidase, which is needed to penetrate the zona pellucida. The additive effect of this enzyme from many sperm cells is needed to break through.

183. **D** If the sperm is carrying the sex-linked (X-linked) allele for color-blindness, the child will be a girl. Since the mother has normal vision, she could be "homozygous normal" or a heterozygous carrier of the color-blindness allele. In the former case, the child will be a carrier for color-blindness. However, if the mother is a carrier, the child has a 50% chance of being a carrier and a 50% chance of being color-blind.

184. **C** The early mitotic divisions after fertilization are the cleavage divisions leading to the blastocyst. Gestation (choice B) refers to the entire time of intrauterine development. No differentiation (choice D) has taken place as yet—all cells are still phenotypically identical.

185. **C** The corpus luteum (the mature ovarian follicle after ovulation) produces estrogen and progesterone to maintain the endometrium until the placenta matures later in development. HCG produced by the maternal-embryonic interface helps keep the corpus luteum active.

186. **A** The hormone that causes uterine contractions during labor, oxytocin, is made in the hypothalamus and stored/released by the posterior pituitary gland.

187. **D** The Rh-negative mother will produce anti-Rh antibodies within 72hr after contact with her child's Rh-positive antigens. Although these antibodies only live approximately 30 days, her activated immune system will continue to replace them throughout her life. This will endanger her *next* Rh-positive child. In these situations, a large concentration of anti-Rh antibodies can be administered to the mother *before* her own immune system is activated. Then, after approximately 30 days, these antibodies will be gone and, since her immune system was never activated, they will not be replaced.

188. **C** According to Markovnikov's Rule, when an acid, HX, adds to a double bond, the hydrogen atom bonds to the carbon atom that already is attached to the most hydrogen atoms. Thus the H in HBr bonds to C-1 and the Br to C-2 of 1-butene.

189. **B** In this case, the H adds to C-2 to produce the more stable cation H_2C^+-CH_2-CF_3. Applying Markovnikov's Rule would produce the less stable H_3C–$\overset{+}{\underset{H}{C}}$–$CF_3$ in which an electron-withdrawing group –CF_3 is bonded to an electron deficient carbon atom. Such a species is of high energy and therefore does not form to any extent.

190. **C** If one applies Markovnikov's Rule then the usual carbocation would form. However carbocations sometimes rearrange to give a more stable species. In this case a methide ion (:CH_3^-) would shift to yield the more stable carbocation.

191. **A** The addition of HX to alkenes proceeds through an open carbocation. With a p orbital at the electron-deficient carbon, the electrophile can attack equally as well from the top or bottom. Thus, the enantiomers are produced in equal amounts creating an optically inactive, racemic solution.

192. **D** When the alkene is protonated the activated complex will resemble the carbocation intermediate. Because the primary carbocation is less stable, its associated activation energy will be greater and its rate constant smaller according to the Arrhenius equation:

$$k = Ae^{-Ea/RT}$$

The tertiary carbocation will thus form more readily and lead to more product.

193. **C** For both classes of acyl compounds, the first step involves the addition of a nucleophile (:Nu) that forms a tetrahedral intermediate:

$$R\text{–}\overset{\overset{\displaystyle O}{\|}}{C}\text{–}X + :Nu \longrightarrow R\text{–}\overset{\overset{\displaystyle O^-}{|}}{\underset{\underset{\displaystyle X}{|}}{C}}\text{–}Nu$$

$$R\text{–}\overset{\overset{\displaystyle O}{\|}}{C}\text{–}R + :Nu \longrightarrow R\text{–}\overset{\overset{\displaystyle O^-}{|}}{\underset{\underset{\displaystyle R}{|}}{C}}\text{–}Nu$$

The ability of X to leave depends on its basicity: the weaker the base the better the leaving group. In the case of an aldehyde or ketone, the very strong bases, the hydride ion (:H^-) or alkide ion (:R^-) would have to leave in order for substitution to occur. Thus, the carboxylic acids tend to undergo substitution reactions while aldehydes and ketones tend to undergo addition reactions.

194. **A** The tetrahedral intermediate is favored by electron withdrawing groups that delocalize the negative charge, and hindered by bulky groups that cause crowding.

195. **D** Nucleophilic attack on a tetrahedral alkyl carbon generates a crowded transition state and a partially broken sigma bond.

196. **B** In the hydrolysis of an ester, an alcohol is displaced by a nucleophile. In the same way, one alcohol can displace another alcohol from an ester. This cleavage by an alcohol (alcoholysis) of an ester is called transesterification. Transesterification is catalyzed by acid or base.

197. **B** Both electronic factors (the tendency of oxygen to acquire electrons) and steric factors (relatively unhindered transition state associated with the trigonal acyl reactant becoming the tetrahedral intermediate) make the carbonyl group susceptible to nucleophilic attack at the carbonyl carbon. In the presence of acid, H+ attaches to the carbonyl oxygen, making the carbonyl carbon even more susceptible to attack by a nucleophile: Oxygen can acquire the π electrons of the carbonyl group without developing a negative charge.

198. **C** The basicity of the leaving group: $Cl^- < R'COO- < OR'- < NH_2^-$

199. **D** D-(+)- Glucose does not undergo some reactions typical of aldehydes: Although it is readily oxidized it does not form a bisulfite addition product and it gives a negative Schiff test. Also, when D-(+)- glucose (mp = 146° C) is dissolved in water, the specific rotation drops from 112° to 52.7° while crystals (mp = 150°C) are dissolved in water, specific rotation rises from 19 to 52.7°. α-D-(+) Glucose is the form with the higher positive rotation while β-D-(+) glucose is the form with the lower rotation. When each form is dissolved in water, the specific rotation will change to the equilibrium value (mutarotation).

200. **C** When D-(+)- glucose reacts with methanol and HCl, methyl D-glucoside forms in which only one –CH$_3$ group is added; however its properties resemble a full acetal. Only the structures below are consistent with this data.

Methyl β–D-glucoside

Methyl α–D-glucoside

201. **D**

Methyl α–D-glucose

Methyl β–D-glucose

202. **B** See the answer to number 201.

203. **D** Both cellulose and starch consist of chains of D- glucose units, each unit connected by a glycoside linkage to C-4 of the next:

204. **B** Epimers are a pair of diastereomeric aldoses that differ only in configuration about C-2. Epimers have the same configuration about C-3, C-4, and C-5.

(+)–Glucose   (+)–Mannose

205. **D** 150 nucleotides would be present to form the 50 codons needed to encode 50 amino acids. The additional three nucleotides would be present to encode STOP!

206. **A** Absorbing sea water would make the blood hypertonic to the tissues. Therefore, the tissues would become hypotonic (having less solute, but more water than the blood) and lose water to the blood. The tissues would dehydrate.

207. **C** Parathyroid hormone (parathormone) helps increase calcium levels in the blood. Calcitonin (Answer B) is produced by the thyroid gland and <u>decreases</u> calcium levels in the blood.

208. **B** Each muscle cell in the biceps brachii muscle must contract completely if it is stimulated. Individual cells cannot partially contract (all-or-none principle). A whole muscle can give a graded response, depending <u>on how many</u> individual cells are stimulated to perform the job at hand.

209. **B** Autonomic motor circuits extend only to our involuntary effectors (smooth muscle, cardiac muscle, and glands). Motor signals to our voluntary effectors (skeletal muscle) would be considered part of the body's somatic circuits.

210. **D** The cerebellum coordinates the body's motor activities. To do this, it receives input from the voluntary motor centers in the cerebrum, from proprioceptors in the muscles, tendons and joints, and from the balance/equilibrium receptors of the inner ear.

211. **B** The middle ear ossicles, the malleus, incus, and stapes, amplify the sound vibrations between the tympanum and oval window. Vibrations usually <u>decrease</u> with distance (Answer A), and amplification is no longer needed after the sound receptors in the cochlea have been stimulated (Answer C).

212. **C** Macrophages and neutrophils are both phagocytes that can engulf invading cells and "display" their antigens. Lymphocytes (appropriate B-cells and T-cells) will subsequently arrive, recognize the displayed foreign antigen, bind to it, and eventually form clones of additional protective cells.

213. **D** The chance of two heterozygotes having an offspring that is double recessive is 1/4. The chance of having two such offspring in a row is the product of each event ($1/4 \times 1/4 = 1/16$).

214. **C** The physical changes in albumin during heating reflect the temperature sensitivity of all proteins. The temperature specificity of enzymes (all of which are proteins) is due to physical changes that may occur affecting the active site and catalytic capability of each enzyme molecule.

215. **D** The macula densa senses if the level of sodium is low and renin is secreted. Angiotensin II is formed, which acts on the adrenal cortex to increase the secretion of the hormone aldosterone, which regulates the conservation of sodium.

216. **C** With the structural formula, you can ascertain the chiral carbons and draw enantiomers as well as determine the existence of a meso compound. Fischer projections for a meso compound all contain a plane of symmetry. The actual optical activity of an enantiomer must be experimentally measured.

217. D An equilibrium exists between the enol and keto structures, but it usually lies in favor of the keto form:

$$-\overset{\displaystyle |}{C}=\overset{\displaystyle |}{C}-OH \quad \rightleftharpoons \quad -\overset{\displaystyle |}{\underset{\displaystyle H}{C}}-\overset{\displaystyle |}{C}=O$$

Enol structure   Keto structure

Phenol is an exception because the enol form (phenol) is stabilized by the aromatic ring.

218. B Tertiary amines do not react with acid chlorides to form amides because tertiary amines cannot lose a proton after attacking the carbon. The alkylation of amines by alkyl halides is a nucleophilic substitution reaction in which the organic halide is attacked by the nucleophilic amine. Peptides are formed by the reaction between the carboxyl group of an amino acid and the amino terminal of another amino acid to form an amide linkage:

219. A Fats are triacylglycerols :

$$
\begin{array}{l}
CH_2-O-\overset{\displaystyle }{\underset{\displaystyle \overset{\|}{O}}{C}}-R \\
CH-O-\overset{\displaystyle }{\underset{\displaystyle \overset{\|}{O}}{C}}-R \\
CH_2-O-\overset{\displaystyle }{\underset{\displaystyle \overset{\|}{O}}{C}}-R
\end{array}
$$

All three ester linkages are to acyl groups. Phosphoglycerides contain only two acyl groups: a phosphate group replaces the third acyl group:

A Phosphoglyceride

$$
\begin{array}{l}
R-\overset{\|}{\underset{O}{C}}-O-CH_2 \\
R-\overset{\|}{\underset{O}{C}}-O-C-H \\
\qquad\qquad CH_2-O-\overset{\displaystyle }{\underset{\displaystyle OH}{\overset{\displaystyle O}{P}}}-OH
\end{array}
$$

NOTES

NOTES

NOTES

NOTES

NOTES

NOTES

NOTES

NOTES

NOTES

NOTES

NOTES

NOTES

NOTES

NOTES

NOTES

NOTES

NOTES

NOTES

The Graduate Channel at Petersons.com

—Your One-Stop Online Destination for Information on Degree Programs, Financial Aid, and More

Explore the Graduate Channel today!

To visit the Graduate Channel, simply go to **www.petersons.com** and select the Graduate Programs navigation bar located in the upper left-hand corner of your screen.

Whether you want to pursue an academic career or use grad school as a springboard to professional success, the Graduate Channel offers a wealth of information and services that can help you reach your goals. Search an extensive database of more than 36,000 graduate and professional programs, practice with simulated GRE® CAT tests, and discover financial resources that can help you pay for your degree. You can even apply online!

PETERSON'S
™
THOMSON LEARNING